VASCULAR RECONSTRUCTIONS

Springer
New York
Berlin
Heidelberg
Barcelona
Hong Kong
London
Milan
Paris
Singapore
Tokyo

VASCULAR RECONSTRUCTIONS

Anatomy, Exposures, and Techniques

Jamal J. Hoballah, MD

Department of Surgery
University of Iowa Hospitals and Clinics

With 961 Illustrations

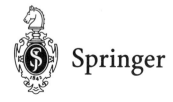

Springer

Jamal J. Hoballah, MD
Department of Surgery
University of Iowa Hospitals and Clinics
200 Hawkins Drive
Iowa City, IA 52242
USA
jamal-hoballah@uiowa.edu

Illustrations by Sheri Pressler.

Library of Congress Cataloging-in-Publication Data
Hoballah, Jamal J.
    Vascular reconstructions : anatomy, exposures, and techniques / Jamal J. Hoballah.
        p.   cm.
    Includes bibliographical references and index.
    ISBN 0-387-98500-X (hardcover : alk. paper)
    1. Blood-vessels—Surgery Handbooks, manuals, etc. I. Title.
    [DNLM: 1. Anastomosis, Surgical—methods.   2. Vascular Surgical
Procedures—methods.   WG 170 H68lv 2000]
RD598.5.H83 2000
617.4' 13—dc2l
DNLM/DLC
                                                        99-29750

Printed on acid-free paper.

Production managed by MaryAnn Brickner; manufacturing supervised by Joe Quatela.
Typeset by A Good Thing, Inc., New York, NY.
Printed and bound by Maple-Vail Book Manufacturing Group, York, PA.
Printed in the United States of America.

9 8 7 6 5 4 3 2 1

ISBN 0-387-98500-X Springer-Verlag New York Berlin Heidelberg SPIN 10671934

This book is dedicated to my mother and father with love and appreciation.

Preface

"Practice makes perfect," and time spent in the operating room should be used most efficiently. In an attempt to comply with these two principles, I designed a vascular anastomoses workshop for our surgical residents at the University of Iowa. The workshop introduced the basic steps of constructing various vascular anastomoses in a relaxed environment outside the operating room. During the workshop, the residents expressed the need for a manual that outlines and describes the various vascular reconstructions in a step-by-step manner from beginning to end. Most textbooks usually include a picture of a vascular anastomosis during or after the completion of the reconstruction without detailing the beginning and conduct of the procedure. The usefulness of including sections that address commonly asked or unasked questions was also apparent. These questions pertain to vascular instruments, grafts, and sutures, as well as vascular anatomy and exposures. It is with these thoughts in mind that this book was conceived. This book is not intended to be a substitute for traditional atlases of specific vascular procedures; rather, it was written to focus on the technical aspects of vascular reconstructions and to better prepare the surgical residents before they start their vascular rotation.

This book is divided into four parts. The first part starts with a review of commonly used vascular instruments and an overview of grafts and sutures used in vascular reconstructions. A detailed chapter on vascular anatomy and exposures is provided to serve as a quick reference before starting a vascular procedure. The remaining chapters in the first part of this book review the basic steps usually performed before and after constructing a vascular anastomosis in addition to thrombectomy and endarterectomy. The second part of this book focuses on the various methods used to conduct a vascular reconstruction, which include primary closure, closure with a patch angioplasty, end-to-end, end-to-side, and side-to-side anastomoses. The various possible modifications used are outlined. The third part of this book reviews the various adjunctive methods used when constructing the proximal or distal anastomoses of an infrainguinal bypass. The fourth part of the book reviews the various modifications that are carried out when constructing the proximal and distal anastomoses of an aortic occlusive or aneurysmal pathology. Finally, the vascular anastomoses workshop that inspired the conception of this book is included as an appendix.

I certainly hope that this book will help make the vascular rotation a pleasant experience for both the surgical residents and the vascular faculty. I believe this book can also be very useful to recent graduates embarking on conducting vascular reconstructions independently as well as healthcare providers who wish to be familiar with the various steps involved in conducting of a vascular procedure.

We hope you enjoy this book as much as we enjoyed putting it together. We are eager for your comments, feedback, and suggestions for future editions. You may write directly to the medical editorial department at Springer-Verlag New York, Inc., 175 Fifth Avenue, New York, New York 10010. Send your comments to the attention of the Editor, General Surgery Book Program.

Jamal J. Hoballah
Iowa City, Iowa

Contents

ix

Acknowledgments

I am indebted to many for the completion of this book. I thank Dr. Frank C. Spencer and the faculty of the Department of Surgery at New York University for my training in General Surgery and for igniting my interest in Vascular Surgery. I also thank Dr. John D. Corson, Dr. Steve G. Friedman, Dr. Anthony M. Imparato, Dr. Gary Giangola, Dr. Ismael M. Khalil, Dr. Timothy F. Kresowik, Dr. Patrick J. Lamparello, Dr. Thomas S. Riles and Dr. William J. Sharp for their contribution to my training in Vascular Surgery. I am very grateful to my Department head, Dr. Carol Scott-Conner for her encouragement and support. I am also very grateful to the remarkable efforts of the illustrator Sheri Pressler. I am thankful to the surgical residents and fellows who were the impetus for the conception of this work. I am again thankful to Dr. John D Corson and Dr. Timothy Kresowik and the surgical residents who provided me with valuable suggestions while writing this book. I am greatly appreciative of the assistance and thoroughness of the staff at Springer-Verlag (Laura Gillan, MaryAnn Brickner). I am also very grateful to all those who helped and were not recognized in this section. Finally, this book could not have been completed without the support of my wife Leila and my sons Jawad and Nader.

I

Basic Principles in Vascular Reconstruction

Vascular Instruments

Vascular surgery can be performed with the addition of only a few instruments to the standard surgical tray. This chapter provides an overview of commonly used instruments during vascular reconstructions. Following is a list of commonly used instruments with suggestions for possible sites of application.

Instrument	Common use
Scalpel blades	
Number 10; 20	Skin incision
Number 15	Dissection in scarred tissue
Number 11; microknife	Incision of blood vessels
Scissors	
Metzenbaum scissors	All purpose dissection
Church scissors (Fig. 1.1)	Dissection of medium vessels (popliteal)
Stevens tenotomy scissors (Fig. 1.2) (sharp tip; curved blades)	Dissection of small vessels (tibial)
Potts scissors (Fig. 1.3)	Extension of incisions in medium vessels
Castroviejo scissors (Fig. 1.4)	Extension of incisions in small vessels
Tissue forceps	
Russian tissue forceps	Removal of aortic plaque
Debakey tissue forceps (Fig. 1.5) (tip 1; 1.5; 2 mm)	Medium and large blood vessels
Debakey–Diethrich	Medium and large blood vessels
Microsuture ring tip forceps (Fig. 1.6)	Small blood vessels
Microsuture tying forceps	Small blood vessels
Bishop–Harmon serrated iris forceps (Fig. 1.7)	Removal of fine fibers from an endarterectomized surface
Jeweler's forceps (fine tip)	Removal of fine fibers from an endarterectomized surface
Hemostatic forceps	
Right-angle forceps	Passing silastic loops around vessels
Right-angle forceps (Fig. 1.8) (fine tip)	Passing silk ties around small vessels (venae comitantes)

Needle holders

Mayo Hegar needle holder (Fig. 1.9)	<4-0 sutures
Ryder needle holder (Fig. 1.10)	5-0; 6-0 sutures
Castroviejo needle holder (Fig. 1.11) (with or without locking handle)	5-0; 6-0; 7-0 sutures

Totally occluding vascular clamps

Debakey aortic aneurysm clamp (Fig.1.12)(side-to-side apposition of aortic wall)	Supraceliac; infrarenal aorta
Debakey-Bahnson aortic aneurysm clamp (Fig.1.13a)	Infrarenal aorta
Howard-Debakey aortic aneurysm clamp with reverse curve shafts (Fig.1.13b) (side-to-side apposition of aortic wall)	
Fogarty aortic clamp (Fig.1.14) (side-to-side apposition of aortic wall)	Infrarenal aorta; aortic grafts, calcified aorta
Debakey aortic aneurysm clamp) (Fig.1.15) (apposition of anterior and posterior walls together)	Infrarenal aorta
Lambert-Kay aortic clamp (Fig.1.16a) (apposition of anterior and posterior walls together)	Infrarenal aorta
A rubber tube is inserted along the lower jaw of the Lambart-Kay clamp. (Fig.1.16b)	
A curved clamp is passed around the aorta to retrieve the free end of the rubber tube.	
Gentle traction on the rubber tube will guide the application of the Lambart-Kay clamp. (Fig.1.16c)	
Wylie hypogastric clamp (Fig.1.17)	Iliac arteries especially hypogastric arteries
Debakey peripheral vascular clamp (angled handle)	Iliac arteries
Debakey peripheral vascular clamp (angled jaw, 45°) (Fig.1.18)	Iliac and common carotid arteries
Henly subclavian clamp (Fig.1.19)	Subclavian and common femoral arteries

Partially occluding (side-biting) vascular clamps

Lemole-Strong aorta clamp (Fig.1.20)	Aorta, aortic grafts
Satinsky clamp (Fig.1.21)	Aorta, vena cava
Cooley anastomosis clamp	Aorta, aortic grafts
Cooley-Derra clamp	Graft limbs
Cooley pediatric clamp (Fig.1.22)	Common femoral artery, saphenofemoral junction

Self-compressing vascular clamps: do not require an applicator

Gregory carotid "soft" bulldog (Fig.1.23)	Small vessels
Potts bulldog, straight and angled jaw (Fig.1.23)	Small vessels
Debakey bulldog (Fig.1.23)	Small vessels
Diethrich bulldog (Fig.1.23)	Small vessels

Self compressing vascular clamps: require an applicator

Yasargil aneurysm clips (Fig.1.24)	Small vessels and branches
Heifitz clips	Small vessels and branches
Kleinert-Kutz clips-straight, angled, curved	Microvascular anastomoses
Louisville microvessel approximator	Microvascular anastomoses

Retractors (self-retaining)

Balfour abdominal retractors	Abdominal exposures
Poly-tract full abdominal retractor	Abdominal exposures
Omni-tract retractor (Fig.1.25)	Abdominal exposures
Beckman retractor (swing arm)	Deep soft tissue exposures
Gelpi retractor (sharp prongs)	Medium-depth soft tissue exposures
Weitlaner retractor (Fig.1.26)	Superficial soft tissue exposures
Spring retractor (Fig.1.27)	Superficial soft tissue exposures
Adson retractor	Superficial soft tissue exposures

Retractors (handheld)

Deaver retractor	Deep abdominal exposure
Harrington retractor	Liver retraction
Brewster retractor	Superficial soft tissue
Vein retractor	Renal vein

Miscellaneous

Freer double-ended elevator (Fig.1.28)	Starting an endarterectomy
Internal occluders (Fig.1.29)	Small arteries

VASCULAR CLAMPS

The most commonly used jaw design is a single row of serrated teeth opposing a double row of serrated teeth. This design allows for occluding the vessel with minimal damage to the vessel walls. In one variation, a double row of serrated teeth is opposing a triple row. In another variation, a special soft insert is applied to the clamp jaws (Fogarty clamps). These variations are specially designed for use with calcified diseased arteries. Vascular clamps with straight jaws are usually used to completely interrupt the blood flow. (Diagram 1) Vascular clamps with curved jaws can be used to provide total or partial interruption of blood flow. (Diagram 2) In the latter situation, they are used as side-biting clamps providing control of a segment of the vessel wall and yet maintaining distal perfusion.

VALVULOTOMES

Several instruments have been designed to produce effective valve destruction of venous conduits. These valvulotomes include the Mills, Hall, Lemaitre, Bush, and Gore Eze-Sit valvulotomes. The Retrograde Mills valvulotome has the shape of a nerve hook. (Fig. 1.30a; 1.30b) It is made of a rigid thin metallic wire with the tip bent at a 90° angle. The tip has a cutting edge to incise the valves. The instrument can be a retrograde or an antegrade valvulotome, depending on the location of the cutting edge. The retrograde Mills valvulotome has the cutting edge along the inner aspect of the tip. In the antegrade variety, the cutting edge is along the outer aspect of the tip. The retrograde valvulotome is 24 cm long and is usually introduced in the vein lumen through the distal end of the vein or through a side branch; this facilitates its use in small-diameter veins. However, the use of this valvulotome usually requires exposure of the entire vein. Valve cutting is achieved by withdrawing the valvulotome in the arterialized vein from proximal to distal. (Diagram 3) The valvulotome is first advanced proximal to the valve to be disrupted. It is then withdrawn until the valve is engaged. The engaged valve leaflet is incised by pulling the valvulotome. The valvulotome is then readvanced and rotated 180° to engage the remaining opposite valve leaflet. The Mills retrograde valvulotome is one of the safest valvulotomes because of the limited contact area between the instrument and the endothelium(1). Nevertheless, injury to the vein can occur, especially if the valvulotome engages a side branch inadvertently. In the remaining valvulotomes (Hall, Le Maitre, Bush, Gore), a cylindrical valve disrupter-cutter is introduced through the distal end of the vein and then withdrawn through the valves. The Hall Valve Stripper consists of two metal cylinders which are attached to a wire. The head cylinder has the negative imprint of a venous valve. The second metal cylinder is located 5 mm below the head cylinder and serves to stretch the vein. As the instrument is retracted, the lower end of the head cylinder engages the valve and rips it apart. The Hall Valve Stripper has been criticized for lacking a cutting edge which could inflict significant injury to the endothelium when the valve is being disrupted. The Expandable LeMaitre valvulotome has a self-centering head with four blades, one at each quadrant. The head is mounted on a 110-cm-long catheter. The Gore Eze-Sit valvulotome has a circular head with four serrated blades on each quadrant. This valvulotome comes with three head sizes (2, 3, 4 mm) and is mounted on a 95-cm-long catheter. The Bush retrograde valvulotome has three heads (2, 3, 4 mm) with shark-tooth-shaped blades. These valvulotomes do not require complete exposure of the vein conduit. However, injury to the vein wall can occur as these instruments are advanced in the nondistended vein, especially if the vein diameter is less than 4 mm(1). Valves can be inadequately incised or missed with the use of any valvulotome. Valvulotomy can also be performed under angioscopic guidance. However, angioscopy can result in fluid overload, potential endothelial injury from the angioscope, and added cost. When valve disruption is carried under angioscopic guidance, the Olympus retrograde valvulotome is commonly used. This instrument consists of a long flexible wire. A round metal head can be screwed to the tip of the wire. The wire is introduced through the distal end of the vein and guided proximally until it emerges from the proximal end of the vein. The round metal head is then unscrewed and replaced with the valvulotome head which is similar in shape to the Mills valvulotome. The Fogarty Valvulotome (Baxter) is a new valvulotome that is also designed to disrupt the venous valves under direct vision. This instrument is an optical valvulotome that incorporates within it an angioscope and also allows for coil embolization of the venous side branches.

CAROTID SHUNTS

Several carotid shunts are available to maintain cerebral perfusion during carotid endarterectomy. The proximal end of the shunt is placed in the common carotid artery and the distal end in the internal carotid artery. Shunts can be either inlying or outlying. The inlying shunt is straight and lies entirely in the lumen of the common and internal carotid arteries (Diagram 4). The outlying shunt is longer than the inlying shunt. It is inserted with only the ends lying in the vessel lumen while the remainder of the shunt extrudes as a loop outside the vessel (Diagram 5a). Performing the endarterectomy is usually easier with an outlying shunt (Diagram 5b). However, the limbs of the shunts extruding from the lumen can make closure of the arteriotomy more demanding than with an inlying shunt. Surgeons should be familiar with the various shunts available and should use the one with which they feel most confortable.

The shunts most commonly used include the Javid, the Sundt, and the Inahara Pruit shunts (Fig.1.31). The Javid shunt has two ends of different calibers with small bulges on either end of the shunt. These bulges serve to stabilize the shunt and prevent bleeding around it; this is achieved by applying special clamps on the common and internal carotid arteries at the level of the bulges. The Javid shunt is an outlying shunt. It is simple to use, but it is relatively rigid. The Sundt shunt is made of silastic and is fairly soft. It has a metallic skeleton incorporated in its wall to help maintain its tubular shape. This metallic skeleton prevents clamping the shunt. The Sundt shunt also has a bulbous portion on either end to help its stabilization, which is usually achieved with the use of Rumel tourniquets. The Sundt shunt is available in various sizes with an outlying or inlying configuration. The Inahara Pruit shunt (Fig.1.31) has inflatable balloons at each end to stablize the shunt with a side arm that allows flushing the lumen. A Rummel tourniquet is usually used to stablize the proximal part of the shunt. The distal end may be stabilized with balloon inflation only. The shunt is provided with two syringes to inflate the balloons. A good habit is to fill each syringe with just the amount of saline necessary to inflate the balloon to the desired size. This practice can help avoid accidental overinflation of the balloons which could result in balloon rupture or intimal damage. In the new shunts, the distal balloon is also attached to another small safety balloon placed along the distal arm of the shunt. The safety balloon will inflate if the pressure in the distal balloon exceeds the acceptable limit.

Reference

1. Leather RP, MD, Chang BB, MD, Darling CR III, MD, and Shah DM, MD. Not all in situ bypasses are created equal. In Yao JST, Pearce WH, editors: The ischemic extremity, advances in treatment. Connecticut, 1998. Appleton and Lange, pp. 391-404.

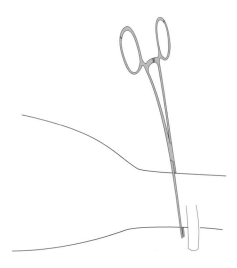

Diagram 1: Straight jaw vascular clamp completely interrupting blood flow.

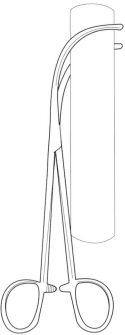

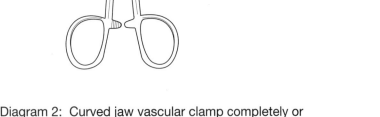

Diagram 2: Curved jaw vascular clamp completely or partially interrupting blood flow.

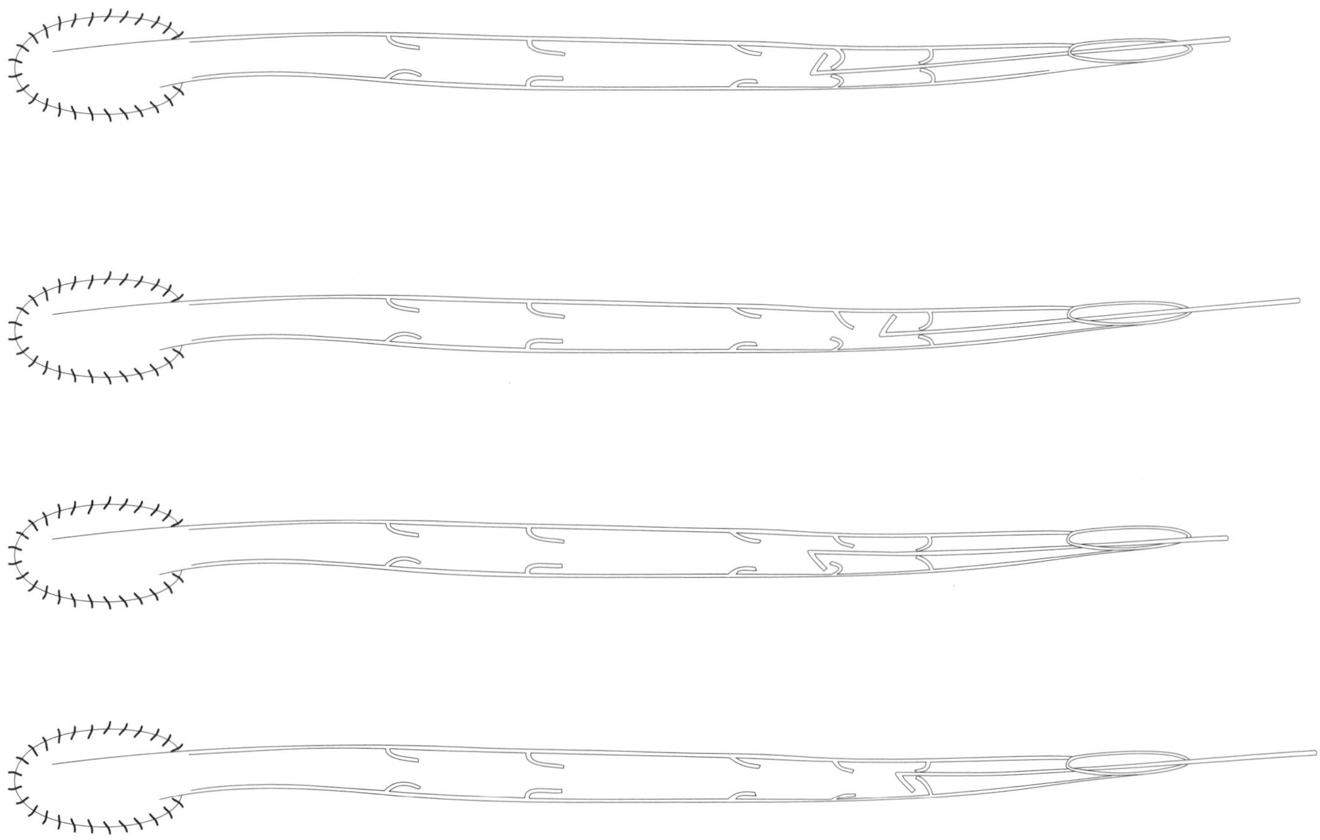

Diagram 3: Mills retrograde valvulotome disrupting valve leaflets.

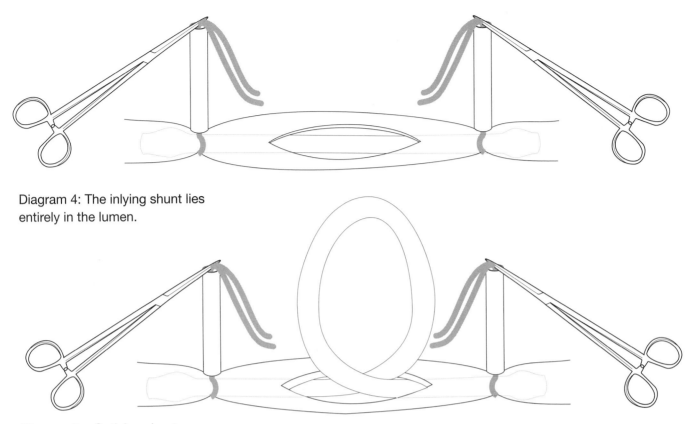

Diagram 4: The inlying shunt lies
entirely in the lumen.

Diagram 5a: Outlying shunt.

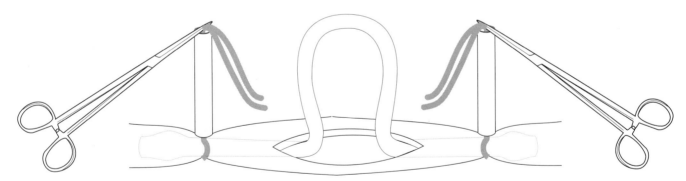

Diagram 5b: The outlying shunt can be adjusted to
facilitate the endarterectomy.

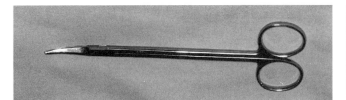

Figure 1.1 Church scissors

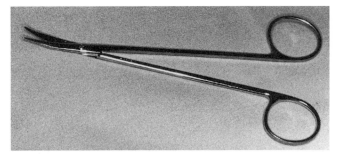

Figure 1.2 Stevens tenotomy scissors

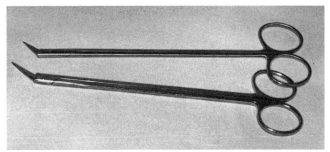

Figure 1.3 Potts scissors

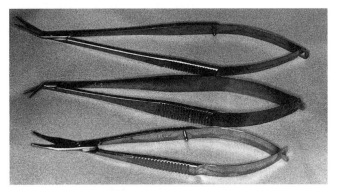

Figure 1.4 Castroviejo scissors

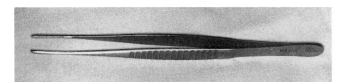

Figure 1.5 Debakey tissue forceps

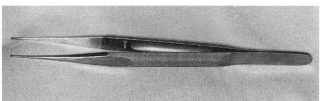

Figure 1.6 Microsuture ring tip forceps

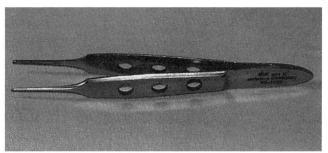

Figure 1.7 Bishop-Harmon forceps

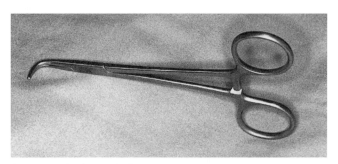

Figure 1.8 Right-angle forceps

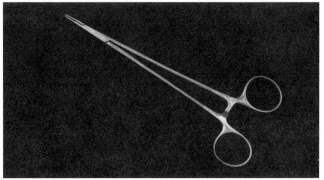

Figure 1.9 Mayo Hegar needle holder

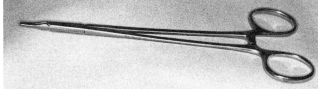

Figure 1.10 Ryder needle holder

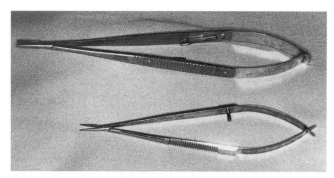

Figure 1.11 Castroviejo needle holder

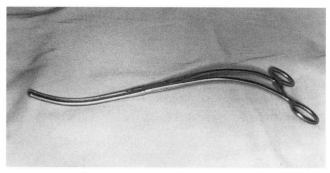

Figure 1.13a Debakey-Bahnson aortic aneurysm clamp

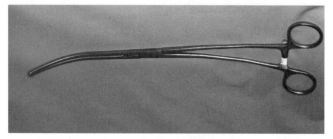

Figure 1.12a Debakey aortic aneurysm clamp

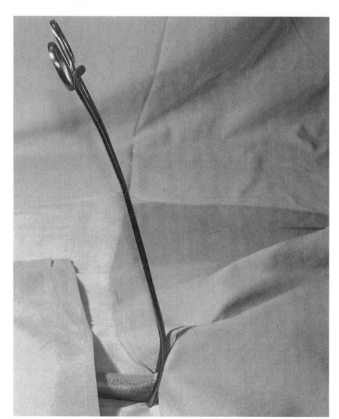

Figure 1.12b

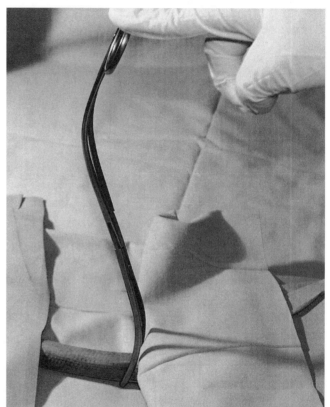

Figure 1.13b

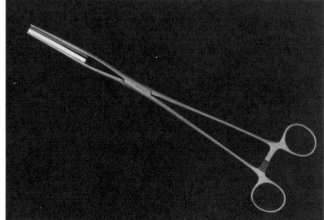

Figure 1.14 Fogarty clamp

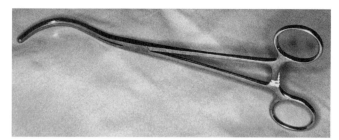

Figure 1.15 Debakey aortic aneurysm clamp

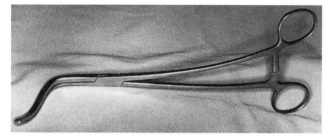

Figure 1.16a Lambert-Kay aortic clamp

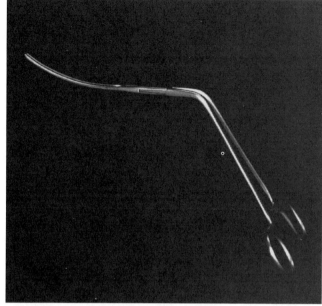

Figure 1.17a Wylie hypogastric clamp

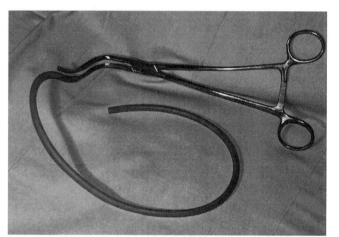

Figure 1.16b

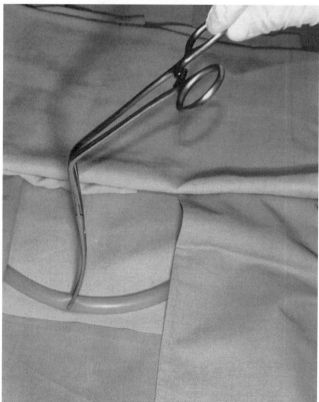

Figure 1.17b

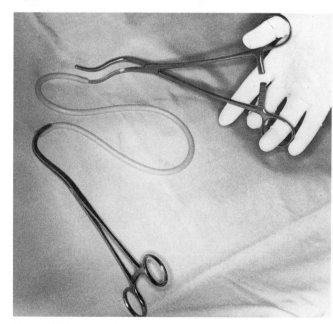

Figure 1.16c

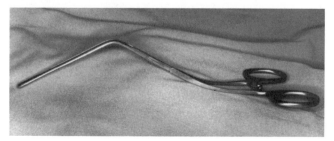

Figure 1.18 Debakey peripheral vascular clamp

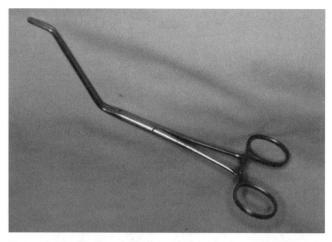

Figure 1.19a Henly subclavian clamp

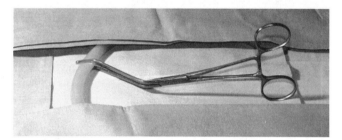

Figure 1.19b

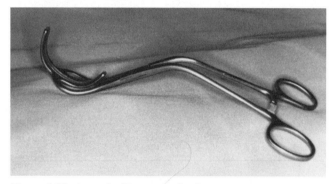

Figure 1.20a Lemole-Strong aortic clamp

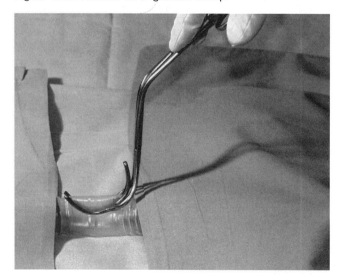

Figure 1.20b

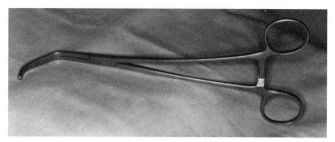

Figure 1.21 Satinsky clamp

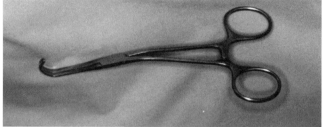

Figure 1.22 Cooley Pediatric clamp

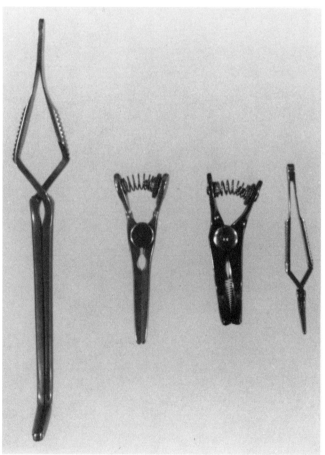

Figure 1.23 Bulldog clamps (Gregory, Potts, Debakey, Diethrich)

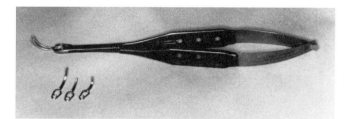

Figure 1.24 Yasargil aneurysm clips and applicator

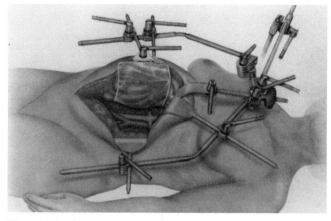

Figure 1.25 Omni-tract retractor

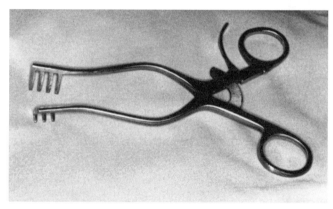

Figure 1.26 Weitlaner retractor

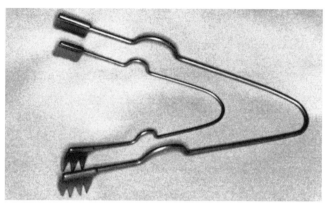

Figure 1.27 Spring retractors

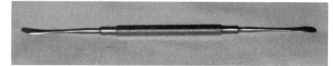

Figure 1.28 Freer double-ended elevator

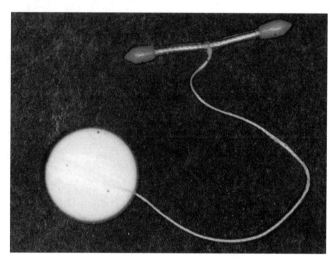

Figure 1.29 Internal occluder

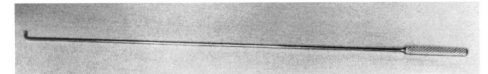

Figure 1.30a Mills valvulotome

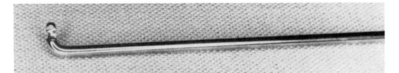

Figure 1.30b

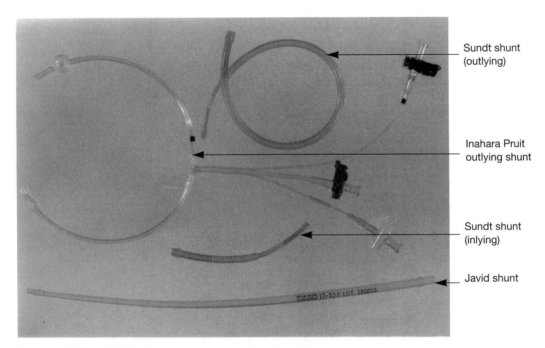

Figure 1.31 Carotid shunts

Vascular Grafts, Patches, and Sutures

VASCULAR GRAFTS

Modern vascular surgery became possible with the development of acceptable arterial substitutes. The usefulness of an arterial substitute is determined by several essential qualities. These qualities include porosity, durability, tissue reactivity, and flexibility. The ideal conduit should be impermeable to blood and capable of lasting the duration of the recipient's life. Graft durability is dependent on its ability to maintain its characteristics and strength over time, resisting dilatation and degeneration. Graft durability is also related to its short- and long-term patency rates. The ideal conduit should be able to resist thrombosis even in low flow states. In addition, its compliance, which measures its volume change with variations in pressure, should match that of the replaced arterial segment. Compliance mismatch has been identified as a possible cause of neointimal hyperplasia, which is a leading cause of graft failure. The graft should also stimulate minimal antigenicity and should not induce significant tissue reaction. The conduit should be flexible with good handling characteristics. It should be resistant to infection and easily available for elective or emergency use. Finally, the graft should be affordable. Vascular grafts can be classified according to their source of origin into autogenous, homologous, bovine, and synthetic (prosthetic) grafts. It is hard to find, in the currently available vascular grafts, one conduit that possesses all the characteristics of the ideal arterial substitute; this explains why the ultimate arterial substitute is still to be developed. In general, in high-flow situations such as aortic reconstructive surgery, large-caliber prosthetic grafts perform well and are the conduits of choice. In infrainguinal reconstructions, the best performance has been achieved with autogenous conduits.

AUTOGENOUS CONDUITS

Veins are the most commonly used autogenous conduits. The veins used as conduits include the greater and lesser saphenous veins, the superficial femoral-popliteal vein, and the cephalic and basilic veins. Arterial segments have also been used as autogenous grafts; these include the internal iliac artery, the radial artery, and the internal mammary artery. The latter two have been predominantly used for coronary revascularization and are not reviewed in this chapter. Autogenous conduits should be handled gently to minimize their injury during the harvesting process. One obvious mechanism of injury is crushing the vessel wall with the forceps during the dissection. This can be avoided by grasping only the adventitia of the conduit. Trauma to the conduit can also occur when a silastic loop is used to retract the vessel and excessive traction is applied on the loop. Another form of injury occurs when small branches are inadvertently avulsed during the dissection or when branches are ligated very close to the body of the conduit, resulting in impingement on the lumen. Another important mechanism of trauma is overdistension of the conduit, leading to considerable endothelial injury. The endothelium can be protected by keeping the intraluminal pressure below 300 mmHg and using chilled whole blood to distend the graft. A cold solution of Ringer's lactate (1 L) or Dextran 40 (1 L) mixed with 5000 units of heparin and 60 mg of papaverine can also be used to distend a vein graft. The vein should also be protected from desiccation injury during its exposure by keeping the vein covered with gauze soaked with warm saline. Papaverine (60 mg/500 mL) can be added to the saline solution in an attempt to decrease spasm in the conduit.

Autogenous veins can be evaluated preoperatively with B-mode ultrasonography. This useful noninvasive method for assessing the availability, size, and quality of the venous conduit can also determine the presence of a duplicate system or other anatomical variations. A duplex surveillance program is recommended to routinely evaluate any autogenous vein bypass postoperatively. This test can identify failing grafts, resulting in graft revision before graft occlusion. Autogenous bypass failure during the first postoperative month is usually the result of technical reasons or poor choice of the inflow or outflow vessels. After the first postoperative month and for the following 2 years, neointimal hyperplasia becomes the most common cause of graft failure. Progression of atherosclerosis is the predominant cause of graft failure after the second postoperative year. Duplex surveillance is usually recommended every 3 months in the first postoperative year, every 6 months in the second year, and yearly thereafter.

Greater Saphenous Vein

In infrainguinal reconstructions, the greater saphenous vein (GSV) is considered the gold standard against which all other conduits are compared. When used as a bypass, the GSV can be harvested or kept in its bed after disrupting its valves (in situ vein bypass). A harvested GSV is either reversed (reversed vein graft), or used in a nonreversed fashion after disrupting the valves (translocated nonreversed vein graft). A learning curve is expected when the valves of a venous conduit are disrupted with a valvulotome. Incomplete disruption of valve leaflets or vein damage can occur with improper manipulation of any valvulotome. A duplicate venous system can be found in the thigh in 35% of the population. (11) When the GSV is of a good size (>3 mm) and quality, it is expected to perform equally well whether used as a reversed, nonreversed, or in situ bypass. However, vein utilization appears to be greatest with the in situ vein bypass, especially when the vein diameter is less than 3 mm. The patency rates of GSV bypasses to the above-knee popliteal artery have been reported to be comparable to those obtained with prosthetic bypasses at 4-year follow-up. However, the long-term patency of GSV infrainguinal bypasses is superior to that of prosthetic grafts, especially when the bypass extends below the knee. The patency rates of infrainguinal bypasses at various levels performed with the GSV and other conduits are shown in Table 2.1.

Lesser Saphenous Vein

The lesser saphenous vein serves as a good alternative source of autogenous vein grafts when the GSV is not available. Due to its limited length, the lesser saphenous vein is ideal for usage as a short bypass or for bypass revisions.

Superficial Femoral-Popliteal Vein

Although the superficial femoral vein belongs to the deep venous system, it can be harvested and used as a conduit for infrainguinal revascularization. (10) In addition, it has been successfully used to replace infected aortic grafts. (8)

TABLE 2.1. Patency rates of infrainguinal reconstructions at 4 years

	ABOVE-KNEE POPLITEAL	BELOW-KNEE POPLITEAL	REFERENCE #
Greater saphenous vein			
(primary)	70	65–75	1, 2, 3, 4, 6, 13, 14
(secondary)		81	
Arm vein			
(primary)	60	70	3, 7
Umbilical vein			
(primary)	70	60	5
PTFE			
(primary)	60	40	1, 14

When additional length is needed, the harvesting is extended to include the popliteal vein. Following harvesting of the superficial femoral-popliteal vein, the incidence of long-term postoperative swelling does not appear to be of clinical significance. (8,10) This is noted especially if the patient has a normal deep venous system preoperatively and an intact greater saphenous vein, and if the junction with the profunda femoris vein is preserved. Nevertheless, the use of this conduit for infrainguinal revascularization has not gained wide acceptance, especially when other sources of vein conduits are available.

Arm Veins (Basilic and Cephalic)
The basilic and the cephalic veins can also be used as vein bypasses. These veins are relatively thin and delicate and can be challenging to use. They have a limited length and may also have unsuspected intraluminal pathology related to scarring from previous venipuncture. Arm veins can be used for bypass revisions or as grafts when the greater or lesser saphenous veins are unavailable. They can also be used as segments of composite bypasses. A duplex surveillance is essential to assist the long-term patency of arm vein bypasses. (3)

Composite Bypass
When two conduits are joined together to achieve the required length for a revascularization, the bypass is referred to as a composite graft. The conduits are usually joined using an end-to-end or an end-to-side reconstruction. When an end-to-side reconstruction is used, the second segment usually arises from the distal part of the first conduit and the graft is described as a sequential bypass. The composite bypass is usually constructed from a prosthetic and a vein segment. The prosthetic part is usually kept above the knee with the vein segment crossing the knee joint to the popliteal or the infrapopliteal arteries. The patency of this type of conduit is limited by the prosthetic component, and its value remains controversial. The composite bypass can also be constructed from two vein segments (composite vein bypass). The vein segments may be harvested from the upper or lower extremity. This composite vein bypass is usually used for infrapopliteal bypasses when the greater saphenous vein is inadequate. The performance of such bypass usually depends on the quality of the veins used.

Internal Iliac Artery
The internal iliac artery has been recommended for usage as a conduit in young patients suffering from renovascular hypertension. (9) Unlike the greater saphenous vein, the internal iliac artery does not appear to develop aneurysmal dilatation when used in children to construct an aortorenal bypass. Aneurysmal dilatation of saphenous vein aortorenal bypasses in children has been noted in 20% of the patients on long-term follow-up. (9, 19)

HOMOLOGOUS GRAFTS

Umbilical vein grafts (UVG)

The source of these grafts are umbilical cord veins that are treated with glutaraldehyde. Despite their reinforcement with a dacron mesh, UVG grafts can develop aneurysmal dilatation on long-term follow-up. They are mainly used for infrainguinal revascularization. Their superiority over prosthetic grafts remains controversial.

Cryopreserved Veins

Cryopreserved veins are greater saphenous veins procured from cadaveric donors. Each donor is supposed to be extensively tested for any infectious disease. The harvested vein is preserved in a special solution and then stored in liquid nitrogen freezers. The veins are available in lengths varying from 50 to 80 cm with the inner diameter ranging from 3 to 6 mm. The veins are usually matched to the patient's ABO blood group. Cryopreserved vein grafts are costly, and their superiority over commonly used prosthetic grafts is not proven. Rejection may play a role in delayed failure.

Aortic Allograft

Before the development of prosthetic grafts, aortic segments harvested from cadavers were used to replace the diseased aorta. However, on late follow-up, aortic allografts were noted to suffer from a significant rate of occlusion or aneurysmal degeneration. With the evolution and availability of the current prosthetic grafts, the use of aortic allografts was abandoned. However, an interest in these grafts has been resurrected recently as new studies advocate their utilization for the in situ replacement of infected aortic grafts. (15)

BOVINE GRAFTS

Bovine grafts such as Artegraft (Artegraft, Inc. North Brunswick, NJ) are collagen conduits. They are usually composed of a selected section of a bovine carotid artery that has been subjected to enzymatic treatment with ficin and tanned with dialdehyde starch. These grafts have been mainly used for hemodialysis access. The ease of handling of these grafts was originally tempered by the early recognition of a high incidence of complications such as thrombosis, aneurysmal formation, and infection. However, the incidence of these complications has been reported to be comparable to that seen with other prosthetic dialysis conduits. Nevertheless, these grafts are not used frequently.

PROSTHETIC GRAFTS

The currently available prosthetic grafts can be generally classified into either textile or nontextile grafts. After the implantation of a prosthetic graft, the graft material is infiltrated by connective tissue that grows through the pores of the wall to reach the luminal surface. The inner lining becomes an organized layer of blood coagulum partially supported by the invading strands of connective tissue. This layer is referred to as pseudointima because it lacks endothelium, except at the level of the anastomoses to the native vessel where some endothelial cells may be found. The pseudointima has a very poor resistance to clotting and does not possess the highly specialized qualities of the true endothelium. The connective tissue forms an outer shell or a "capsule" around the prosthesis, which may vary in thickness depending on the reactivity of the prosthesis and the characteristics of the surrounding tissues. Ideally, the graft should be well incorporated without an overwhelming connective tissue invasion.

Textile Grafts

Textile vascular prostheses such as Dacron (Dupont, Inc.) are made of polyester. They are usually constructed by extruding polyester fibers and then twisting them together to form a yarn. The polyester yarn is then woven or knitted to produce the graft fabric. Textile grafts are porous. Healing and tissue ingrowth into textile grafts tend to increase with the porosity of the fabric. However, bleeding through the interstices of the grafts will also increase with the porosity of the graft. Textile grafts are usually crimped to provide some degree of elasticity and support across curvatures or joints. However, the elasticity is usually lost after the graft is implanted.

In woven polyester grafts, straight yarns are interlaced in an over-and-under pattern. Depending on the tightness of the weaving process, woven vascular grafts do not necessarily need to be preclotted. These grafts are stiff and do not tend to stretch. Their tissue incorporation is the least among the polyester grafts. They tend to fray or unravel if transected with a regular knife, which can be reduced by cutting with a hot knife or cautery. These grafts were mainly used during thoracic aortic replacements and when preclotting was not possible. Currently, they are less frequently used as more desirable grafts have become available.

In knitted polyester grafts, loops of yarn are interlaced in various patterns that allow stretching of the graft. These are more porous than the woven grafts. The porosity of these grafts allows good tissue ingrowth into the graft after implantation. Preclotting of the graft with nonheparinized blood is necessary, however, to prevent bleeding through the fabric.

A velour polyester graft is produced by adding supplementary loops of yarns that project outward from the fabric, giving the surface a look and feel of velvet. The velour surface can be added to a woven or knitted core. A double velour graft has velour on the inner and outer surface of the graft fabric. The configuration of the velour surface is designed to allow for more efficient preclotting and strong tissue ingrowth into the graft. These features explain why knitted double velour grafts are popular and very frequently used in aortic reconstructive procedures.

Textile grafts can also be impregnated or coated with sealants such as collagen, albumin, or gelatin to eliminate the need for preclotting before their implantation. This feature is very desirable even though it increases the cost of the graft. "Hemashield" is impregnated with collagen and manufactured by Meadox (Boston Scientific); "Intervascular" (Bard Cardiovascular) is coated with albumin, and "Gelseal" (Vascutek) is coated with gelatin.

Polyester grafts are the most commonly used aortic prostheses. They are available in a tube or a bifurcated configuration. They have also been used for infrainguinal reconstruction procedures; however, they remain less popular in the infrainguinal position than other available prosthetic conduits. The main concern with polyester grafts is their tendency to dilate with time, which is more commonly seen with the knitted variety. The long-term significance and clinical consequences of such dilatation remains undetermined.

Expanded Polytetrafluoroethylene (PTFE)

PTFE grafts are nontextile grafts. They are produced by extrusion of the Teflon polymer, which is then mechanically stretched to produce a microporous tube. This tube is composed of solid nodes of PTFE interconnected by PTFE fibrils. The space between the fibrils represents the pores of the PTFE tube. Stretching the PTFE tube tends to lengthen the fibrils and widen the space between the nodes. PTFE grafts are microporous and do not require any preclotting. Tissue incorporation does occur despite the microporosity of the graft. Some of the first-generation PTFE grafts were noted to develop aneurysmal dilatation on follow-up. Gore-Tex, the PTFE graft produced by W.L. Gore, Inc., has an extra layer of PTFE added to its outer surface. In the other grafts, the manufacturing process has been modified to rectify this concern.

PTFE grafts are available in various lengths and diameters permitting their utilization in aortic or peripheral reconstructions. They have become the conduit of choice for dialysis access when a primary fistula is not possible. They are also the grafts most commonly used for infrainguinal revascularization when autogenous veins are unavailable. The results of aortic PTFE grafts have been very favorable. They do not tend to dilate on long-term follow-up, as noted in the polyester grafts. Nevertheless, their use for aortic reconstructions has not gained wide acceptance yet. The main concerns have been the handling characteristics of the graft in the aortic location and needle-hole bleeding from the suture line. Nonaortic PTFE grafts can be externally supported by rings placed on the outer surface of the conduit. Wall thickness varies from 0.6 to 0.4 mm in the thin wall grafts.

Several modifications have been accomplished in PTFE grafts in an attempt to further improve their patency and handling characteristics. W.L. Gore has produced a stretch PTFE variety to decrease the compliance mismatch between grafts and native vessels. Modifications in the luminal surface of PTFE grafts have been recently achieved by incorporating carbon particles in the graft in an attempt to further decrease its thrombogenicity (Carboflo graft, Impra). Another new modification by Impra has been the creation of a special hood configuration at the distal end of the graft to simulate the effect of vein cuffs or patches. Vein cuffs and patches have been advocated as a method to decrease the neointimal hyperplastic response that develops at the distal anastomosis of prosthetic infrainguinal bypasses. The hood configuration is now available for hemodialysis grafts (Venoflo) or infrainguinal grafts (Distoflo). The effectiveness of all these modifications on the patency of PTFE grafts is not proven yet. PTFE grafts for nonaortic use are now produced by several manufacturers including W.L. Gore, Impra (Bard), Meadox (Boston Scientific), and Atrium (Atrium Medical Inc.). Aortic PTFE grafts are currently only manufactured by W.L. Gore.

VASCULAR PATCHES

Patches used in vascular reconstructions are also classified as autogenous or prosthetic. Autogenous patches can be obtained from arm or leg veins. The jugular and facial veins have also served as sources of vein patches. One concern with using vein patches relates to their potential risk of rupture. This risk has been mainly reported with the use of the ankle segment of the greater saphenous vein during carotid endarterectomy. Vein patch rupture has also been reported when the thigh segment of the saphenous vein has been used during carotid endarterectomy. Greater saphenous vein patch rupture is more likely to result from the quality of the vein rather than its site of origin. Another concern with the use of a segment of the greater saphenous vein as a patch is the fate of the remaining part of the vein. Thrombosis of the vein will eliminate its potential use in the future as a bypass conduit for coronary or infrainguinal revascularization. Another source for autogenous patches is the occluded superficial femoral artery. After harvesting the occluded artery, an endarterectomy is performed and the endarterectomized vessel is incised longitudinally and used as a patch.

Table 2.2. Non Autogenous Patches

PATCHES	DESCRIPTION	MANUFACTURERS	THICKNESS
Gore-Tex	Expanded polytetrafluoroethylene	W.L. Gore	0.40 mm
Gore-Tex Acuseal	Expanded polytetrafluoroethylene combined with fluoropolymer	W.L. Gore	0.50 mm
Hemashield	Knitted double velour polyester	Meadox (Boston Scientific)	0.76 mm
Hemashield Finesse	Knitted, non velour polyester impregnated with collagen		
Intervascular	Knitted velour polyester coated with collagen	Impra (Bard, Inc)	0.65 mm
Sulzer Vascutek	Polyester bonded with fluoropolymer and sealed with gelatin	Sulzer Vascutek USA	0.38 mm
Vascugard	Bovine pericardium cross linked with glutaraldehyde	(Biovascular, Inc, St. Paul, MN USA)	0.35 mm

Prosthetic patches are usually made of polyester or PTFE. They share the same characteristics as their graft counterparts. The main concerns with the use of prosthetic patches relate to the possibility of infection, future dilatation, needle-hole bleeding, and handling characteristics. The infection rate of prosthetic patches used during carotid endarterectomy is less than 1%. Although the standard PTFE patches have very desirable handling characteristics, the disturbing needle-hole bleeding noted when used during carotid endarterectomy has curtailed their use in carotid procedures. This led to the recent introduction by W.L. Gore of the Acuseal patch where the expanded PTFE is combined with an elastometric fluoropolymer to minimize needle-hole bleeding. The old generation of polyester patches had a propensity to dilate, which led to the development of a newer generation with average handling characteristics. Currently, polyester patches are available in various thicknesses and have very desirable characteristics. Needle-hole bleeding is minimal with the newest generation patches, especially when impregnated with collagen or coated with albumin. The long-term results of these patches with respect to dilatation and neointimal hyperplasia are not available yet. A list of the commercially available patches is outlined in Table 2.2.

VASCULAR SUTURES

Vascular reconstructions are conducted with nonabsorbable sutures. These sutures are needed to provide the tensile strength essential to secure the walls of the vessels together until healing is completed. This provision is especially important when prosthetic material is used because these grafts never completely heal and the tensile strength provided by the sutures is needed for the duration of the patient's life. The suture material available for vascular reconstructions include multifilament sutures such as silk and braided polyester, or monofilament sutures such as polypropylene, polybutester, and polytetrafluoroethylene.

SILK SUTURES

Although silk is nonabsorbable, it is biodegradable and tends to lose its tensile strength over time. Silk has been incriminated in the late development of anastomotic pseudoaneurysms. Silk sutures are very rarely used nowdays to construct vascular anastomoses.

BRAIDED POLYESTER SUTURES (MERSILENE, DACRON, ETHIBOND)

These sutures are nonabsorbable and made of braided fibers of polyester. They maintain their great tensile strength over time and elicit minimal tissue reaction. Mersilene and Dacron are uncoated, resulting in a rough surface. When these sutures are pulled through tissues or tied, a drag feeling is noted, limiting their handling characteristics.

POLYPROPYLENE SUTURES (PROLENE, SURGIPRO, SURGILENE)

Although some surgeons use polyester sutures because of their superior tensile strength, polypropylene sutures have gained a wider popularity and are probably the most commonly used suture material in vascular reconstructions. Made of a monofilament strand of a synthetic linear polyolefin, these polypropylene sutures tend to maintain their tensile strength over time. In addition, they have a low coefficient of friction and excellent handling characteristics. They maintain their tensile strength in vitro and elicit a minimal transient acute inflammatory tissue reaction. Polypropylene sutures are very smooth. Seven throws are usually placed to secure the knot and avoid unraveling.

POLYBUTESTER SUTURES

The polybutester suture (Novofil; Davis & Geck) is a new type of monofilament nonabsorbable suture. This suture is advertised as being stronger than polypropylene with increased flexibility and little memory. It is coated with polytribolate to reduce drag and improve tissue passage during suturing. The experience in using these sutures in vascular reconstructions remains limited because most surgeons are used to polypropylene.

POLYTETRAFLUOROETHYLENE SUTURES

Polytetrafluoroethylene (PTFE) sutures also have excellent handling characteristics. They have been developed with the intention of minimizing needle-hole bleeding, which is often seen when polypropylene sutures are used with PTFE grafts or patches. They are designed to have a very minimal difference in the diameter of the needle and the suture line. Thus, theoretically, the PTFE thread should fill all the space created by the penetration of the needle and the leak around the PTFE thread should be minimal. However, needle-hole bleeding still occurs with PTFE sutures, especially when the needle has been inadvertently subjected to lateral movements when penetrating the vessel wall.

Monofilaments usually have a low tissue friction and a low drag coefficient, which makes them ideal for usage as a continuous suture line. Despite these properties, inappropriate pulling on the thread may result in tearing and longitudinal slits in the vessel walls that could also result in an excessive amount of suture line bleeding. A careful use of a nerve hook could result in tightening of the suture line without tearing the vessel wall.

All sutures are susceptible to fraying and breakage if poorly handled. Suture breakage can develop intraoperatively or postoperatively, resulting in catastrophic complications. Following are some tips in handling suture material.

1. Avoid crushing the suture line with the tissue forceps or the needle holder.

2. Use rubber clamps or plastic-shod clamps to stabilize the unused part of a suture line.

3. Apply the rubber-shod clamps close to the needle rather than in the middle of the suture line.

4. Avoid excessive friction between both ends of the suture line while tying as this can lead to fraying.

5. If tying was started with a sliding or granny knot, crossing the hands with the following throws is essential to achieve square knots with the remaining throws and avoid the possibility of unraveling or slipping of the knot.

6. Use sutures appropriately sized for your reconstruction. The following guidelines are suggested for the choice of suture size:

> 2-0, 3-0; aorta
> 4-0; iliac arteries
> 5-0; axillary, common carotid, common femoral, and superficial femoral arteries
> 5-0, 6-0; internal carotid, popliteal and brachial arteries
> 7-0, 8-0; tibial or inframalleolar arteries

NEEDLE SIZE

Sutures used for vascular reconstructions are usually double armed with a needle on each end of the suture. The suture thread is enclosed in the eye of the needle. Thus the hole in the vessel wall is determined by the size of the needle and the smoothness of introducing the needle through the vessel wall. Several needle shapes are available. Cutting needles have a sharp pyramidal shape and are used for tough tissues such as the skin. They are not used in vascular reconstructions to avoid excessive tears in the vessel wall. Taper needles have a round smooth shape. They are most favored in vascular reconstructions as they puncture the vessel wall with minimal cutting. In very calcified vessels, a hybrid of the taper and cutting needle is available to allow penetration of the needle through the vessel wall. These hybrid needles are called tapercut needles because the tip has a cutting profile while the rest of the needle has a round design. Unfortunately, the same needle shape and size may be given a different name by a different manufacturer. Surgeons should be familiar with the shapes and names of needles available at their institutions. Choosing the appropriate needle shape and size during a vascular reconstruction is very important. The following guidelines are suggested for choosing the appropriate needle. All the following needles are taper point needles except for the V7 and CC (Ethicon), which are tapercut.

VESSEL SIZE	ETHICON	U.S.S.C.	DAVIS AND GECK	GORE-TEX
Small (calcified tibial)	CC	KV-1	CV-311/DTE-10	PT-9
Small (tibial, internal carotid)	BV-1	CV-1	CV-310/TE-10, 11	TT-9
Small (tibial)	BV	CV	CV-309/TE-9	TT-12
Medium (common carotid, femoral, popliteal)	C-1	CV-11	CV-301/TE-1	TT-13
Large (common iliac)	RB-1	CV-23	CV-331/T-31	TH-18
Large (aorta)	V7	V-20	CV-305/T-5	TH-26
Large (posterior wall of aorta)	MH	V26	CV-C00/T-10	TH-35

REFERENCES

1. Bergan JJ, Veith FJ, Bernhard VM, et al. Randomization of autologous vein and polytetrafluoroethylene grafts in femoral-distal reconstructions. Surgery 1982;92:921–930.

2. Bush HL, Nabseth DC, Curl GR, et al. In situ saphenous vein bypass grafts for limb salvage. A current fad or a viable alternative to reversed vein bypass grafts? Am J Surg 1985;149:477–480.

3. Chalmers RTA, Hoballah JJ, Kresowik TF, Sharp WJ, Synn AY, and Corson JD. The impact of color duplex surveillance on the outcome of lower limb bypass with arm veins. J Vasc Surg 1994;19:279–288.

4. Corson JD, Hoballah JJ, Kresowik TF, Sharp WJ, Worsey MJ, Synn AY, Martinasevic M, Kury Neto W, and Brummer M. Technical aspects and results of the open in situ saphenous vein bypass technique. Int Angiol 1993;12:162–163.

5. Dardick H, Miller N, Dardick A, et al. A decade of experience with the gluteraldehyde tanned human umbilical cord vein graft for revascularization of the lower limb. J Vasc Surg 1988;7:336–346.

6. Fogle MA, Whittemore AD, Couch NP, Mannick JA. A comparison of in situ and reversed saphenous vein grafts for infrainguinal reconstruction. J Vasc Surg 1987;5:46–52.

7. Harris RW, Andros G, Salles-Cunha SX. Alternative autogenous vein grafts to the inadequate saphenous vein. Surgery 1986;100:822–827.

8. Kakish HB, Clagett GP. Replacement of infected aortic prostheses with lower extremity deep veins. Perspectives in Vascular Surgery 1998;9:21–39.

9. Lawson JD, Boerth R, Foster JH, et al. Diagnosis and management of renovascular hypertension in children. Arch Surg 122:1307–1316.

10. Schulman ML, Badhey MR, Yatco R. Superficial femoral-popliteal veins and reversed veins as primary femoropopliteal bypass grafts: A randomized comparative study. J Vasc Surg 1987;6:1–10.

11. Shah DM, Chang BB, Leopold PW, et al. The anatomy of the greater saphenous venous system. J Vasc Surg 1986;3:273–283.

12. Stanley JC, Ernst CB, Fry WJ. Fate of ibo aortorenal vein grafts: Characteristics of late graft expansion, aneurysmal dilatation, and stenosis. Surgery, 1973;74:931–944.

13. Taylor LM, Edwards JM, Porter JM, Phinney ES. Reversed vein bypass to infrapopliteal arteries: Modern results are superior or equivalent to in-situ bypass for patency and for vein utilization. Ann Surg 1987;205:90–97.

14. Veith FJ, Gupta SK, Ascer E, et al. Six-year prospective multicenter randomized comparison of autologous saphenous vein and expanded polytetrafluoroethylene grafts in infrainguinal arterial reconstructions. J Vasc Surg 1986;3:104–114.

15. Vogt PR, Bruner-La Rocca HP, Carrel T, et al. Cryopreserved arterial allografts in the treatment of major vascular infection: A comparison with conventional surgical techniques. J Thorac Cardiovasc Surg 1998;116:965–72.

3

Vascular Anatomy and Exposures

ARTERIES OF THE NECK AND UPPER EXTREMITY

ANATOMY OF THE SUBCLAVIAN AND VERTEBRAL ARTERIES

The Subclavian Artery

The right subclavian artery (SCA) originates from the innominate (brachio-cephalic) artery at the base of the neck behind the right sternoclavicular junc-tion (Fig. 3.1). It curves upward and laterally to pass behind the right anterior scalene muscle and then crosses underneath the clavicle and over the first rib to become the axillary artery.

The left subclavian artery originates directly from the aortic arch and as-cends in the mediastinum to the base of the neck where it follows, on the left side, a similar course to that of the right subclavian artery (Fig. 3.1).

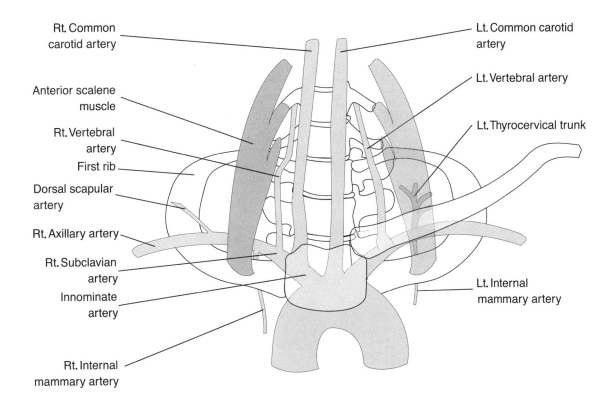

Figure 3.1. Anatomy of the aortic arch vessels.

The subclavian artery is divided into three parts based on its anatomical relationship to the anterior scalene muscle. The first part is medial, the second part is posterior and the third part is lateral to the anterior scalene muscle. The branches of the first part of the subclavian artery are the vertebral artery, the internal mammary artery, and the thyrocervical trunk. Usually no branches originate from the second part of the subclavian artery. The third part of the subclavian artery gives rise to the dorsal scapular artery (Fig. 3.1).

The Vertebral Artery
Each vertebral artery usually originates from the upper posterior part of the subclavian artery as its first branch (Fig. 3.1) Occasionally, the right vertebral artery may originate from the innominate artery and similarly the left vertebral artery may originate directly from the aortic arch. The vertebral artery ascends in the neck posteriorly and usually enters the transverse process foramen of the sixth cervical vertebrae. The vertebral artery then courses cranially through the foramina of the transverse processes of C6–C2. It exits through the transverse foramen of the atlas (C2), and runs in the suboccipital region above the atlas. It then passes through the atlantooccipital membrane, and ascends to join the opposite vertebral artery to form the basilar artery. The vertebral artery is arbitrarily divided into four parts: V1 represents the artery from its origin until its entrance into the transverse foramen, V2 is the part that runs between C6 and C2, V3 is from C2 to the atlantooccipital membrane, and V4 is from the atlantooccipital membrane to the basilar artery.

EXPOSURE OF THE INNOMINATE AND SUBCLAVIAN ARTERIES

A median sternotomy is necessary to expose the origin of the innominate and right subclavian arteries. (19, 26, 27, 35) A left anterior thoracotomy through the third or fourth intercostal space is needed to expose and control the origin of the left subclavian artery. (26, 27) The remaining parts of the subclavian arteries are usually exposed through a supraclavicular approach. The various possible incisions used for exposing the aortic arch vessels are diagrammed in Fig. 3.2.

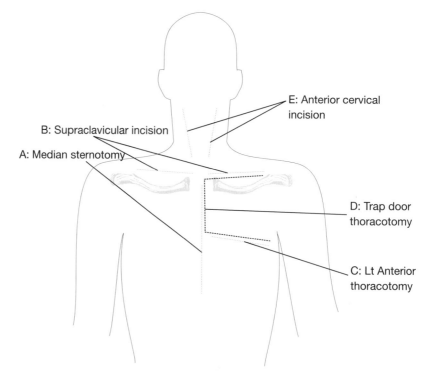

Figure 3.2. Incisions used for exposure of the aortic arch vessels.

Median Sternotomy

A skin incision is performed from the sternal notch to the xiphoid process. The skin incision is deepened through the subcutaneous tissues to the sternum. The clavicular ligament between the sternal heads of the clavicle is divided. The subxiphoid space is carefully dissected to engage an electric sternal saw. The sternum is longitudinally divided in half. A sternal bone spreader is then placed to spread the divided sternum. The thymus remnant is identified in the upper part of the incision and separated in the middle, exposing the left brachiocephalic vein directly beneath it. The left brachiocephalic vein is exposed and circumferentially dissected. A silastic vessel loop is passed around the left brachiocephalic vein and used to retract the vein superiorly, exposing the innominate artery and the origins of the right subclavian and both common carotid arteries (Fig. 3.3). The innominate artery can be mobilized and traced up to its bifurcation. Care should be taken to avoid any iatrogenic injury to the right recurrent laryngeal nerve as it arches around the origin of the right subclavian artery (Fig 3.4).

The median sternotomy can be extended along a right supraclavicular incision if more distal exposure of the right subclavian artery is necessary. It can also be extended along the anterior border of either sternocleidomastoid muscle if further exposure of either common carotid artery is required(see Fig. 3.2). The left subclavian artery is hard to expose through a median sternotomy because of the posterior path of the aortic arch. If the need to expose the left subclavian artery becomes apparent during a median sternotomy,

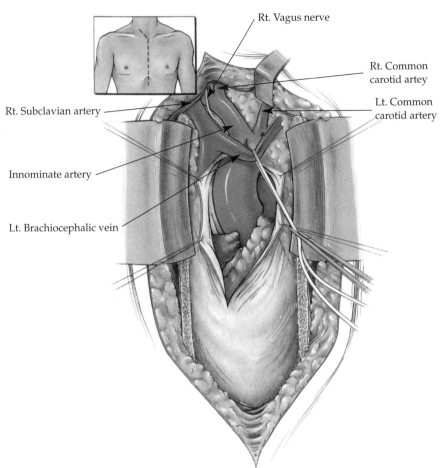

Figure 3.3 A median sternotomy is necessary for exposure of the aortic arch and the origin of the innominate, right subclavian, and right and left common carotid arteries. (From Berguer R., Kieffer E. Surgery of the Arteries to the Head. Springer-Verlag, 1992, with permission.)

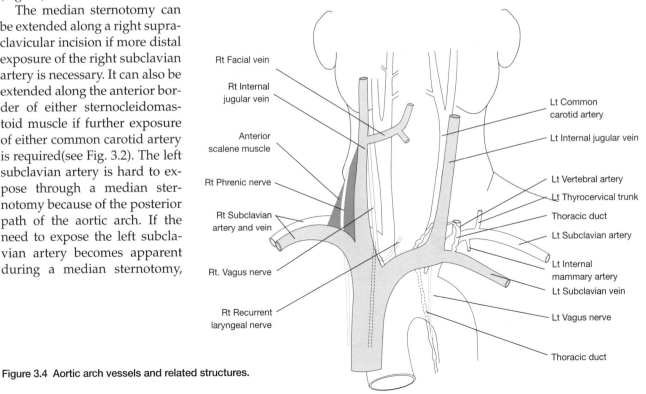

Figure 3.4 Aortic arch vessels and related structures.

division of the left brachiocephalic vein has been reported to allow access to the origin of the left subclavian artery. Furthermore, the addition of a supraclavicular incision to the median sternotomy has also been reported to provide adequate access to the left subclavian vessels. However, traditionally a left anterior thoracotomy is recommended to control the origin of the left subclavian artery. If distal exposure of the subclavian artery and vein is needed in an unstable trauma patient, the median sternotomy and left anterior thoracotomy are converted into a trapdoor thoracotomy.(26, 27, 35)

Trapdoor Thoracotomy

In this approach, the median sternotomy is connected to an anterior thoracotomy and to a supraclavicular incision (Fig. 3.5). The supraclavicular incision is started 1–2 cm above the sternal notch and carried parallel to the clavicle. The sternocleidomastoid and the anterior scalene muscles are divided close to the clavicle. The sternal spreader is repositioned to expose the left subclavian vessels. It is important to note that the exposure achieved by the combination of a supraclavicular incision and a median sternotomy may be sufficient, eliminating the need and morbidity of the additional thoracotomy (14). If the exposure is deemed inadequate, an anterior thoracotomy is started by an infraareolar incision and carried through the fourth intercostal space. The incision is extended into the sternum resulting in a trap door thoracotomy. Dividing the clavicle in its middle third can allow further lateral reflection of the thoracic trap door providing an unhindered exposure of the entire left subclavian artery.

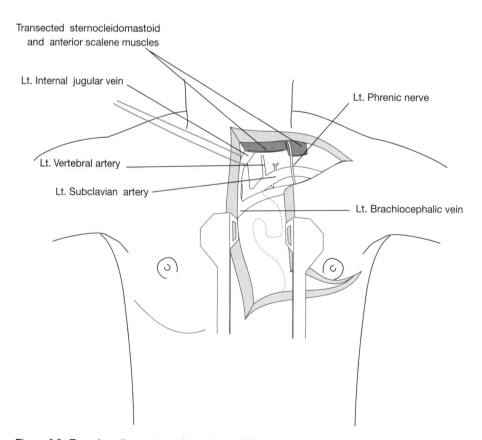

Transected sternocleidomastoid
and anterior scalene muscles

Lt. Internal jugular vein

Lt. Phrenic nerve

Lt. Vertebral artery

Lt. Subclavian artery

Lt. Brachiocephalic vein

Figure 3.5 Trap door thoracotomy is performed by connecting a median sternotomy to a left supraclavicular incision and a left anterior thoracotomy.

Left Anterior Thoracotomy

In elective procedures, a double-lumen endotracheal tube is preferentially used to secure the airways. The skin incision is performed over the left fourth rib from the left sternal edge to the mid axillary line. The incision is deepened through the subcutaneous tissues exposing the rib cage and the intercostal muscles. Either the third or fourth intercostal space can be used to enter the chest cavity. The intercostal muscles are divided and the pleural space is entered. The left lung is deflated and retracted inferiorly, allowing access to the aortic arch, which is exposed by incising its overlying pleura (Fig. 3.6). The origin of the left subclavian artery is identified as the most distal branch originating from the aortic arch. This approach allows for additional distal exposure of the left subclavian artery through a supraclavicular incision should it become necessary. A left posterolateral thoracotomy can also provide a good exposure of the origin and proximal part of the left subclavian artery (2) (Fig. 3.7). However, this approach is usually reserved for elective conditions where the pathology is limited to the very proximal part of the left subclavian artery. The patient's position in this approach does not allow for additional exposure of the left subclavian artery through a supraclavicular incision.

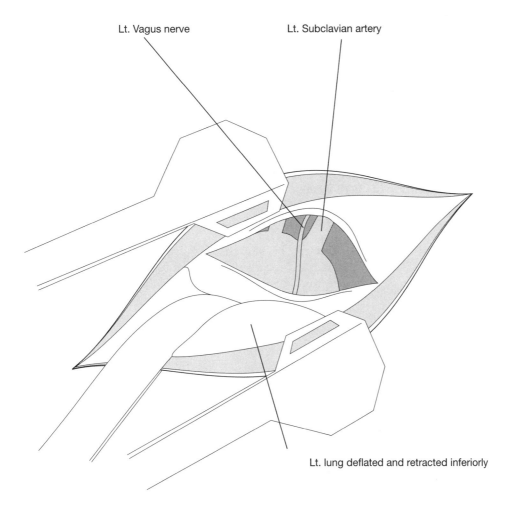

Lt. Vagus nerve

Lt. Subclavian artery

Lt. lung deflated and retracted inferiorly

Figure 3.6. A left anterior thoracotomy is necessary for exposure of the origin of the left subclavian artery. This approach allows for additional exposure of the left subclavian artery through a supraclavicular incision.

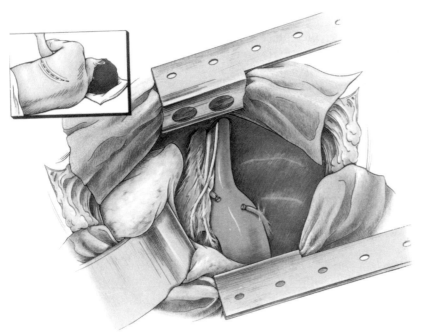

Figure 3.7 A left posterolateral thoracotomy provides exposure of the origin of the left subclavian artery. The patient's position does not allow for additional exposure of the left subclavian artery through a supraclavicular incision. (From Berguer R., Kieffer E. Surgery of the Arteries to the Head. Springer-Verlag, 1992, with permission.)

Supraclavicular Exposure of the Subclavian Artery
The main steps in the supraclavicular approach to the SCA are

1. Skin incision
2. Division of the platysma muscle
3. Mobilization of the scalene fat pad
4. Division of the anterior scalene muscle

Important structures that can be injured during exposure of the subclavian artery include the phrenic and recurrent laryngeal nerves, the brachial plexus and lymphatic structures such as the thoracic duct on the left side (see Fig. 3.4).

Details of the Supraclavicular Exposure of the Subclavian Artery A supraclavicular incision is made starting 1–2 cm above the clavicle between the heads of the sternocleidomastoid muscle. The incision extends laterally and parallel to the clavicle for 10–12 cm and is deepened through the subcutaneous tissues to expose the platysma muscle (Fig. 3.8). The platysma muscle is divided with electrocautery to expose the scalene fat pad. The fat pad is mobilized from inferior to superior, starting at the level of the clavicle, to expose the anterior scalene muscle. The phrenic nerve is identified as it lies anterior to the anterior scalene muscle crossing from its lateral to medial side. The scalenus anterior muscle is divided close to its insertion onto the first rib while retracting and protecting the phrenic nerve. Any lymphatics encountered in the line of the incision are ligated to avoid the complication of postoperative lymph leak. Once the anterior scalene muscle is divided, the subclavian artery can be identified by palpation or insonation with a handheld doppler probe. The subclavian artery is then dissected and encircled with a silastic loop. This exposure provides full access to the second part of the subclavian artery. Gentle tension on the vessel loop will facilitate additional proximal and distal arterial exposure. Division of the clavicular head of the sternocleidomastoid muscle can help to provide additional proximal exposure.(22) Further mobilization of the distal segment of the first part of the subclavian artery will expose the origins of the thyrocervical trunk, the internal mammary, and the vertebral arteries (Fig. 3.8). The mobilization of this part of the subclavian artery may be facilitated by dividing the internal mammary artery. However, division of the internal mammary artery should be avoided as this will prohibit its use for possible future coronary artery revascularization.

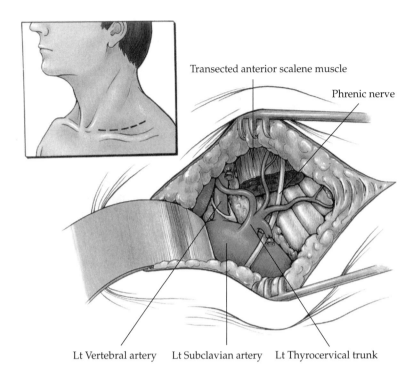

Figure 3.8 A supraclavicular incision is ideal for exposure of the second part and distal segment of the first part of the subclavian artery. It also allows for exposure of the proximal segment of the vertebral artery. (From Berguer R., Kieffer E. Surgery of the Arteries to the Head. Springer-Verlag, 1992, with permission.)

Further medial exposure of the subclavian artery can be obtained by subperiosteal resection of the medial third of the clavicle. The skin incision is extended toward the sternoclavicular junction. The incision is deepened directly over the clavicle to expose the periosteum. The edges of the clavicle are defined. A right-angle clamp is then passed around the clavicle to grab a Gigli saw, which is used to divide the clavicle laterally. The divided clavicle is then grasped with a towel clip and dissected further posteriorly and anteriorly until the head of the clavicle is released from all its ligamentous and fibrous attachments. For more proximal access, a median sternotomy will be necessary to provide additional exposure.(14) In elective procedures, an attempt can be made at dividing the clavicle and reflecting it medially without severing all the ligamentous and fibrous attachments of the sternal head. The reflected medial portion of the clavicle can be replaced in its position at the completion of the vascular procedure and stabilized with a plate for cosmetic purposes and to prevent possible future shoulder discomfort.

EXPOSURE OF THE VERTEBRAL ARTERY

Although the vertebral artery can be accessible at all four segments, V2 and V4 are relatively hard to expose as they are covered by bony structures. The origin of the vertebral artery and the V1 segment can be exposed using a supraclavicular approach as described in the exposure of the first and second parts of the subclavian artery (see Fig. 3.8). Transection of the clavicular head of the sternocleidomastoid muscle usually facilitates the exposure. Division of the sternal head may also be necessary. The vertebral artery can also be exposed through an anterior cervical incision. This incision can be extended to expose all the segments of the vertebral artery. The incision can be started along the anterior border of the sternocleidomastoid muscle and extended to the sternal notch. The sternocleidomastoid is retracted laterally exposing the carotid sheath. The anterior cervical incision can also be modified to run between the heads of the sternocleidomastoid muscle. The muscle heads are separated, retracting the clavicular head laterally and the sternal head medially, exposing the carotid sheath. The carotid sheath is then mobilized medially and the dissection is continued posteriorly through its bed exposing the thyroidal branches crossing from the thyrocervical trunk. Division of these branches is usually necessary to expose the underlying sympathetic chain, stellate ganglion, and vertebral vein. Mobilization of the vertebral vein will expose the first segment of the vertebral artery. Division of the vertebral vein may enhance the exposure.

When a transposition of the V1 segment into the common carotid artery is contemplated, the approach to the vertebral artery through the anterior cervical incision is slightly modified after exposing the carotid sheath. In this situation, instead of mobilizing the carotid sheath medially, it is incised to expose the carotid artery. The carotid artery is then mobilized and retracted medially. The vagus nerve is kept out of harm's way and left adjacent to the jugular vein, which is retracted laterally. The posterior aspect of the carotid sheath is incised, exposing the thyroidal branches of the thyrocervical trunk. The exposure is then continued as previously described (Figs. 3.9, 3.10). This modification provides a new path for the vertebral artery between the common carotid artery and the internal jugular vein. This new and direct path facilitates the transposition of the vertebral artery into the common carotid artery.

Exposure of V2 will require unroofing of the bony canal in which the vertebral artery runs from C6 to C2. This is performed with the use of a bone rongeur. The vertebral artery is found surrounded by a rich vertebral venous plexus. Exposure of V3 is also obtained through a high cervical incision anterior to the sternocleidomastoid. The part of the vertebral artery between C1 and C2 is usually the segment exposed. The spinal accessory nerve is identified and preserved. The C1 transverse process is palpated, and the muscles inserting in the lower aspect of C1 are resected, exposing V3. This exposure may be facilitated by dividing the attachment of the sternocleidomastoid to the skull. The approach to V4 requires a posterior craniotomy to obtain exposure in the posterior fossa.

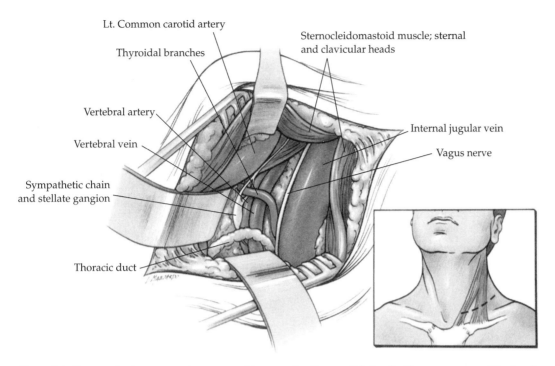

Figure 3.9 The vertebral artery can be accessed by exposing the carotid sheath. The common carotid artery is retracted medially and the jugular laterally. Dissection in the plane posterior to the carotid sheath will reveal the crossing thyroidal branches of the thyrocervical trunk. (From Berguer R., Kieffer E. Surgery of the Arteries to the Head. Springer-Verlag, 1992, with permission.)

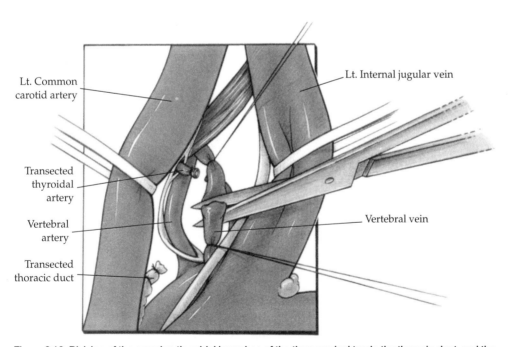

Figure 3.10 Division of the crossing thyroidal branches of the thyrocervical trunk, the thoracic duct, and the vertebral vein will provide exposure of the V1 segment of the vertebral artery along with the stellate ganglion (From Berguer R., Kieffer E. Surgery of the Arteries to the Head. Springer-Verlag, 1992, with permission.)

ANATOMY OF THE AXILLARY AND BRACHIAL ARTERIES

The Axillary Artery

The axillary artery is the continuation of the subclavian artery after it crosses over the first rib (Fig. 3.11). It runs over the apical part of the chest wall and travels behind the pectoralis minor muscle toward the axillary fossa. The axillary artery is divided by the pectoralis minor muscle into three parts. The first part is the segment between the lateral border of the first rib and the medial border of the pectoralis minor muscle. The second part is the segment posterior to the pectoralis minor muscle. The third part is the segment distal to the lateral border of the pectoralis minor muscle. It extends to the lower border of the teres major muscle.

The Brachial Artery

The brachial artery is the continuation of the axillary artery. It starts at the lower border of the teres major muscle. The brachial artery travels down the arm starting medial to the humerus. It progressively moves into an anterior location and terminates into the radial and the ulnar arteries approximately 1 cm distal to the elbow crease (Fig. 3.11).

Exposure of the Axillary Artery

The main steps in exposing the axillary artery are

1. Skin incision
2. Incision of the pectoralis major muscle fascia
3. Separation of the pectoralis major muscle fibers
4. Division of the pectoralis minor muscle
5. Mobilization of the axillary vein

Details of the Exposure: The skin incision is placed 2 cm below the clavicle and extends in a parallel direction to the clavicle for 10–12 cm (Fig. 3.12). After incising the skin and the subcutaneous tissues, the fascia of the pectoralis major muscle is encountered. The fascia is incised, and the incision is deepened toward the chest wall by splitting the pectoralis major muscle bluntly along the length of its fibers to expose the areolar tissue over the chest wall (Fig. 12). The medial part of the pectoralis minor muscle is identified toward the lateral aspect of the incision. Digital palpa-

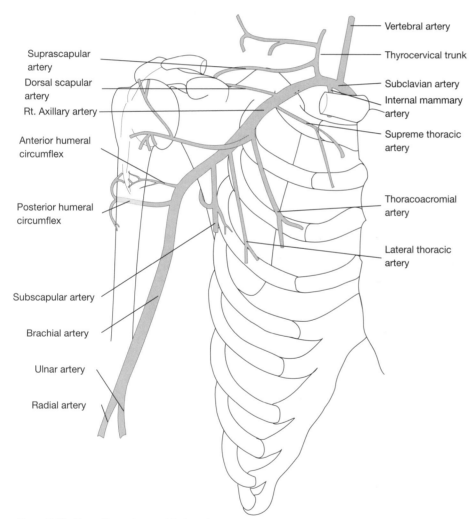

Figure 3.11. The axillary artery and its branches.

Vertebral artery
Thyrocervical trunk
Subclavian artery
Internal mammary artery
Supreme thoracic artery
Thoracoacromial artery
Lateral thoracic artery

Suprascapular artery
Dorsal scapular artery
Rt. Axillary artery
Anterior humeral circumflex
Posterior humeral circumflex
Subscapular artery
Brachial artery
Ulnar artery
Radial artery

tion or Doppler auscultation over the chest wall medial to the pectoralis minor muscle will reveal the location of the axillary artery. The axillary vein is seen partially covering the axillary artery as it lies anterior and superior to it. The axillary vein is mobilized caudally to better expose the axillary artery. Occasionally, the cephalic vein or other venous branches draining into the axillary vein may need to be divided along with branches of the thoracoacromial artery to better expose the axillary artery. The lateral pectoral nerve supplying the pectoralis major muscle lies near the thoracoacromial artery and should be protected.

The first part of the axillary artery can be exposed without having to divide the pectoralis minor muscle. However, division of the pectoralis minor muscle close to its insertion greatly facilitates the exposure of the axillary artery. When the second and third parts of the axillary artery need to be exposed, complete division of the pectoralis minor muscle is necessary. The distal part of the axillary artery is usually hard to expose from this approach because of the overlying pectoralis major muscle and its attachment on the shoulder. Exposure of the most distal part of the axillary artery from this approach then requires division of the lateral portion of the pectoralis major and the coracobrachialis muscles. Alternatively, the third part of the axillary artery can be exposed via an axillary incision along the lateral border of the pectoralis major muscle. The pectoralis muscle is mobilized laterally and the axillary fossa is entered. The median nerve and the axillary vein will be first exposed. By dissecting superior to these structures, the distal segment of the axillary artery is identified.

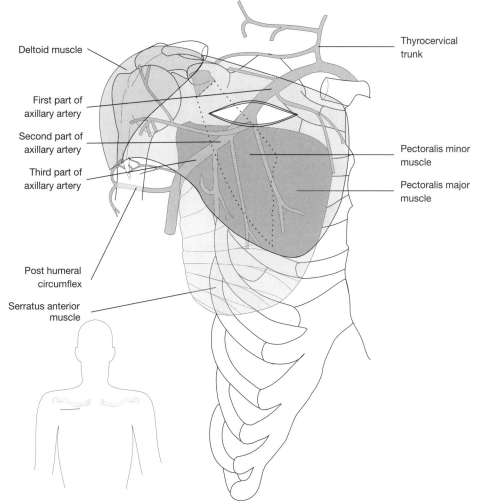

Figure 3.12. Exposure of the axillary artery.

Exposure of the Brachial Artery

In the upper arm, the brachial artery is exposed using a longitudinal incision parallel to the humerus. The incision is placed along the medial border of the biceps brachii muscle. After incising the subcutaneous tissues, the sheath covering the brachial neurovascular bundle is incised. The incision is guided by digital palpation of the brachial pulse or by insonating the artery with a Doppler probe if the pulse cannot be felt. The basilic vein is identified and mobilized posteriorly, exposing the brachial artery lying between the medial cutaneous nerve of the arm and the median and ulnar nerves.

At the elbow level, the brachial artery is exposed using a transverse incision or an S-shaped curvilinear incision. Division of a portion of the biceps brachii aponeurosis will expose the artery as it lies immediately beneath the aponeurosis and medial to the biceps brachii muscle and tendon (Fig. 3.13).

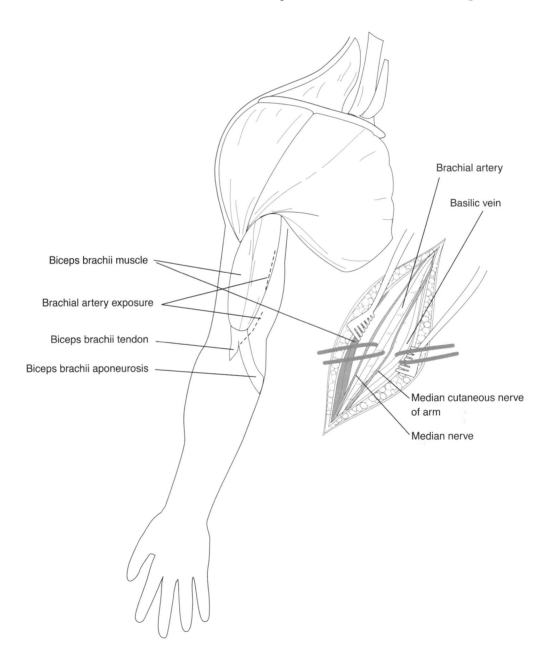

Figure 3.13. Exposure of the brachial artery.

ANATOMY OF THE RADIAL AND ULNAR ARTERIES

The Radial Artery

The radial artery starts at the bifurcation of the brachial artery just below the elbow joint. It continues along the radial side of the forearm to the wrist (Fig. 3.14). It then crosses around the outer side of the wrist to continue behind the extensor tendon of the thumb. The radial artery then connects with the deep branch of the ulnar artery to form the deep palmar arch.

The Ulnar Artery

The ulnar artery starts just distal to the elbow joint as the larger of the two terminal branches of the brachial artery. It crosses along the inner side of the forearm and continues down toward the wrist along the ulnar border of the forearm (Fig. 3.14). It crosses the wrist to divide into two branches that form the superficial and deep palmar arches.

EXPOSURE OF THE RADIAL AND ULNAR ARTERIES

Exposure of the Radial Artery

At the elbow level, the radial artery is accessed by exposing the brachial artery and tracing it distally until it bifurcates. Distally, the radial artery is exposed by performing a 3-cm transverse or longitudinal skin incision a few centimeters proximal to the wrist joint (Fig. 3.14). After incising the skin and the underlying fascia, the radial artery can be identified running between the tendons of the flexor carpi radialis and supinates longus muscles. The former is the most prominent tendon when the wrist is flexed while the latter is the most radial tendon in the incision.

Exposure of the Ulnar Artery

At the elbow, the ulnar artery is accessed by exposing the brachial artery and tracing it distally. At the wrist, the ulnar artery is exposed by performing a longitudinal incision along the ulnar aspect of the forearm (Fig. 3.14). The artery is identified just below the skin and the underlying fascia.

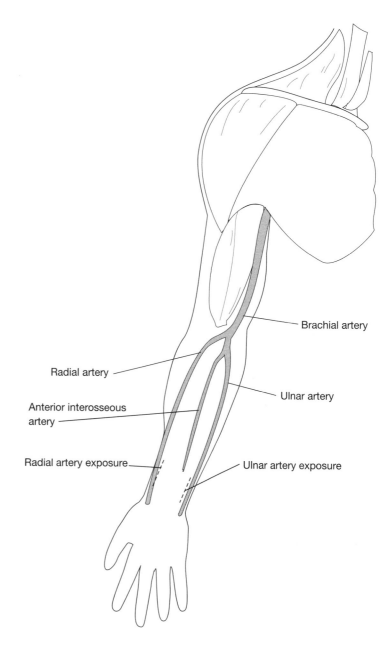

Figure 3.14. Exposure of the radial and ulnar arteries.

ANATOMY OF THE CAROTID ARTERY

The right common carotid artery originates from the innominate artery at the base of the neck behind the right sternoclavicular junction. The left common carotid artery usually originates directly from the aortic arch. The left common carotid artery can share a common ostium with the innominate artery in 16% of the population.(3) It can also originate directly from the trunk of the innominate artery in 8% of individuals.(43) One anomaly of the arch vessels is the retroesophageal subclavian artery, which occurs in 0.5% of the population(3). In this anomaly, the innominate artery does not exist and each carotid and subclavian artery originate directly and separately from the aortic arch. The right common carotid artery is the first branch. The left common carotid artery is the second branch and is followed by the left subclavian artery, with the right subclavian artery being the last branch.

Each common carotid artery ascends in the neck in the carotid sheath. The carotid sheath also contains the internal jugular vein, which lies lateral to the carotid artery, and the vagus nerve, which lies deeply between the carotid and the internal jugular vein. At the base of the neck, the common carotid artery lies deep behind the strap muscles and the sternocleidomastoid muscle. However, as the common carotid artery ascends in the neck, it becomes more superficial and is separated from the skin by the carotid sheath, platysma, and partially by the sternocleidomastoid muscle (Fig. 3.15). At the level of the hyoid bone or the fourth cervical vertebra, the common carotid artery bifurcates into the external and internal carotid arteries.

The External Carotid Artery

As it originates from the common carotid artery, the external carotid artery lies anteromedial to the internal carotid artery. The first branch of the external carotid artery is the superior thyroid artery, which on occasion may arise directly from the common carotid artery. The other branches that originate from the external carotid artery are, in ascending order: the ascending pharyngeal, the lingual, the facial, the occipital and the posterior auricular arteries (Fig. 3.16). The two terminal branches of the external carotid artery are the superficial temporal artery and the internal maxillary artery. Branches of the external carotid artery can provide important collateral circulation to the brain when the ipsilateral internal carotid artery is occluded (Fig. 3.17).

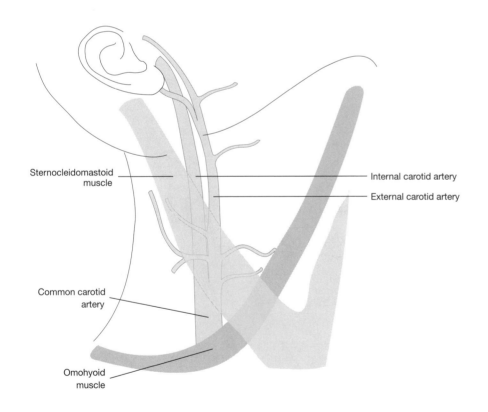

Sternocleidomastoid
muscle

Internal carotid artery

External carotid artery

Common carotid
artery

Omohyoid
muscle

Figure 3.15. The common carotid artery and adjacent muscles.

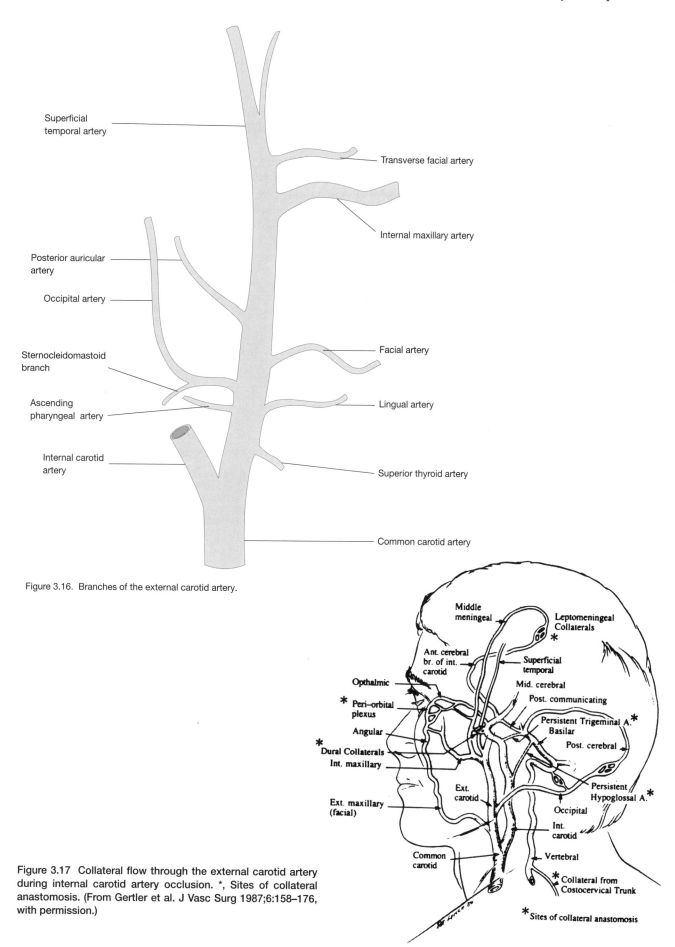

Figure 3.16. Branches of the external carotid artery.

Figure 3.17 Collateral flow through the external carotid artery during internal carotid artery occlusion. *, Sites of collateral anastomosis. (From Gertler et al. J Vasc Surg 1987;6:158–176, with permission.)

The Internal Carotid Artery

The internal carotid artery originates from the common carotid artery, usually at the level of the fourth cervical vertebra, lying posterior and lateral to the external carotid artery. The internal carotid artery is divided into three segments: the cervical, petrous, and intracranial segments. The cervical segment extends from the carotid bifurcation to the origin of the carotid canal at the base of the skull. It is crossed anteriorly by the hypoglossal nerve, the occipital artery, the digastric muscle, the stylohyoid muscle, and the posterior auricular artery (Fig. 3.18). The petrous segment represents the internal carotid artery as it advances in the carotid canal to lie in the petrous portion of the temporal bone. The intracranial segment represents the remaining part of the internal carotid artery as it courses on the lateral body of the sphenoid bone, continuing through the cavernous sinus before it pierces the dura to contribute to the cerebral circulation.

The internal carotid artery does not give off any branches in the neck. In the carotid canal, the internal carotid artery gives the caroticotympanic branches to the middle ear. Further up in the cavernous sinus the internal carotid artery gives off several branches. These branches include the inferior hypophyseal artery, small branches to the dura, a small branch to the middle meningeal branches, an anastomotic branch to the artery of the pterygoid canal, and anastomotic channels with the ascending pharyngeal artery and branches of the maxillary artery. Just after it penetrates the dura, the internal carotid artery gives rise to the ophthalmic artery, which is its first major branch. The internal carotid artery (ICA) then gives rise to the posterior communicating artery just before dividing into the anterior and middle cerebral arteries. The posterior communicating artery communicates with the posterior cerebral artery. The anterior cerebral arteries are joined by the anterior communicating artery, completing the circle of Willis (Fig. 3.19). The branches of the internal carotid artery play an important role in providing collateral cerebral pathways in the presence of occlusive disease of the internal carotid artery.

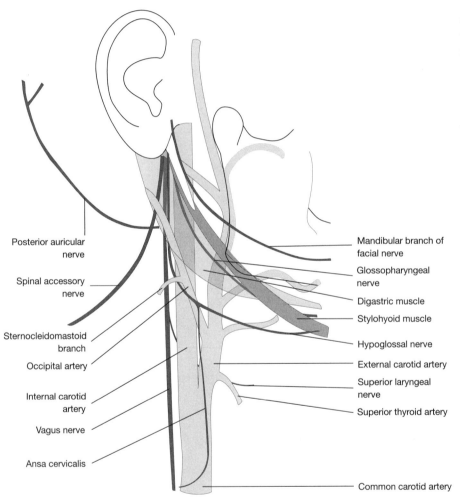

Posterior auricular
nerve

Spinal accessory
nerve

Sternocleidomastoid
branch

Occipital artery

Internal carotid
artery

Vagus nerve

Ansa cervicalis

Mandibular branch of
facial nerve

Glossopharyngeal
nerve

Digastric muscle

Stylohyoid muscle

Hypoglossal nerve

External carotid artery

Superior laryngeal
nerve

Superior thyroid artery

Common carotid artery

Figure 3.18. The carotid bifurcation and related structures.

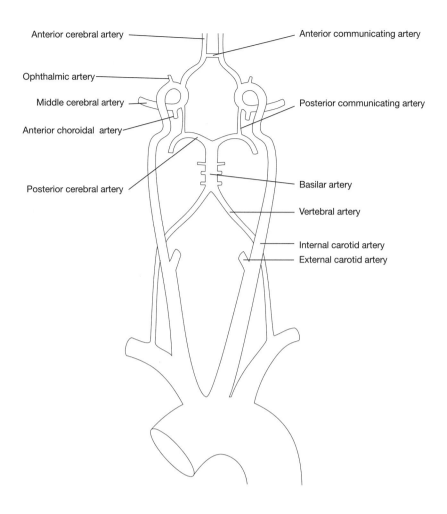

Anterior cerebral artery

Ophthalmic artery

Middle cerebral artery

Anterior choroidal artery

Posterior cerebral artery

Anterior communicating artery

Posterior communicating artery

Basilar artery

Vertebral artery

Internal carotid artery

External carotid artery

Figure 3.19. Circle of Willis.

Carotid Artery Exposure

To expose the origin and the first few centimeters of the common carotid artery, a median sternotomy is necessary. More distally, the common carotid artery is exposed through a neck incision. The main steps in exposing the common, external, and internal carotid arteries in the neck are

1. Skin incision
2. Division of platysma muscle
3. Mobilization of the sternocleidomastoid laterally
4. Incising the carotid sheath
5. Mobilization of the internal jugular vein
6. Division of the facial vein

Details of the Neck Exposure of the Common Carotid Artery and Its Bifurcation: Most commonly, a longitudinal incision along the anterior border of the sternocleidomastoid muscle is used to expose the common carotid artery and its bifurcation (Fig. 3.20). Transverse neck incisions along a flexion skin crease starting 5 cm below the angle of the mandible can also be used; however, they require the creation of skin flaps and can be cumbersome if high exposure of the internal carotid artery becomes necessary. The longitudinal incision starts two fingers breadth above the sternal notch and extends along the anterior border of the sternocleidomastoid muscle. If necessary, the incision can be extended posteriorly behind the ear toward the mastoid process to aid in distal exposure. (17) The subcutaneous tissues and the platysma muscle are incised, exposing the sternocleidomastoid muscle. The dissection is carried out throughout the length of the incision along the upper and medial border of the sternocleidomastoid dividing the small vessels that supply it. A self-retaining retractor is placed to retract the sternocleidomastoid muscle laterally, thus exposing the anterior aspect of the internal jugular vein.

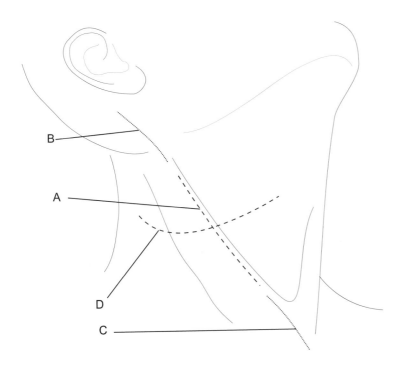

Dissection is now performed along the medial edge of the internal jugular vein. The attachments of the lateral aspects of the carotid sheath to the sternocleidomastoid are left undisturbed so that, when the sternocleidomastoid muscle is retracted laterally, the jugular vein will be retracted along with it. The dissection is carried along the medial border of the internal jugular vein throughout the length of the incision. The facial vein is identified as it usually marks the level of the carotid bifurcation (see Fig. 3.4). The facial vein is divided and suture ligated, thus exposing the carotid bifurcation. Any other venous branches draining facial structures into the medial aspect of the jugular vein that are identified are also ligated and divided. Occasionally, the facial vein is replaced by two smaller

Figure 3.20. Exposure of the carotid bifurcation. (A): Incision anterior to sternocleidomastoid muscle. (B): Extension behind the ear towards the mastoid process for high exposure of the internal carotid artery. (C): Extension towards the sternal notch for proximal common carotid exposure. (D): Transverse cervical incision; extension of exposure is limited.

veins located superior and inferior to its usual location.

Once the internal jugular vein has been mobilized laterally, the carotid artery is easily identified. A "minimal touch" technique is very important during the dissection of an atherosclerotic carotid artery to prevent distal embolization. If additional proximal exposure of the common carotid artery is needed, the incision can be extended to the sternal notch and the omohyoid muscle overlying the carotid sheath is divided. The ansa cervicalis or some of its branches are often noted crossing over the common carotid artery. The ansa cervicalis can be divided without any significant sequelae. The proximal segment of the ansa usually leads to the hypoglossal nerve. The carotid dissection is continued superiorly until the carotid bifurcation is reached. Dissection along the medial aspect of the common carotid artery at the level of the carotid bifurcation will first identify the superior thyroid artery. Further dissection superiorly exposes the external carotid artery and its branches.

Dissection along the lateral border of the common carotid artery leads to the internal carotid artery. The upper set of the deep cervical lymph nodes are often encountered between the carotid bifurcation and the digastric muscle. These lymphatic structures can obscure the location of the internal carotid artery and the hypoglossal nerve. It is thus important to proceed very carefully at this level to avoid any iatrogenic nerve injury. The lymphatics are carefully mobilized, exposing the areolar tissues overlying the internal carotid artery up to the level of the digastric muscle.

It is prudent to avoid using electrocautery in the vicinity of nerves in the neck as this can cause iatrogenic nerve damage. The nerves that can be injured during a carotid exposure are the vagus nerve, the hypoglossal nerve, the glossopharyngeal nerve, the mandibular branch of the facial nerve, and the posterior auricular nerve (23) (Fig. 3.21). The vagus nerve is usually lying posteriorly between the carotid artery and the jugular vein. It is the nerve most commonly injured during carotid endarterectomy. It can be injured by the dissecting scissors during mobilization of the carotid artery or by the vascular clamps if inadvertently clamped while occluding the common or internal carotid arteries.

The hypoglossal nerve is usually seen running inferior and parallel to the digastric muscle. Occasionally, the hypoglossal nerve can lie in a more inferior location or closer to the edge of the external carotid artery. It can be injured during the mobilization of the internal carotid artery, especially if the exposure is compromised by inadequate hemostasis. This injury will result in deviation of the extended tongue toward the affected side. The mandibular branch of the facial nerve can be injured as a result of direct compression by a handheld retractor applied below the angle of the mandible to improve the carotid exposure. This injury will result in drooping of the ipsilateral lower lip when the patient is asked to show the teeth. The posterior auricular nerve can be injured when the dissection is carried out along the anterior border of the upper part of the sternocleidomastoid.

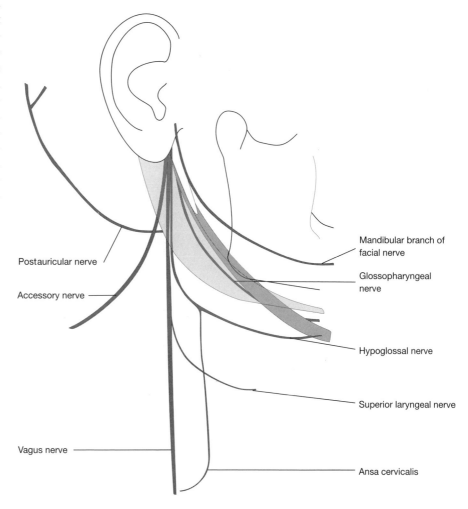

Figure 3.21. Regional nerves at risk during exposure of the common carotid artery and its branches.

High Exposure of the Internal Carotid Artery
High exposure of the internal carotid artery can be achieved by dividing its overlying muscles and mobilizing the hypoglossal nerve (Fig. 3.22). The hypoglossal nerve is mobilized by dividing the ansa cervicalis close to the hypoglossal nerve. The divided distal segment of the ansa cervicalis can be used to provide gentle traction on the hypoglossal nerve. (29) A branch of the occipital artery to the sternocleidomastoid muscle usually acts as a sling that tethers the hypoglossal nerve. Bleeding from this branch can compromise the exposure, whereas its ligation and division along with its accompanying vein allow considerable mobilization of the hypoglossal nerve. Further cephalad, division of the occipital artery aids in additional mobilization of the hypoglossal nerve. Division of the digastric muscle provides further exposure above the level of the hypoglossal nerve (Fig. 3.23).

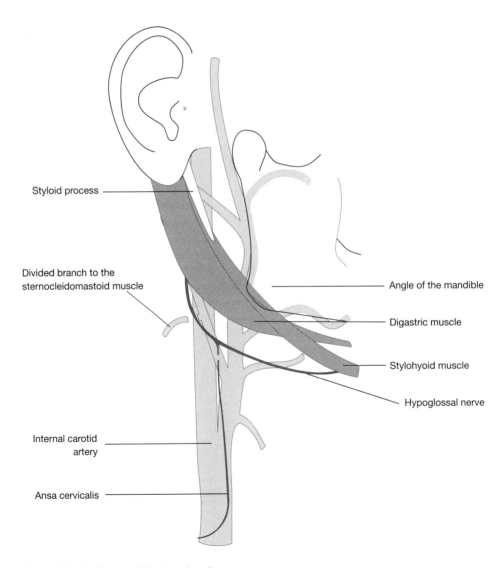

Figure 3.22. Mobilization of the hypoglossal nerve.

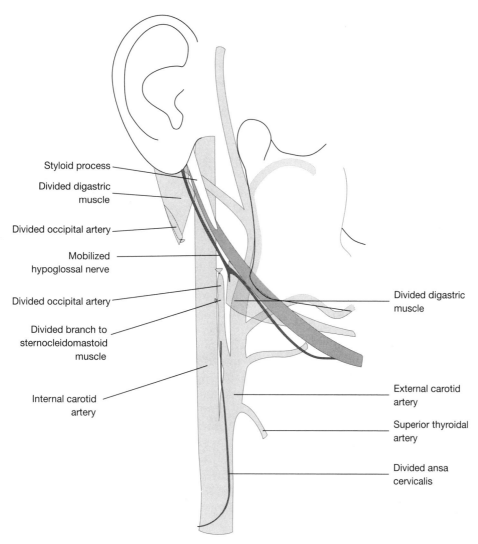

Styloid process

Divided digastric
muscle

Divided occipital artery

Mobilized
hypoglossal nerve

Divided occipital artery

Divided branch to
sternocleidomastoid
muscle

Internal carotid
artery

Divided digastric
muscle

External carotid
artery

Superior thyroidal
artery

Divided ansa
cervicalis

Figure 3.23. High exposure of the internal carotid artery.

If the exposure provided by these methods is inadequate, a mandibular subluxation may be necessary to achieve a higher dissection of the internal carotid artery.(16) Mandibular dislocation should be avoided as it can cause permanent damage to the temporomandibular joint. Various mandibular osteotomies have also been described to achieve high exposure of the internal carotid artery at the level of C1. However, such procedures are very infrequently performed as they are usually needed for the management of rare aneurysmal or traumatic pathology. When the need for high exposure is anticipated, nasotracheal intubation can be very helpful as this widens the space behind the angle of the mandible, thus facilitating higher internal carotid artery exposure (4) (Fig. 3.24).

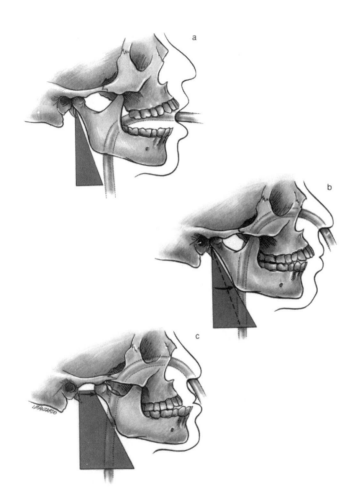

Figure 3.24 High exposure of the internal carotid artery. (a) Orotracheal intubation. (b) Nasotracheal intubation improves high exposure of the internal carotid artery. (c) Mandibular subluxation allows additional exposure. (From Berguer R., Kieffer E. Surgery of the Arteries to the Head. Springer-Verlag, 1992, with permission.)

ABDOMINAL AORTA AND ITS BRANCHES

ANATOMY OF THE ABDOMINAL AORTA AND ITS BRANCHES

The Abdominal Aorta

The aorta enters the abdominal cavity through the aortic hiatus at the level of the 12th thoracic vertebra. At that level, the aorta is surrounded by the right and left crura of the diaphragm and lies on the anterior aspect of the vertebral column. The aorta runs distally in the retroperitoneum anterior to the spine until the level of the fourth lumbar vertebra, where it bifurcates into the right and left common iliac arteries. Throughout its course in the abdomen, the aorta gives off several branches. These include the inferior phrenic arteries, the celiac artery, the superior mesenteric artery, the right and left renal arteries, the inferior mesenteric artery, the gonadal arteries, the lumbar arteries, and the middle sacral artery. The surgical anatomy and exposure of the major branches that may require revascularization are reviewed next.

The Celiac Artery

The celiac artery originates from the anterior aspect of the aorta shortly after it enters the abdominal cavity at the level of the upper part of the first lumbar vertebra. The celiac artery is a short trunk surrounded by a plexus of sympathetic nerves. The celiac artery runs for 1–2 cm before it gives off the left gastric, the splenic, and the common hepatic arteries (Fig. 3.25).

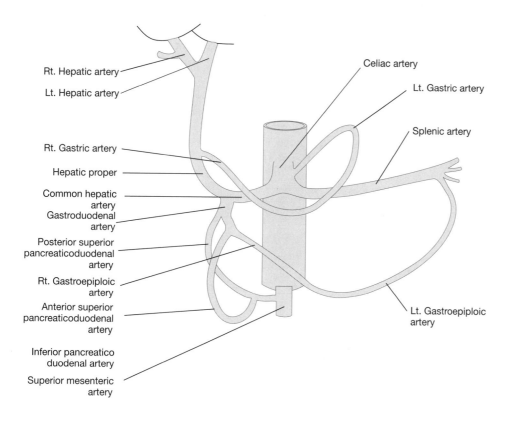

Figure 3.25. The celiac artery and its branches.

The Common Hepatic Artery

The common hepatic artery arises from the celiac artery behind the posterior wall of the lesser sac and continues to the right along the upper border of the pancreas before it divides into the gastroduodenal artery and the proper hepatic artery. The proper hepatic artery continues into the hepatoduodenal ligament usually giving off the right gastric artery before dividing into the right and left hepatic arteries (Fig. 3.25). The proper hepatic artery lies anterior to the portal vein and lateral to the common bile duct.

The Superior Mesenteric Artery

The superior mesenteric artery arises from the aorta 1–2 cm below the origin of the celiac artery about the level of the midpart of the first lumbar vertebra. It starts behind the neck of the pancreas and then passes between the pancreas and the duodenum to enter the root of the mesentery. The superior mesenteric artery gives off several important branches. These include the inferior pancreaticoduodenal artery (which represents a main communicating vessel to the celiac artery), the middle colic artery, the right colic artery, the ileocolic artery, and numerous jejunal branches(18) (Fig. 3.26).

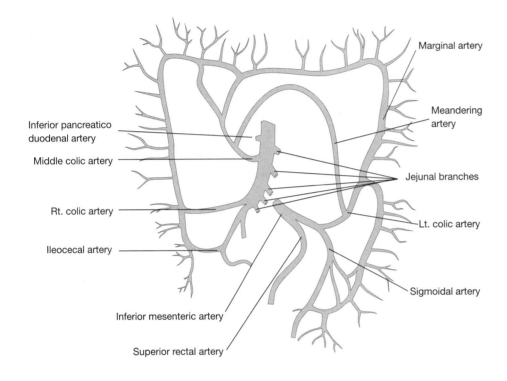

Figure 3.26. The superior and inferior mesenteric arteries and their branches.

The Renal Arteries

The right and left renal arteries originate at the level of the upper part of the second lumbar vertebra from the posterolateral aspect of the aorta. The left renal artery continues inferiorly and posteriorly behind the left renal vein toward the left kidney giving off the inferior adrenal artery and then dividing into the anterior and posterior segmental arteries. On the right side, the renal artery runs behind the vena cava and then posterior to the junction of the right renal vein and the vena cava. The right renal artery then runs for 2–3 cm before it divides into the segmental branches. Multiple renal arteries originating from the aorta are commonly encountered.

The Inferior Mesenteric Artery

The inferior mesenteric artery originates at the level of the lower part of the third lumbar vertebra from the left anterolateral aspect of the aorta. Its origin is surrounded by sympathetic nerves. Transection or injury to these sympathetic nerves can lead to sexual dysfunction, most commonly retrograde ejaculation. (15) The inferior mesenteric artery runs for 1–2 cm before it divides into the superior rectal artery, the sigmoidal artery, and the left colic artery (Fig. 3.26).

The Common Iliac Artery

At the level of the fourth lumbar vertebra, the aorta usually lies slightly to the left of the midline as it bifurcates into the right and left common iliac arteries. Each common iliac artery runs downward and laterally to the pelvic brim before dividing into the internal iliac and external iliac arteries. The right common iliac artery is usually longer than the left common iliac artery. Proximally, the right common iliac artery runs over the inferior end of the vena cava and the termination of the left common iliac vein and is crossed anteriorly by the terminal portion of the ileum. The left common iliac artery has a similar course to the right common iliac artery and is crossed anteriorly by the root of the sigmoid mesocolon. At the level of the iliac bifurcation, each common iliac artery is crossed by a ureter. The internal iliac artery continues medially to enter the pelvis, giving origin to the middle and inferior rectal arteries. The external iliac artery continues in the retroperitoneum along the pelvic brim crossing underneath the inguinal ligament to become the common femoral artery. The external iliac artery gives off the inferior (deep) epigastric and the deep iliac circumflex branches.

Exposure of the Abdominal Aorta and Its Branches

The abdominal aorta and its branches can be exposed through a transperitoneal or retroperitoneal approach.

Transperitoneal Approach to the Abdominal Aorta and Its Branches (Figs. 3.27-3.29)
The main steps in exposing the abdominal aorta and its branches after entering the peritoneal cavity are

1. Retract the transverse colon anteriorly and to the right
2. Retract the splenic flexure posteriorly and laterally
3. Divide the peritoneal periaortic attachment of the duodenum
4. Reflect the small bowel and duodenum to the right
5. Incise the retroperitoneum overlying the aorta
6. Identify the left renal vein
7. Transect the inferior mesenteric vein if necessary

The transperitoneal approach can be performed through a midline, paramedian, or transverse incision. Once the abdominal cavity is entered, the transverse colon is reflected upward and to the right (Fig. 3.27). The small bowel is wrapped with a moist towel or placed in a plastic bag and retracted laterally to the right. The ligament of Treitz and the attachment of the duodenum to the paraaortic tissues are sharply incised. The duodenum is dissected off the aorta and retracted along with the small bowel to the right (Fig. 3.28). The aorta is palpated and the overlying peritoneum is incised up to the level of the left renal vein (Fig. 3.29). The inferior mesenteric vein is also identified. Division of the inferior mesenteric vein can provide additional exposure if necessary by allowing further lateral retraction of the left colon. However, it is important to avoid dividing any accompanying arterial branch as it may provide important collateral circulation to the left colon.

Transabdominal Exposure of the Infrarenal Aorta

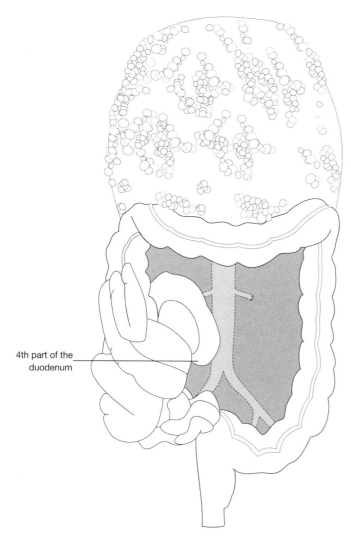

4th part of the duodenum

Figure 3.27. The transverse colon is retracted superiorly and the small bowel is retracted to the right, identifying the duodenum and the ligament of Treitz.

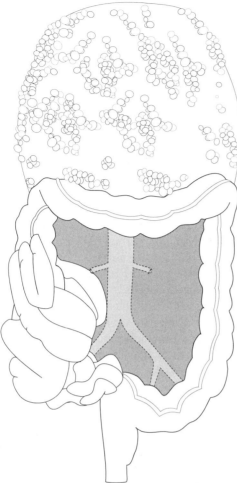

Figure 3.28. The peritoneal attachments of the duodenum are incised and the duodenum is mobilized to the right.

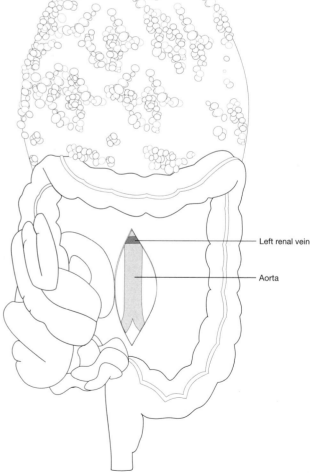

Left renal vein

Aorta

Figure 3.29. The peritoneum over the aorta is incised up to the level of the left renal vein.

Transperitoneal Exposure of the Juxtarenal Aorta and Renal Arteries (Figs. 3.30-3.34): The left renal vein is identified. Dissection on the lateral aspect of the vein will reveal its tributaries, which include the adrenal vein superiorly and the lumbar and the gonadal veins inferiorly (Fig. 3.30). The gonadal and lumbar veins often have a common trunk. It is important to gently dissect, ligate, and divide these branches to obtain free mobilization of the left renal vein. The left renal vein can then be retracted anteriorly and cephalad (Fig. 3.31). Division of the adrenal vein allows retraction of the left renal vein caudally (Fig. 3.32). The exposure of the suprarenal aorta can also be facilitated by the division of the left renal vein. However, when division of the left renal vein is contemplated, the adrenal, lumbar, and gonadal branches must be preserved to maintain collateral venous drainage for the left kidney. (33) The renal vein is divided close to its junction with the vena cava. (Figs. 3.33, 3.34) Resuturing of the divided left renal vein is not usually necessary unless there is evidence of left kidney venous congestion.

Dissection posterior to the left renal vein will reveal the origin of the left renal artery. Posterior attachments of the left crus of the diaphragm can be divided to allow further freeing of the aorta. Lymphatics are frequently noted crossing over the aorta at the level of the left renal vein. These lymphatics are gently dissected, ligated, and transected to prevent the development of postoperative chylous ascites. Dissection on the right lateral aspect of the aorta reveals the origin of the right renal artery under the junction of the left renal vein and the inferior vena cava. Dissection along the medial aspect of the vena cava reveals several venous branches such as the right gonadal and lumbar veins. Division of these branches allows for lateral mobilization of the vena cava; this will improve the exposure of the proximal right renal artery as it passes behind the inferior vena cava.

Dissection around the origins of the right and left renal artery allows for suprarenal aortic exposure. The left renal vein is usually mobilized circumferentially and then retracted caudally or cephalad to expose the pararenal and suprarenal aorta. As aortic dissection is carried out proximal to the renal arteries, sympathetic nerves and ganglia will be encountered. The division of these structures allows identification of the origin of the superior mesenteric artery, which is the most proximal branch of the aorta that can be accessed through this approach.

Transabdominal Exposure of the Juxta-renal Aorta and Renal Arteries

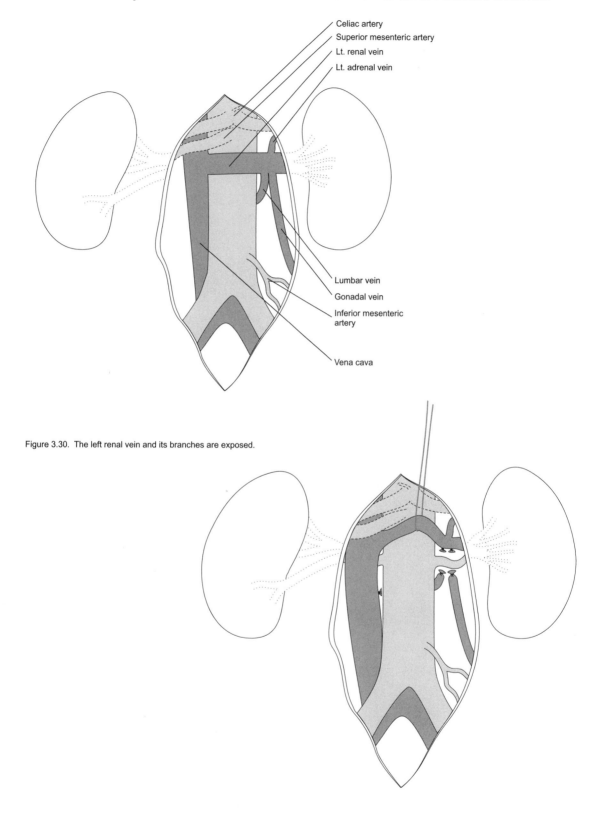

Celiac artery
Superior mesenteric artery
Lt. renal vein
Lt. adrenal vein

Lumbar vein
Gonadal vein
Inferior mesenteric
artery

Vena cava

Figure 3.30. The left renal vein and its branches are exposed.

Figure 3.31. Division of the gonadal and lumbar veins allows cephalad mobilization of the left
renal vein, exposing the left renal artery.

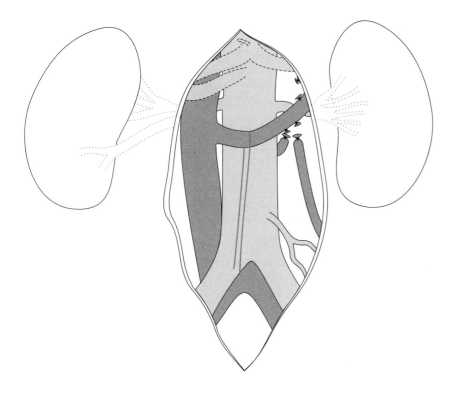

Figure 3.32. Division of the adrenal branch will allow mobilization of the left renal vein caudad for pararenal exposure.

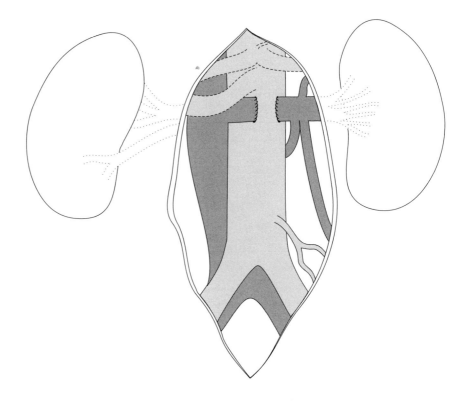

Figure 3.33. When division of the left renal vein is contemplated, the division line is carried close to the junction with the vena cava.

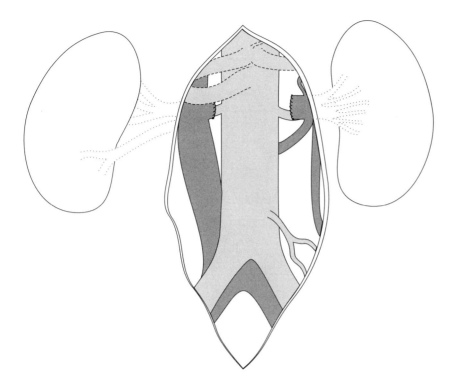

Figure 3.34. Further mobilization of the divided renal vein will facilitate the exposure of the pararenal aorta.

Exposure of the Left Renal Artery (Figs. 3.35, 3.36)
The left renal artery can be approached through the mesentery of the left colon, as already described in the exposure of the juxtarenal aorta, or by reflecting the left colon and splenic flexure downward. (11, 12, 39) In the latter approach, the peritoneal attachment of the left colon and the splenic flexure are taken down (Fig. 3.35). The left colon is reflected medially and caudally (Fig. 3.36). The renal vein branches are identified and the left renal vein is visualized. Dissection along the caudal aspect of the left renal vein will reveal the left renal artery, which can be followed distally to its segmental branches.

Transabdominal Exposure of the Left Renal Artery

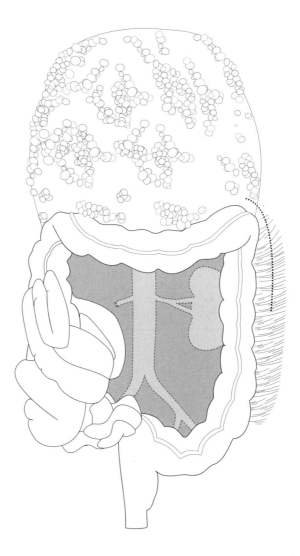

Figure 3.35. The left renal artery can be exposed by reflecting the splenic flexure and the left colon medially.

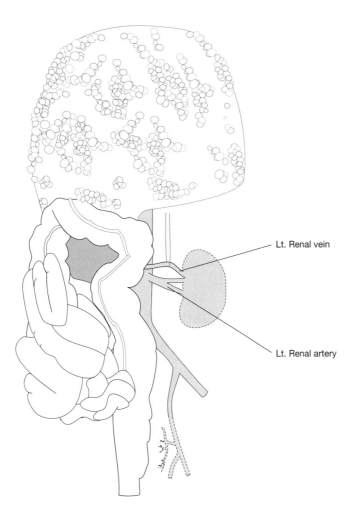

Figure 3.36. The lateral peritoneal attachments of the left colon are incised. The splenic flexure is mobilized carefully to avoid any iatrogenic injury to the spleen. The left renal artery can be exposed beneath the left renal vein.

Exposure of the Right Renal Artery (Figs. 3.37-3.39)
The exposure of the proximal part of the right renal artery is outlined in the section on the exposure of the pararenal aorta (11, 12, 39). The distal part of the right renal artery can be exposed by first mobilizing the second and third part of the duodenum using a Kocher maneuver. The peritoneum lateral to the second part of the duodenum is incised and the duodenum and head of pancreas are reflected medially and anteriorly (Figs. 3.37, 3.38). The inferior vena cava is exposed beneath the duodenum and the right renal vein is identified. Dissection around the caudal aspect of the right renal vein will reveal the right renal artery (Fig. 3.39). The right renal artery can often be palpated as a cord structure as it crosses underneath the vena cava. The right renal artery is then exposed and dissected proximally and distally until it divides into its segmental branches. The division of the adrenal arterial branch usually allows for additional mobilization of the proximal renal artery.

Transabdominal Exposure of the Right Renal Artery

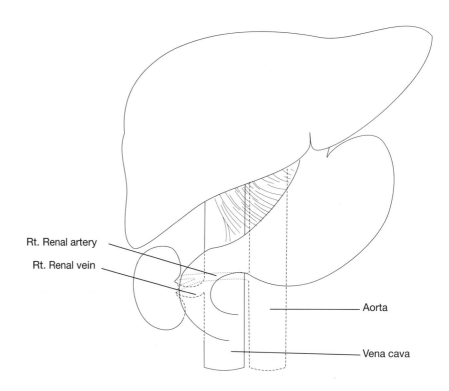

Figure 3.37. The right renal artery and adjacent structures.

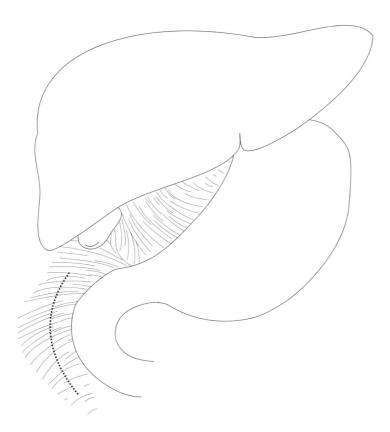

Figure 3.38. The peritoneum lateral to the duodenum is incised and a Kocher maneuver is performed.

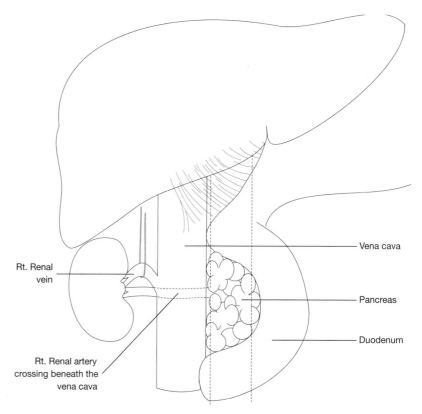

Rt. Renal vein

Rt. Renal artery crossing beneath the vena cava

Vena cava

Pancreas

Duodenum

Figure 3.39. The duodenum is reflected medially. The right renal vein is mobilized superiorly, exposing the right renal artery.

Exposure of the Aorta and Its Branches at the Diaphragm

Transperitoneally, the aorta at the diaphragmatic hiatus can be accessed through the lesser sac using blind dissection or under direct vision. (44) Blind dissection can be utilized for emergency control of the supraceliac aorta during the replacement of a ruptured abdominal aortic aneurysm. Exposure under direct vision can also be used for providing urgent control of the supraceliac aorta during the repair of a ruptured abdominal aortic aneurysm. It is also ideal for the construction of an antegrade aortoceliac or aortomesenteric bypass for chronic visceral ischemia. This exposure usually provides access to 4–5 cm of the aorta proximal to the origin of the celiac artery. It has also been recommended for aortic control in the presence of significant scarring from previous aortic surgery. (21) Furthermore, it is also preferred by some over clamping above the renal or superior mesenteric arteries when aortic control proximal to these vessels is necessary. This approach however is not suitable for replacing aortic aneurysmal pathology involving the superior mesenteric or celiac arteries because of the overlying pancreas and adjacent structures. To expose this segment of the aorta through a transabdominal incision, the viscera of the left-upper quadrant will need to be reflected medially, a procedure referred to as medial visceral rotation. Alternatively, this segment of the aorta can also be exposed using a thoracoabdominal or retroperitoneal approach. The medial visceral rotation can eliminate the morbidity of extending the exposure into a thoracoabdominal approach. The thoracoabdominal approach cannot be avoided when exposure of the thoracic aorta is also required.

Transperitoneal Blind Dissection of the Supraceliac Aorta

The lesser sac is entered and one hand is introduced toward the diaphragm to palpate the aorta as it exits from the aortic hiatus (Fig. 3.40). The presence of a nasogastric tube will help in identifying the location of the esophagogastric junction. Using the index finger, the right and then left crura of the diaphragm

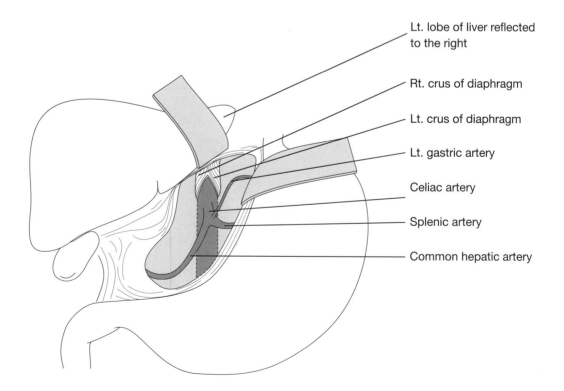

Figure 3.40. Transabdominal exposure of the supraceliac aorta.

are palpated and gently dissected away from the aorta. The aorta is then bluntly dissected on each side along its longitudinal axis down to the vertebral column using a sweeping motion of the index finger. The aorta is then pinched between the index finger and the thumb to ensure adequate dissection. The aorta is then straddled by the second and third fingers. The blades of an aortic clamp are then carefully guided over the fingers to control the dissected part of the supraceliac aorta.

Transperitoneal Exposure of the Supraceliac Aorta

When the supraceliac aorta is exposed under direct vision for elective or emergency control, the triangular ligament of the liver is first divided. Care should be taken to avoid injuring the hepatic veins or vena cava as the medial part of the triangular ligament is being divided close to the diaphragm. The left lobe of the liver is retracted to the right. The lesser omentum is incised. The stomach and esophagogastric junction are then gently retracted to the left. This can be facilitated by the presence of a nasogastric tube. The right crus of the diaphragm is identified. Using a right-angle clamp, the fibers of the right crus of the diaphragm are engaged and then divided. This will provide good visualization of the right edge of the supraceliac aorta. The left aspect of the aorta is exposed next. The dissection is carried inferiorly and then superiorly, dividing the medial arcuate ligament and exposing the most distal part of the thoracic aorta. This provides an adequate space for cross-clamping the aorta under direct vision. Ligation and division of the phrenic arteries may be necessary to enhance the exposure.

Transperitoneal Exposure of the Celiac Artery

To expose the celiac artery, the supraceliac aorta is exposed under direct vision as previously described. The dissection is extended inferiorly on the anterior aspect of the supraceliac aorta. (45, 47) Fibrous bands, sympathetic nerves, and the celiac ganglia are usually lying anterior to the celiac artery. Division of these structures will expose the celiac artery (Fig. 3.40).

Exposure of the Hepatic Artery
The lesser omentum is incised. The stomach is reflected inferiorly. Palpation along the upper border of the pancreas will reveal the location of the hepatic artery. A 2×3 cm lymph node is often noted in that area. Mobilization of the lymph node will usually reveal the common hepatic artery directly inferior to it. The common hepatic artery is dissected and encircled with a silastic vessel loop. Gentle traction of the vessel loop will facilitate the exposure of the common hepatic artery as it divides into the proper hepatic and the gastroduodenal arteries (Figs. 3.41, 3.42).

Transabdominal Exposure of the Common Hepatic Artery

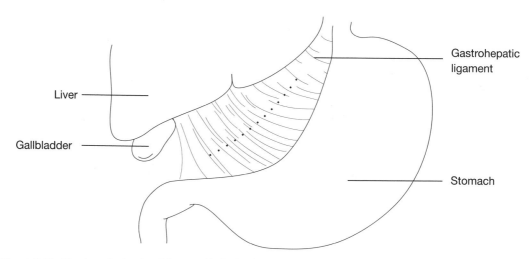

Figure 3.41. The hepatoduodenal ligament is incised.

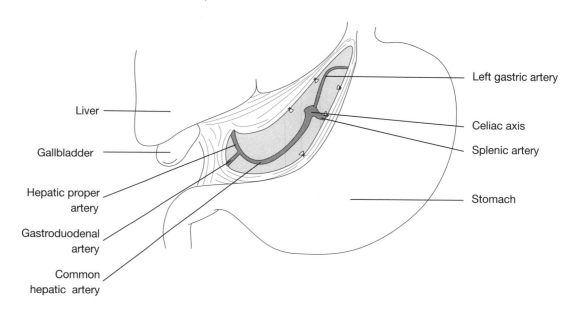

Figure 3.42. The common hepatic artery is dissected.

Transperitoneal Exposure of the Superior Mesenteric Artery (SMA)
The origin of the superior mesenteric artery can be accessed through the lesser sac by exposing the aorta at the level of the celiac artery and then carrying the dissection distally on the anterior aspect of the aorta. (45, 47) The upper border of the pancreas is mobilized to allow for exposure of the origin of the superior mesenteric artery as it lies just underneath it. Further distal exposure of the superior mesenteric artery from this approach is limited by the overlying pancreas. Thus, 3–5 cm distal to its origin from the aorta, the superior mesenteric artery is best exposed by an incision at the root of the small bowel mesentery. The transverse colon is retracted anteriorly and cephalad and the small bowel is reflected caudally (Fig. 3.43). The root of the small bowel mesentery is palpated revealing the location of the vascular pedicle. The peritoneum overlying the root of the mesentery is incised. The superior mesenteric vein and artery are exposed. The superior mesenteric artery is identified and mobilized to the patient's left side (Fig. 3.44). The superior mesenteric artery is further dissected distally exposing its branches. This approach allows for the exposure of the superior mesenteric artery from the level of the middle colic to the ileocolic branch.

Transabdominal Exposure of the Superior Mesenteric Artery

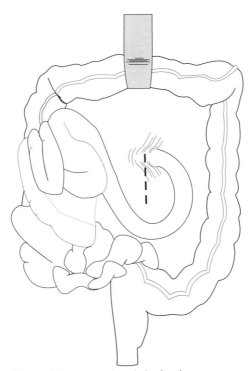

Figure 3.43. The peritoneum in the base of the mesentery is incised.

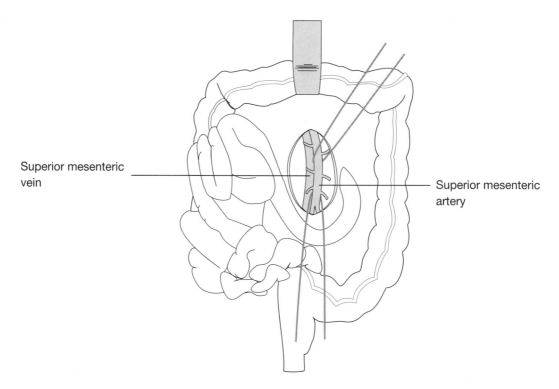

Superior mesenteric vein

Superior mesenteric artery

Figure 3.44. The artery is dissected and identified, usually to the left of the superior mesenteric vein. This approach allows the exposure of the superior mesenteric artery up to the level of the origin of the middle colic artery.

Exposure of the Suprarenal Abdominal Aorta and Its Branches Through a Medial Visceral Rotation

The suprarenal aorta and its branches can also be exposed through a transabdominal incision up to the level of the diaphragm by performing a medial visceral rotation. (40, 41) In this approach, the left colon, the spleen, the pancreas, and the stomach are mobilized and reflected medially. The left lateral peritoneal reflection is incised, mobilizing the descending colon. The incision is carried cephalad and around the spleen through the phrenocolic and lienorenal ligaments. The plane of the dissection can be either anterior or posterior to the left kidney. In the former, the kidney and adrenal gland are left undisturbed, and the plane of dissection is carried between the pancreas and Gerota's fascia. In the latter, the kidney and adrenal gland are rotated anteriorly and reflected medially along with the spleen, the pancreas, and the stomach (Fig. 3.45). At this stage, the aorta is well exposed along with the origin of the celiac and superior mesenteric arteries. Although this exposure can avoid the addition of a thoracic incision, it can be challenging in overweight patients or in the presence of a narrow costal angle. Furthermore, care should be taken to avoid avulsing the splenic capsule during this exposure.

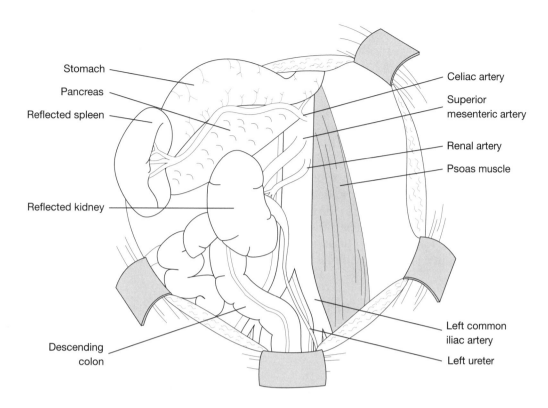

Figure 3.45. Medial visceral rotation.

Retroperitoneal Exposures of the Abdominal Aorta and its Branches

The abdominal aorta can be exposed through a right or left retroperitoneal approach. (34, 37, 38) The left-sided approach is the most commonly used because of its versatility. Unlike the right retroperitoneal approach, the left retroperitoneal approach is ideal for celiac or superior mesenteric artery revascularization procedures or for exposure of the juxtarenal or suprarenal abdominal aorta. The right retroperitoneal approach can be useful in selected situations such as left retroperitoneal exposures and scarring or if there is a need for right renal revascularization.

The main steps in exposing the aorta through a retroperitoneal approach are

1. Skin incision
2. Division of the external oblique, internal oblique, and transversus muscles
3. Entering the retroperitoneal space
4. Mobilization of the peritoneal contents
5. Identifying the lumbar vein
6. Exposing the abdominal aorta
7. Identification of the left renal artery

Details of the Left Retroperitoneal Exposure

The patient is positioned with the left side of the chest rotated almost at a 90°
angle and the pelvis at a 30° angle to the horizontal (Fig. 3.46). The skin incision
is performed from the lateral edge of the rectus muscle to the tip of the 11th rib.
Extension of the skin incision beneath the 12th rib or into the 11th interspace
may be needed to improve the exposure. This may also be achieved by resecting the 12th rib. The incision is deepened through the subcutaneous tissues.
The external oblique is then incised followed by the internal oblique and the
transverse oblique muscles. The retroperitoneum is entered posteriorly at the
lateral aspect of the incision. The peritoneum is mobilized cranially and caudally, allowing the peritoneal contents to be retracted medially. The peritoneum
is mobilized anterior to the psoas muscle toward the aorta. Cephalad, the plane
of the dissection can be either anterior (Fig. 3.47) or posterior to the left kidney.
In the former, the aortic exposure is similar to that obtained through a transabdominal approach with the left renal vein crossing over the aorta.

Retroperitoneal Exposure of the Abdominal Aorta

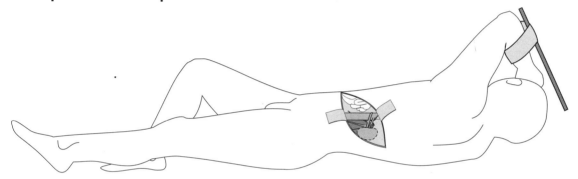

Figure 3.46. Patient's position for the left retroperitoneal approach to the abdominal aorta.

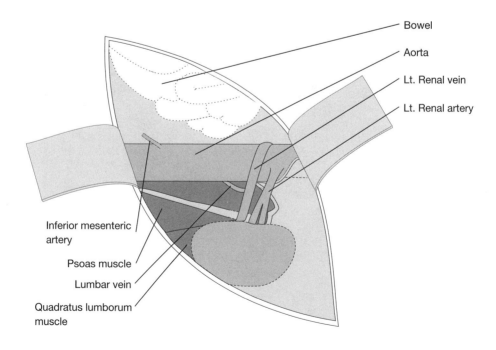

Figure 3.47. Retroperitoneal exposure of the infrarenal aorta with the left kidney undisturbed.

When the plane of the dissection is posterior to the kidney, the kidney is elevated from its bed and reflected anteriorly and medially (Fig. 3.48). This approach facilitates the exposure of the pararenal aorta without having to mobilize the left renal vein. The aorta is palpated anterior to the lumbar vertebrae. The dissection is carried superiorly over the aorta. Dissection is facilitated by dividing the periaortic tissues on the most posterior and lateral aspect of the aorta. At that level, there are no significant branches or structures that can be injured. Dissection of the aorta is then extended superiorly until the left crus of the diaphragm is encountered. Anteriorly, a large lumbar vein crossing over the aorta to join the left renal vein is noted (Fig. 3.48). This lumbar vein usually marks the level just below the origin of the left renal artery. The left renal artery can be easily palpated and then exposed and dissected as needed (Fig. 3.48). Division of the left crus of the diaphragm at that level will provide additional proximal exposure. The right renal artery cannot be exposed from this approach unless the aorta is transected at the infrarenal level. In this situation, the proximal part of the right renal artery can be exposed from beneath the stump of the transected aorta.

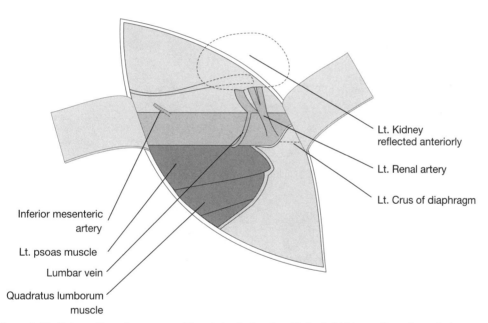

Figure 3.48. Retroperitoneal exposure of the abdominal aorta with the left kidney reflected anteriorly.

Distally, the aorta can be dissected down to its bifurcation. Frequently, exposure of the common iliac arteries is also necessary during the same procedure. The exposure of the left common and external iliac arteries can be performed bluntly or sharply by extending the dissection distally from the aorta. The exposure of the right common and proximal external iliac arteries is more demanding. However, division of the inferior mesenteric artery at its origin from the aorta permits additional retraction of the peritoneum and its content to allow further exposure and dissection of the right common iliac artery. If the main reason for exposing the right common iliac artery from this approach is to secure distal vascular control, this step can be facilitated by occluding the right common iliac artery from within the aortic wall using a balloon occluding catheter.

Retroperitoneal Approach to the Suprarenal Aorta and Its Branches

If supraceliac control is anticipated, the skin incision is usually carried out to the level of the 10th rib and into the 9th interspace. The infrarenal aorta is exposed as previously described up to the level of the left crus of the diaphragm. The left crus of the diaphragm is completely divided exposing the supraceliac aorta. The celiac and the superior mesenteric arteries can be exposed and circumferentially dissected at their origin (Fig. 3.49). In this approach, the aorta can be exposed up to a few cm above the origin of the celiac artery. The pleural cavity is not usually entered and the diaphragm is left intact except at the hiatus. If more proximal exposure is necessary, a thoracoabdominal approach will become necessary.

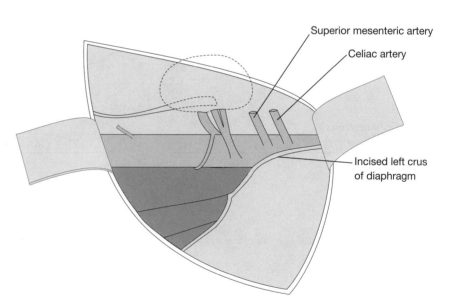

Figure 3.49. Retroperitoneal exposure of the suprarenal aorta.

Thoracoabdominal Exposure of the Thoracic and Upper Abdominal Aorta

Exposure of the thoracic and upper abdominal aorta is achieved through a thoracoabdominal approach. (6, 13) The abdominal portion of the thoracoabdominal exposure can be through a transperitoneal approach or retroperitoneal approach. In the former, a vertical midline abdominal incision is carried into the chest, usually in the sixth or eighth intercostal space depending on the extent of the proximal exposure needed (Fig. 3.50). The sixth intercostal space can provide exposure to the level of the origin of the left subclavian artery. The thoracic incision is usually carried back posteriorly to the level of the latissimus dorsi muscle. Once the pleural cavity is entered, the diaphragm can be divided radially or circumferentially. The circumferential incision has the advantage of preserving the phrenic nerve's attachments to the diaphragm. The stomach, spleen, and distal pancreas are then mobilized medially exposing the origin of the celiac and superior mesenteric arteries. In the retroperitoneal thoracoabdominal approach, it is usually easier to start with the thoracic part of the incision, divide the diaphragm, and then progress into the retroperitoneal space, starting at the level of the left crus of the diaphragm. This will facilitate developing the retroperitoneal plane and extending the exposure into the abdomen through an oblique or left paramedian incision (Fig. 3.51).

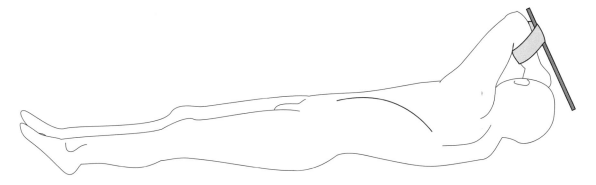

Figure 3.50. Patient's position for the thoracoabdominal retroperitoneal approach to the abdominal and thoracic aorta.

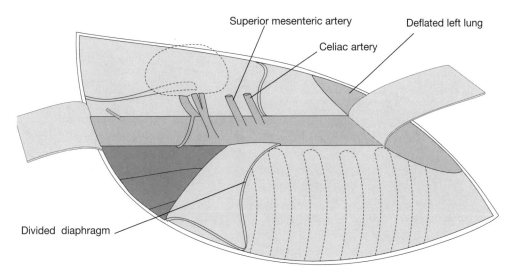

Figure 3.51. Thoracoabdominal retroperitoneal approach.

Transperitoneal Exposure of the Iliac Arteries
The origin of the common iliac arteries can be accessed by exposing the aorta as previously described and carrying the dissection distally to the aortic bifurcation. On the right side, the cecum and the small bowel are usually retracted superiorly and laterally. The peritoneum overlying the aorta is incised and the incision is extended along the right common iliac artery. The right common iliac artery is then dissected distally to the level of the iliac bifurcation. At that level, the right ureter is noted crossing the iliac bifurcation. Exposure of the right external iliac artery can be achieved by incising the peritoneum over the artery distal to the ureter toward the inguinal ligament. On the left side, frequently only a few centimeters of the proximal common iliac artery can be dissected because of the overlying sigmoid mesocolon. Further exposure can be obtained by reflecting the sigmoid colon medially. The peritoneal attachments of the sigmoid colon to the lateral abdominal wall are incised. The left psoas muscle is identified and the external iliac artery is palpated medially. Dissection of the external iliac artery at that level is performed and extended distally and proximally toward the common iliac artery. The internal iliac artery can be identified along the medial and inferior aspect of the left common iliac artery (Fig. 3.52).

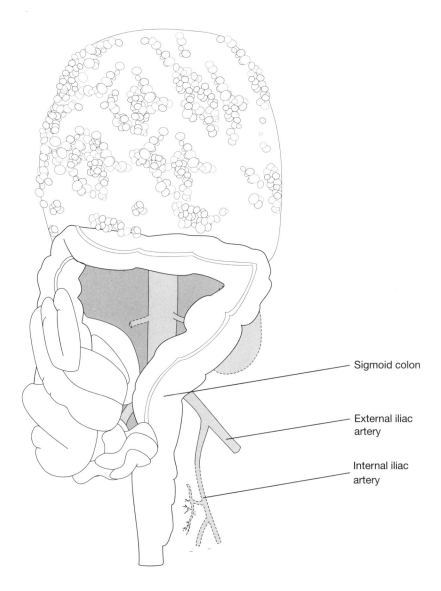

Sigmoid colon

External iliac artery

Internal iliac artery

Figure 3.52. Transabdominal exposure of the left iliac arteries.

Retroperitoneal Exposure of the Iliac Arteries
The retroperitoneal exposure of the iliac vessels is very similar to the retroperitoneal approach to the aorta with the main variation being the location of the incision. Most commonly, a curvilinear incision is used starting from the lateral border of the left rectus muscle and extending to the midaxillary line. For the common iliac artery, the incision starts approximately 5 cm above the symphysis pubis and is 2–3 cm lower for the exposure of the external iliac artery (Fig. 3.53). The distal part of the external iliac artery can also be exposed using a longitudinal infrainguinal incision placed over the common femoral artery. This latter vessel is exposed proximally. The inguinal ligament is retracted superiorly and anteriorly and may also be divided providing exposure to the distal 5 cm segment of the external iliac artery.

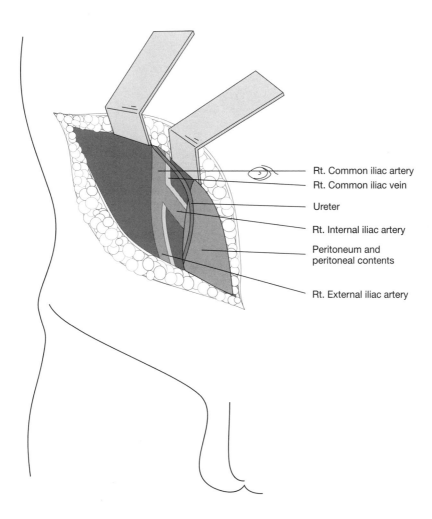

Rt. Common iliac artery
Rt. Common iliac vein
Ureter
Rt. Internal iliac artery
Peritoneum and peritoneal contents
Rt. External iliac artery

Figure 3.53. Retroperitoneal exposure of the iliac arteries.

ARTERIES OF THE LOWER EXTREMITY

ANATOMY OF THE ARTERIES OF THE LOWER EXTREMITIES

The common femoral artery

The common femoral artery is the continuation of the external iliac artery after it passes beneath the inguinal ligament. It is surrounded by the femoral nerve laterally and the common femoral vein medially. Proximally, the common femoral artery and vein are enclosed in a fibrous sheath referred to as the femoral sheath. The femoral artery travels in the femoral triangle, which is made by the sartorius muscle laterally, the adductor longus muscle medially, and the inguinal ligament superiorly. The floor of the triangle is made by the iliopsoas muscle laterally and the pectineus muscle medially. The common femoral artery gives off the superficial iliac circumflex and the superficial epigastric arteries proximally and divides distally into the deep and superficial femoral arteries (Fig. 3.54).

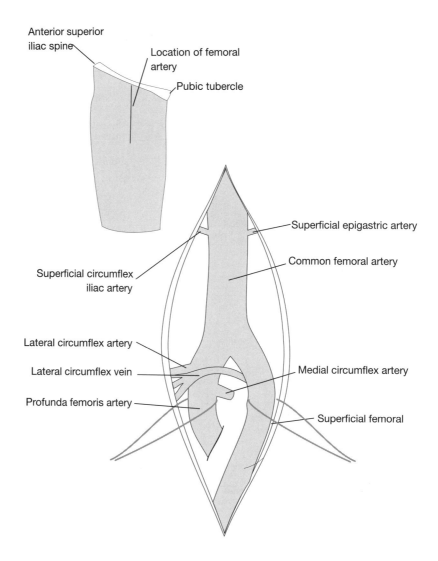

Figure 3.54. Exposure of the common femoral artery and its bifurcation.

The Profunda Femoris Artery

The profunda (deep) femoral artery originates from the posterolateral aspect of the common femoral artery. It follows a posterior and lateral course running parallel and medial to the femur over the pectineus and adductor brevis muscles. The profunda femoris artery ends distal to the femoral triangle between the adductor longus and magnus muscles. The proximal part of the profunda femoris artery gives off the lateral and medial femoral circumflex branches. These branches may also originate directly from the common femoral artery. Awareness of these anatomical variations is important to avoid unexpected retrograde bleeding from these branches upon performing a femoral arteriotomy. More distally the profunda femoris artery gives off three large perforating branches. For the sake of describing surgical exposures, the profunda is divided arbitrarily into three zones. The proximal zone extends from its origin to just distal to the lateral femoral circumflex artery. The distal zone is the part distal to the femoral triangle and is usually distal to the second perforating muscle branch. The middle zone is the segment between the proximal and distal zones (Fig. 3.55).

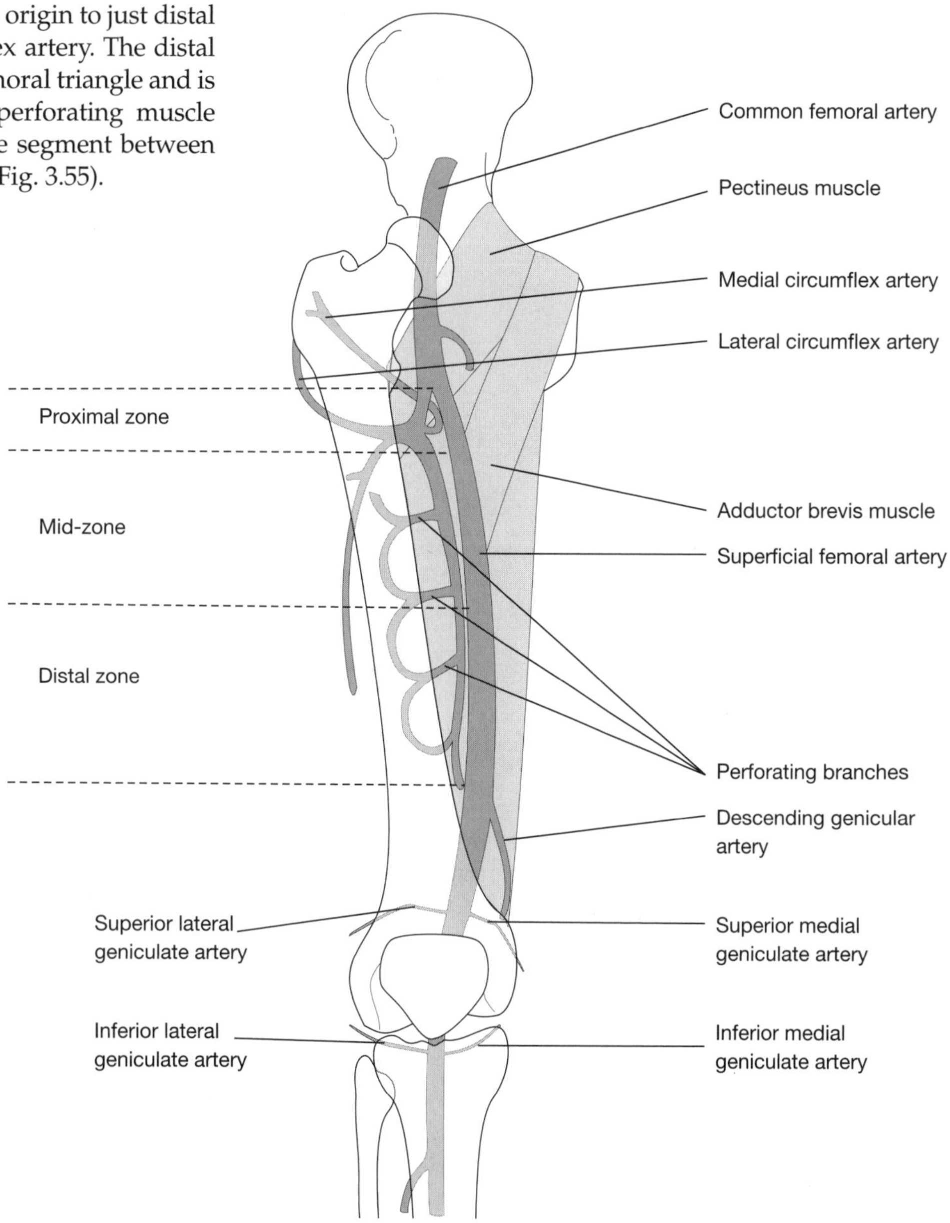

Figure 3.55. Deep femoral artery.

The Superficial Femoral Artery

The superficial femoral artery is the continuation of the common femoral artery. It runs along the anteromedial aspect of the thigh and is bounded laterally by the sartorius muscle and medially by the adductor longus muscle. In the midthigh, it moves medially into a deep and posterior location traveling through the adductor magnus muscle in the adductor (Hunter) canal. It then exits from the adductor hiatus in the distal thigh to become the suprageniculate popliteal artery (Fig. 3.56). During its course, the superficial femoral artery provides several muscular branches as well as the descending genicular artery.

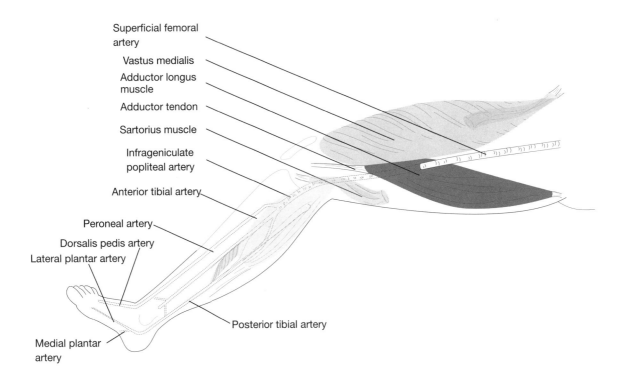

Superficial femoral
artery
Vastus medialis
Adductor longus
muscle
Adductor tendon
Sartorius muscle
Infrageniculate
popliteal artery
Anterior tibial artery
Peroneal artery
Dorsalis pedis artery
Lateral plantar artery
Posterior tibial artery
Medial plantar
artery

Figure 3.56. The superficial femoral artery and adjacent muscles.

The Popliteal Artery

The popliteal artery is the direct continuation of the superficial femoral artery. It has a suprageniculate and infrageniculate component. The suprageniculate (above-knee) popliteal artery starts distal to the adductor canal and travels between the two heads of the gastrocnemius muscle anterior to the popliteus muscle. It continues beyond the knee joint as the infrageniculate (below-knee) popliteal artery for 4–6 cm until it divides into the anterior tibial artery and the tibioperoneal trunk. The popliteal artery gives off several genicular branches. Above the knee, it gives off the superior medial and the superior lateral genicular arteries. Below the knee joint, it gives off the inferior lateral and the inferior medial genicular arteries (Fig. 3.55). These genicular branches provide a rich network between the superficial femoral artery, the profunda femoris artery, and the tibial arteries. This collateral network can be very useful in the presence of chronic occlusive disease of the superficial femoral and popliteal arteries.

The Anterior Tibial Artery

The anterior tibial artery represents the first major branch of the infrageniculate popliteal artery. It curves anteriorly and laterally and penetrates the interosseus membrane to lie between the anterior tibialis muscle and the extensor hallucis longus (Figs. 3.56, 3.57). The anterior tibial artery continues its course in the anterior compartment of the leg, lying on the interosseus membrane down to the ankle level, where it becomes the dorsalis pedis artery.

The Tibioperoneal Trunk

The tibioperoneal trunk is the direct continuation of the popliteal artery. It usually runs for 1–3 cm before bifurcating into the peroneal and the posterior tibial arteries.

The Peroneal Artery

The peroneal artery runs in the deep posterior compartment of the leg as a direct continuation of the tibioperoneal trunk. The peroneal artery runs posterior and medial to the fibula surrounded by the posterior tibialis muscle anteriorly and medially and the flexor hallucis longus posteriorly (Figs. 3.56, 3.57). During its course in the leg, the peroneal artery gives off branches to its adjacent muscles. In the lower leg, the peroneal artery gives off a communicating branch to the posterior tibial artery and another communicating branch that perforates through the interosseus membrane to connect with the anterior tibial artery (Fig. 3.56). The peroneal artery terminates at the ankle as small branches to the lateral malleolus and calcaneus.

The Posterior Tibial Artery

The posterior tibial artery originates from the tibioperoneal trunk and courses medially as it runs in the deep posterior compartment of the leg. The posterior tibial artery is surrounded

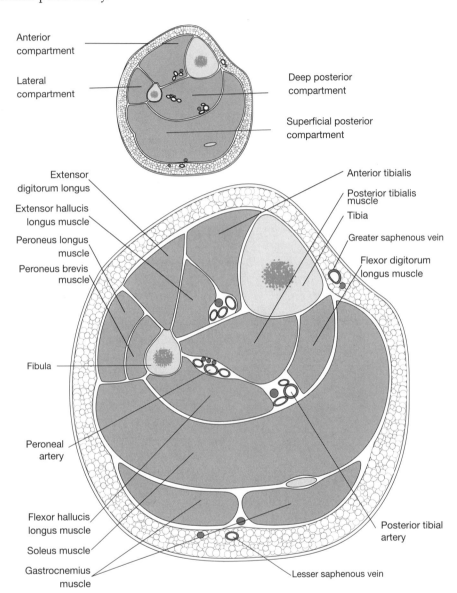

Figure 3.57. Cross section of the leg above midlevel.

by the flexor digitorum longus anteriorly, the flexor hallucis longus posteromedially, and the tibialis posterior muscle posterolaterally (Fig. 56, 57). At the ankle level, the posterior tibial artery continues into the foot and divides into the medial and lateral plantar arteries. The lateral plantar artery is usually the larger branch. It courses in a lateral direction deep to the abductor hallucis muscle and the flexor digitorum brevis muscle to supply the deep plantar arterial arch. The medial plantar artery is the smaller branch of the posterior tibial artery, and it courses in a medial direction to supply the medial forefoot and terminate in the plantar arch.

Exposure of the Common Femoral Artery and Its Bifurcation

A vertical skin incision placed over the femoral pulse is usually used to expose the common femoral artery and its bifurcation. If the femoral pulse is not palpable, the incision is guided by the following anatomical landmarks. The pubic tubercle and the anterior superior iliac spine are palpated and the incision is placed at a point midway between these two structures. In addition, when the femoral pulse is absent, the presence of calcification in the common femoral artery may help to identify its location. The calcified femoral artery can often be palpated by rolling the fingers gently over the femoral region. Occasionally, matted inguinal lymph nodes could give a similar sensation and may be misleading. The incision is deepened through the subcutaneous tissue. If the saphenous vein is encountered during the exposure, this indicates that the dissection is more medial than necessary. If nerves are encountered, the dissection is more lateral than the actual location of the femoral artery. Encountered lymphatics are ligated and divided to avoid postoperative lymph leaks. The femoral sheath is identified and incised. The common femoral artery is then identified and dissected. As the dissection is continued distally, a change in the caliber of the exposed artery will be noted. The change in the vessel caliber marks the origin of the profunda femoris artery and the transition from the common femoral to the superficial femoral artery. The superficial femoral artery can be further exposed and dissected distally by extending the incision inferiorly (see Fig. 3.54).

Medial Exposure of the Proximal Profunda Femoris Artery

The profunda femoris artery can be approached by exposing the common femoral artery at its bifurcation and then proceeding with the dissection along its lateral and posterior aspect to expose the origin of the profunda femoris artery (see Fig. 3.55). Circumferential dissection of the common femoral bifurcation to identify any posterior branches originating from the common femoral artery is important to avoid unexpected retrograde bleeding from these branches upon creating an arteriotomy. Immediately after its origin from the common femoral artery, the profunda femoris is often crossed by venous branches. The first large venous branch is usually the lateral femoral circumflex vein, which crosses over the profunda femoris artery to join the superficial femoral vein (see Fig. 3.54). Division of these veins is essential to expose the profunda femoris artery further distally. The dissection can be carried out distally tracing the profunda femoris artery and its branches for 5–8 cm.

Medial Exposure of the Mid- and Distal Zones of the Profunda Femoris Artery

Mid- and distal zones of the profunda femoris artery can be exposed without exposing the common femoral bifurcation. (31) A 10- to 12-cm skin incision is performed over the medial aspect of the sartorius muscle. The superficial femoral artery and vein are exposed; they are retracted without dissecting them along with the sartorius muscle anteriorly and laterally. The dissection is then continued posteriorly toward the femur. A fibrous layer between the adductor longus muscle and the vastus medialis muscle is noted and incised longitudinally. The location of the profunda femoris artery underneath this layer can be identified by palpation or by using a sterile doppler. Frequently one of the veins accompanying the profunda femoris artery is first visualized. Dissection and mobilization of the accompanying vein will expose the profunda femoris artery.

Medial Exposure of the Superficial Femoral Artery in the Upper Thigh

A longitudinal incision is performed along the course of the inferior border of the sartorius muscle. The incision is deepened through the subcutaneous tissues until the muscular fascia is identified. Care is taken to avoid injuring the greater saphenous vein. The fascia is incised and the sartorius muscle is identified. Dissection along the inferior border of the sartorius muscle is performed, and the sartorius muscle is retracted laterally exposing the superficial femoral artery and vein.

Lateral Exposure of the Common Femoral Artery and its Bifurcation

The common femoral artery can also be exposed through an incision placed lateral to its anatomical location. (5) The incision can be either medial or lateral to the sartorius muscle. In the former, the skin incision is made 4 cm lateral to the femoral pulse. The incision is deepened to the level of the sartorius muscle without creating any skin flaps. The sartorius muscle is mobilized laterally and the incision is deepened medially toward the femoral vessels until the femoral sheath is identified. The femoral sheath is incised along its lateral aspect, exposing the femoral arteries. When the exposure is started lateral to the sartorius muscle, the incision is made approximately 6–8 cm lateral to the femoral pulse. The incision is carried down through the subcutaneous tissues until the fascia lata is identified. The fascia lata is incised and the sartorius muscle identified.

The dissection is then continued posterior to the sartorius muscle in the direction of the femoral vessels. This usually requires mobilization of the proximal part of the sartorius muscle, which often necessitates transection of the first two segmental arterial branches supplying the sartorius muscle. The femoral sheath is then identified from beneath the sartorius muscle as the dissection is being carried medially. The femoral sheath is then incised along its lateral border, exposing the common femoral artery. Extending the incision distally will allow for exposure of the superficial femoral artery as well as the profunda femoris artery. The superficial femoral artery is identified in a plane directly posterior and medial to the sartorius muscle. The profunda femoris artery is identified by dissecting in a deeper plane posterior to the sartorius muscle. This is achieved by incising the connective tissue membrane that extends from the adductor longus to the vastus medialis. The first vessel identified is usually the femoral circumflex artery. After transecting its accompanying vein and dissecting toward its origin, the profunda femoris artery is exposed (30) (Fig. 3.58).

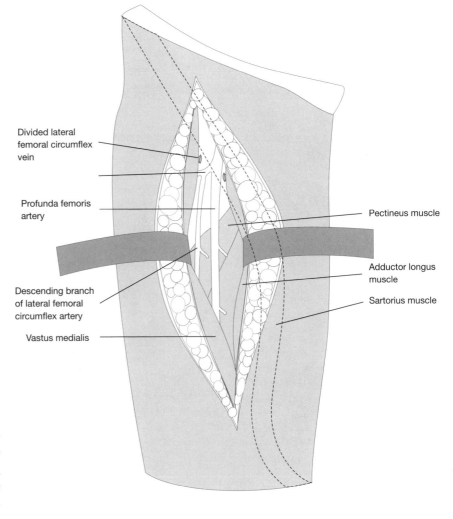

Divided lateral femoral circumflex vein

Profunda femoris artery

Descending branch of lateral femoral circumflex artery

Vastus medialis

Pectineus muscle

Adductor longus muscle

Sartorius muscle

Figure 3.58. Lateral exposure of the profunda femoris artery.

Medial Exposure of the Suprageniculate Popliteal Artery
A longitudinal skin incision is performed from the level of the knee joint extending 10–12 cm proximally (Fig. 3.59). The incision is usually placed along the anticipated location of the anterior border of the sartorius muscle when a prosthetic bypass is being used. If the ipsilateral greater saphenous vein is being utilized as a bypass, the same incision used to expose the vein can also be employed to expose the popliteal artery above the knee. The incision is deepened through the subcutaneous tissue (Fig. 3.60) until the adductor tendon is identified anteriorly and the upper border of the sartorius muscle is noted posteriorly.

Medial Exposure of the Suprageniculate Popliteal Artery

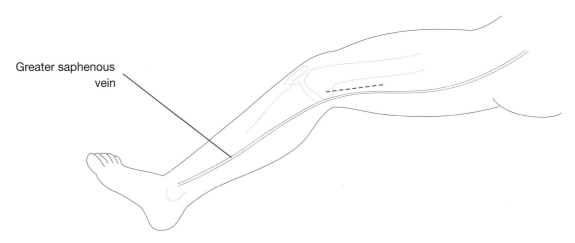

Greater saphenous vein

Figure 3.59.   Incision for exposure of the suprageniculate popliteal artery.

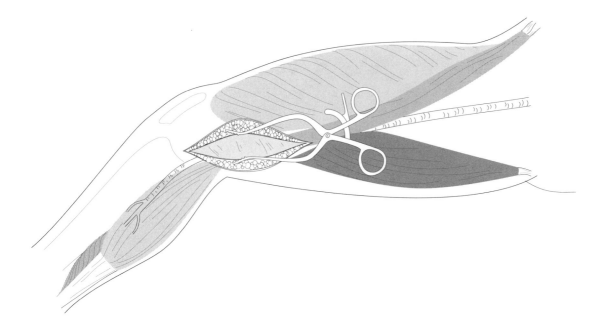

Figure 3.60.   The incision is deepened through the subcutaneous tissues.

The fascia between the adductor tendon and the sartorius muscle is incised and the popliteal fossa is entered (Fig. 3.61). Self-retaining retractors are placed in a deeper plane retracting the adductor tendon anteriorly and the sartorius muscle posteriorly (Fig. 3.62). To improve the exposure, the knee is bent and a rolled towel is placed underneath the proximal thigh; placing the rolled towel directly under the knee can compress the popliteal fossa rather than allowing it to open up for the exposure of the popliteal vessels. In patients with occlusive disease, the hardened calcified popliteal artery can be easily palpated in the popliteal fossa. The popliteal artery can be dissected proximally until it is seen exiting from the adductor canal. Care should be taken at this level to avoid injury to the greater saphenous nerve as it exits from the adductor canal and courses anteriorly to run with the greater saphenous vein. Distally the popliteal artery can be dissected to the level of the knee joint.

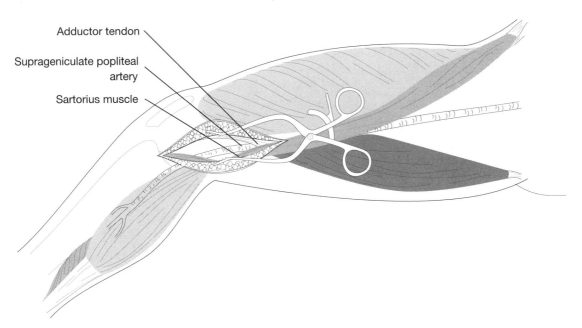

Figure 3.61. The popliteal fossa is entered inferior to the adductor tendon.

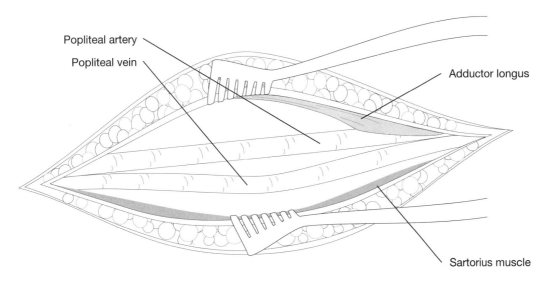

Figure 3.62.   The retractor is placed deeper exposing the popliteal vessels.

Lateral Exposure of the Suprageniculate Popliteal Artery
The suprageniculate popliteal artery can also be exposed through a lateral approach. (24, 32, 43) A 10- to 12- cm longitudinal incision is made from just above the knee joint extending proximally along the lateral aspect of the distal thigh (Fig. 3.63). The incision lies 1 cm posterior to and parallel to the iliotibial tract. Once the deep fascia is incised, the space between the iliotibial tract and biceps femoris muscle is opened exposing the above-knee popliteal artery (Fig. 3.64). The distal superficial femoral artery can be exposed by extending the incision more proximally and incising the adductor magnus muscle.

Lateral Exposure of the Suprageniculate Popliteal Artery

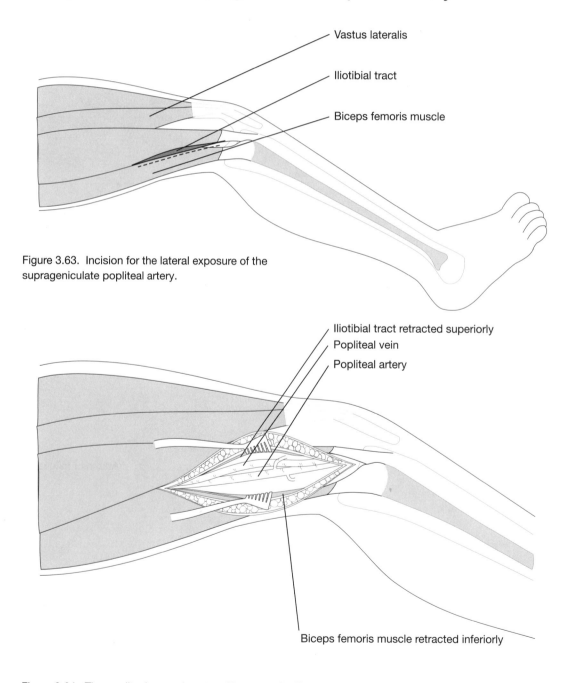

Vastus lateralis

Iliotibial tract

Biceps femoris muscle

Figure 3.63. Incision for the lateral exposure of the suprageniculate popliteal artery.

Iliotibial tract retracted superiorly
Popliteal vein
Popliteal artery

Biceps femoris muscle retracted inferiorly

Figure 3.64. The popliteal space is entered between the iliotibial tract and the biceps femoris muscle.

Medial Exposure of the Infrageniculate Popliteal Artery

A longitudinal skin incision is made from the level of the knee joint and extended distally for 10–12 cm (Fig. 3.65). The incision is deepened through the subcutaneous tissue avoiding injury to the greater saphenous vein at that level. The incision is deepened until the underlying fascia is identified (Fig. 3.66). The fascia is incised and the popliteal space is entered between the gastrocnemius and soleus muscles using a sweeping motion with the index finger. With the knee bent, self-retaining retractors are applied to retract the gastrocnemius muscle posteriorly and laterally, exposing the popliteal space further (Fig. 3.67). The tendons of the semimembranosus and semitendinosus muscles are identified in the upper corner of the incision and divided (Fig. 3.68).

Medial Exposure of the Infrageniculate Popliteal Artery and Its Trifurcation

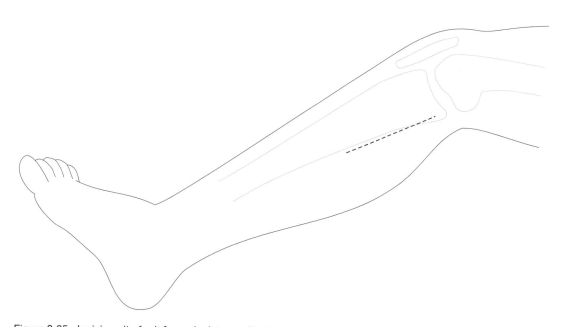

Figure 3.65.   Incision site for infrageniculate popliteal artery.

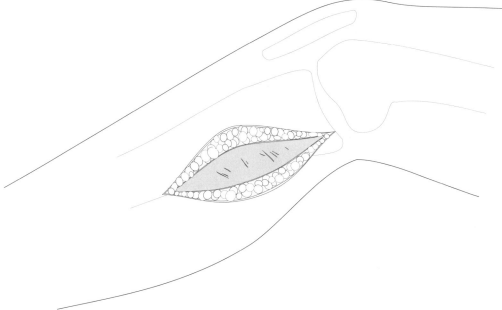

Figure 3.66.   The incision is deepened through the subcutaneous tissues.

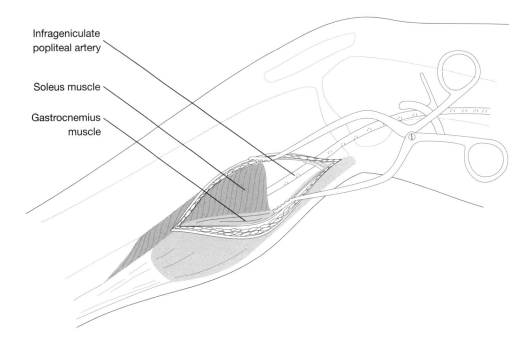

Infrageniculate
popliteal artery

Soleus muscle

Gastrocnemius
muscle

Figure 3.67. The popliteal fossa is entered, retracting the gastrocnemius muscle inferiorly and laterally.

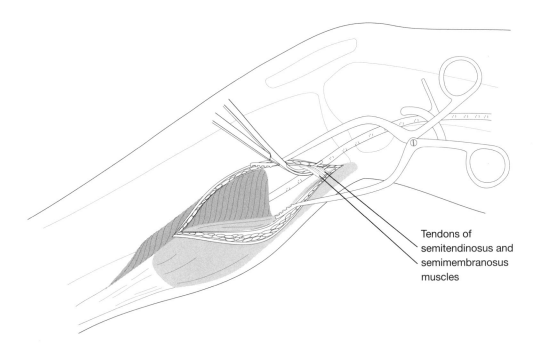

Tendons of
semitendinosus and
semimembranosus
muscles

Figure 3.68. The exposure can be improved by dividing the tendons of the semitendinosus and semimembranosus muscles.

On the distal aspect of the incision, the soleus muscle is usually seen covering the popliteal artery at the level of its trifurcation. Dissection in the areolar tissue will identify the popliteal vascular bundle (Fig. 3.69). The popliteal vein is then identified lying anterior to the popliteal artery. It is not uncommon to find two popliteal veins surrounding the popliteal artery. The anterior popliteal vein is mobilized exposing the popliteal artery. The popliteal artery is then dissected and encircled with a silastic vessel loop. Gentle traction on the vessel loop will assist in the extension of the dissection proximally and distally (Fig. 3.70).

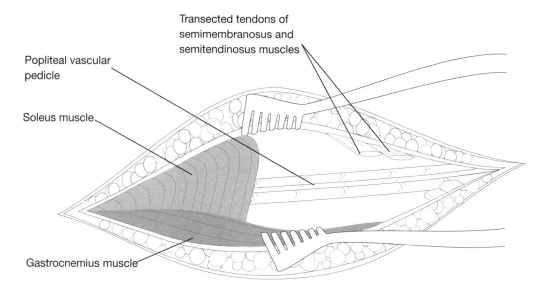

Figure 3.69. The retractor is placed deeper and the popliteal vessels are exposed.

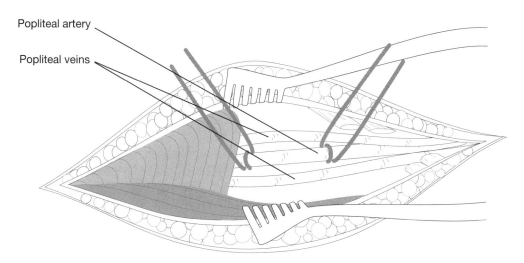

Figure 3.70. The popliteal artery is dissected.

To obtain exposure of the popliteal artery at its bifurcation, the portion of the soleus muscle covering the popliteal artery must be incised. A right-angle clamp can be placed underneath the soleus muscle to guide the transection of the muscle with electrocautery (Fig. 3.71). Soleal veins may be encountered and will need to be suture ligated. The origin of the anterior tibial artery is usually first identified. Very commonly an anterior tibial vein will be seen crossing over the artery and joining the popliteal vein. The anterior tibial vein and other similar crossing veins may need to be ligated and divided to allow for the exposure of the origin of the anterior tibial artery as well as the takeoff of the tibioperoneal trunk (Fig. 3.72). The anterior tibial artery can be further dissected for another 1.0–2.0 cm by incising the interosseous membrane and the muscular fibers beneath it; this allows additional exposure of the anterior tibial artery from the medial aspect of the leg. Exposure of the tibioperoneal trunk is obtained by additional division of the soleus muscle. Care is taken to gently dissect the tibial veins crossing over the tibioperoneal trunk and the origins of the peroneal and posterior tibial arteries.

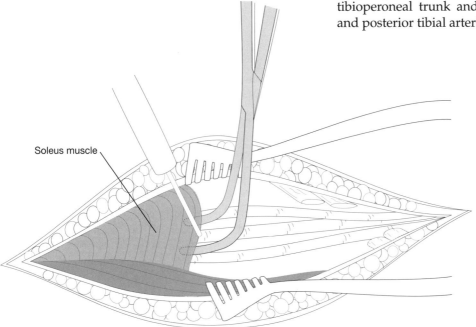

Soleus muscle

Figure 3.71 The soleus muscle is divided to expose the popliteal trifurcation.

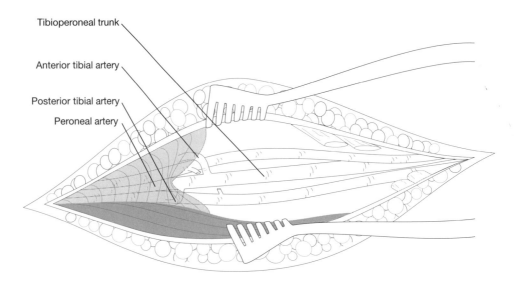

Tibioperoneal trunk
Anterior tibial artery
Posterior tibial artery
Peroneal artery

Figure 3.72. Crossing tibial veins are divided to expose the origin of the tibial vessels.

Lateral Exposure of the Infrageniculate Popliteal Artery

The more commonly used lateral approach to expose the popliteal artery involves resection of the proximal fibula. (7, 8, 24, 42, 43) A longitudinal incision is made starting at the head of the fibula and extending distally for 10–12 cm. The incision is deepened through the subcutaneous tissue. The common peroneal nerve is identified as it crosses over the neck of the fibula and is gently dissected and mobilized. The incision is deepened over the fibula, exposing the periosteum. The periosteum is incised and elevated off the fibula. A right-angle clamp is carefully passed under the fibula and can be used to separate the fibula from its posterior attachments. The fibula is transected approximately 6–8 cm distal to its neck. The proximal segment is lifted up with a bone grasper, and the muscular and ligamentous attachment of the fibula and the biceps femoris tendon are divided. The proximal part of the fibula is removed and the popliteal fossa is entered. The popliteal artery is palpated and dissected (Figs. 3.73, 3.74). The tibial nerve is usually identified crossing the below-knee popliteal artery from the lateral to the medial direction and is separated from it by the popliteal vein. More distal dissection allows a very satisfactory exposure of the trifurcation vessels. Exposure of the infrageniculate popliteal artery through a lateral approach without fibular resection has also been described. However, this exposure is usually more limited than when the proximal fibula is resected.

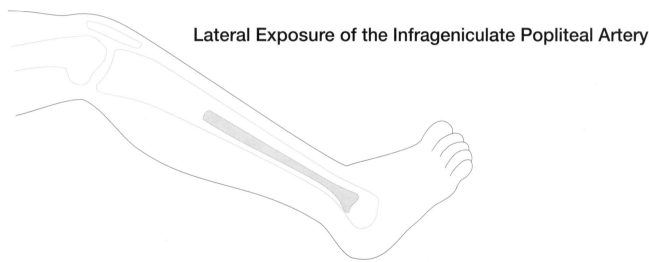

Lateral Exposure of the Infrageniculate Popliteal Artery

Figure 3.73. Lateral exposure of the below-knee popliteal can be achieved by resecting an 8-cm segment of the upper fibula. The common peroneal nerve is dissected as it crosses over the head of the fibula and protected.

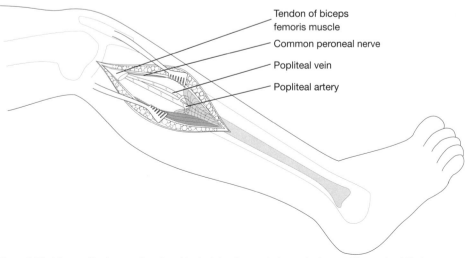

Tendon of biceps femoris muscle
Common peroneal nerve
Popliteal vein
Popliteal artery

Figure 3.74. The popliteal space is entered by incising the posterior periosteum of the excised fibula.

Posterior Exposure of the Popliteal Artery (Fig. 3.75).
The popliteal artery can also be exposed through a posterior approach. This approach has been used in the management of very large popliteal artery aneurysms. The approach, which provides a good exposure of the midpopliteal artery at the level of the knee joint, requires placing the patient in a prone position. An S-shaped incision measuring 12–14 cm is then performed starting along the medial aspect of the distal thigh. The incision is deepened through the subcutaneous tissues exposing the popliteal fascia. The popliteal fascia is incised and the popliteal space is entered. The first structure encountered is usually the tibial nerve, which is protected along with the common peroneal nerve. The popliteal vein is next identified and dissected, exposing the popliteal artery (Fig. 3.75). Proximal exposure is achieved by retracting the biceps femoris muscle laterally and the hamstring muscles medially. Dissection of the distal part of the popliteal artery is achieved by retracting the heads of the gastrocnemius muscle, exposing the origin of the anterior tibial artery as the popliteal artery dips underneath the soleus muscle. The extent of the proximal and distal dissection of the popliteal artery using this approach is limited.

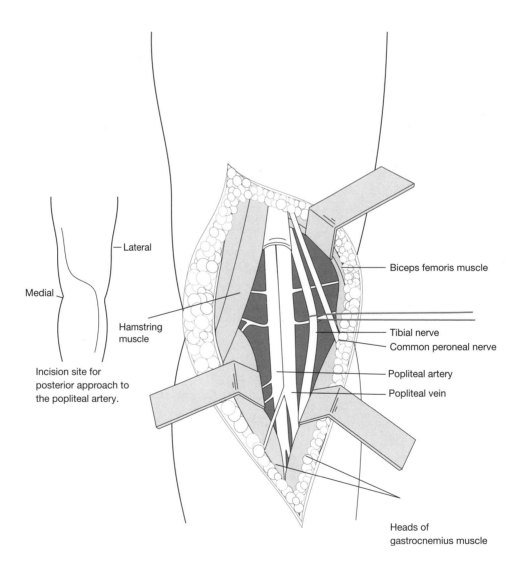

Figure 3.75. Posterior exposure of the popliteal artery.

Exposure of the Posterior Tibial Artery in the Upper Leg (Figs. 3.76-3.81)
A 10- to 12-cm longitudinal skin incision is made along the long axis of the
lower extremity. The skin incision is made 2 cm posterior to the edge of the tibia
(Fig. 3.76, 3.77). Once the incision is deepened through the subcutaneous tissue,
the anterior fascia of the soleus muscle is identified (Fig. 3.78). This fascia and
the soleus muscle fibers are divided along the length of the incision, exposing
the posterior fascia of the soleus muscle. The posterior fascia is then incised
with care to avoid injury to the underlying vascular bundle(25) (Fig. 3.79). After
the fascia is incised, inspection at that level will reveal one muscle attached to
the tibia, which is the flexor digitorum longus muscle (FDL). The second muscle posterior to FDL is the flexor hallucis longus muscle (FHL). The posterior
tibial artery and veins are usually lying in the groove between the FDL and the
FHL muscles (Fig. 3.80). The tibialis posterior muscle is lateral to the posterior
tibial vascular bundle of the leg.

   The exposure of the posterior tibial artery below the middle of the leg is similar to that above the middle of the leg. However, at the lower level of the leg,
the soleus muscle is usually attenuated. The posterior tibial artery and veins
will be seen between the tendons of the flexor digitorum longus muscle and the
flexor hallucis longus muscle (Fig. 3.81).

Exposure of the Posterior Tibial Artery

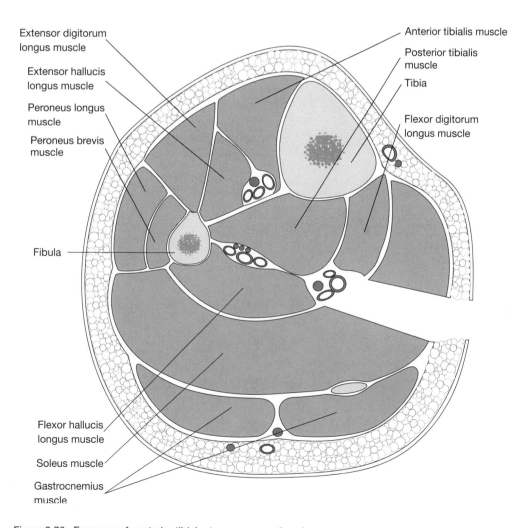

Figure 3.76. Exposure of posterior tibial artery, cross-section view.

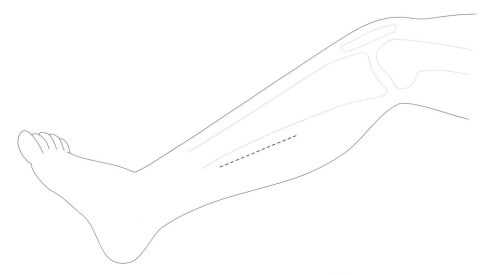

Figure 3.77. Incision site for exposure of the posterior tibial artery in the midleg.

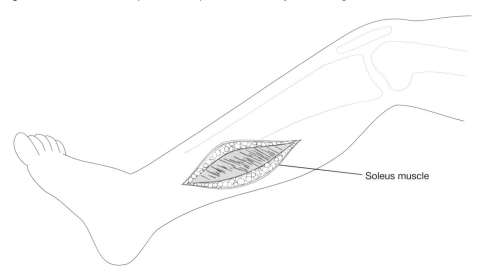

Figure 3.78. The incision is deepened, exposing the fascia overlying the soleus muscle.

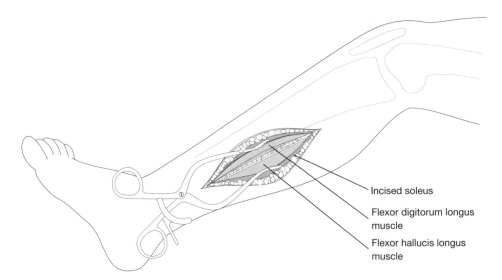

Figure 3.79. The soleus muscle is incised exposing the posterior tibial vessels.

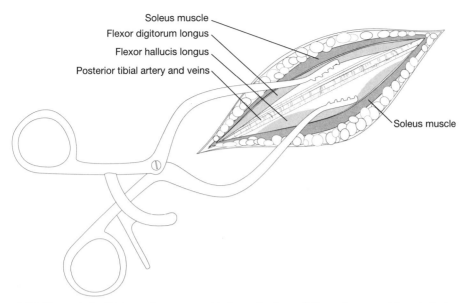

Figure 3.80. The posterior tibial vessels are exposed between the flexor digitorum longus and flexor hallucis longus muscles.

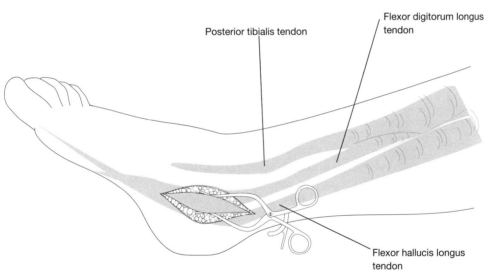

Figure 3.81. Exposure of the posterior tibial artery at the ankle.

Exposure of the Posterior Tibial Artery at the Ankle

A 8- to 10-cm skin incision is performed at the ankle. The incision is deepened through the subcutaneous tissue until the flexor retinaculum is identified. The flexor retinaculum is divided and the posterior tibial artery is identified between the tendons of the flexor digitorum longus and the flexor hallucis longus (Fig. 3.81).

Exposure of the Plantar Arteries (Fig. 3.82)

A 6- to 8-cm skin incision is performed between the medial malleolus and the calcaneous. After deepening the incision through the subcutaneous tissue, the flexor retinaculum is identified. The flexor retinaculum is incised exposing the posterior tibial artery and veins, which are usually surrounded by the tendinous sheath of the flexor digitorum longus superiorly and the flexor hallucis longus inferiorly. The posterior tibial artery is followed distally until it bifurcates into the medial and lateral plantar arteries. (1) The lateral plantar artery can be further exposed by dividing its overlying muscles, mainly the abductor hallucis and the flexor digitorum brevis muscles (Fig. 3.82).

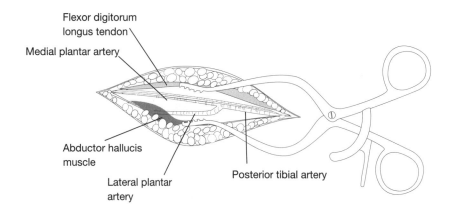

Figure 3.82. Exposure of the posterior tibial and plantar arteries at the ankle.

Medial Exposure of the Peroneal Artery (Figs. 3.83, 3.84)

The medial exposure of the peroneal artery in the upper leg starts by exposing the posterior tibial neurovascular bundle as described earlier. (10, 28) The posterior tibial neurovascular bundle can be retracted anteriorly along with the flexor digitorum longus muscle (Fig. 3.83) or posteriorly along with the flexor hallucis longus muscle (Fig. 3.84). The former approach is preferred in the upper leg and can also be used in the lower leg. The latter approach is preferred by some surgeons in both the mid- and lower leg. (20, 46) After exposing the posterior tibial vessels, the dissection is continued toward the fibula in the tissue plane (intermuscular septum) between the posterior tibialis muscle and the flexor hallucis longus muscle. Deep in the wound, a fascial layer will be identified. Incision of this fascial layer will usually expose one of the veins surrounding the peroneal artery. Further dissection and mobilization of this vein posteriorly exposes the peroneal artery. This usually requires division of a few small and delicate venae comitantes crossing over the peroneal artery. The exposure of the peroneal artery in the lower leg can be challenging in patients with heavy musculature and large-sized legs. In this situation, a lateral approach with resection of a fibular segment may be preferred.

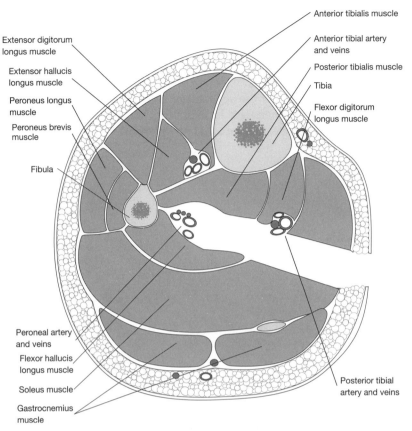

Anterior tibialis muscle

Anterior tibial artery
and veins

Posterior tibialis muscle

Tibia

Flexor digitorum
longus muscle

Extensor digitorum
longus muscle

Extensor hallucis
longus muscle

Peroneus longus
muscle

Peroneus brevis
muscle

Fibula

Peroneal artery
and veins

Flexor hallucis
longus muscle

Soleus muscle

Gastrocnemius
muscle

Posterior tibial
artery and veins

Figure 3.83. Medial approach to peroneal vessel, cross-section view. In the upper leg, the posterior tibial vessels can be retracted anteriorly.

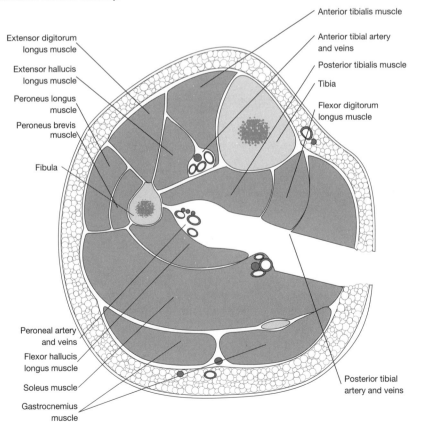

Anterior tibialis muscle

Anterior tibial artery
and veins

Posterior tibialis muscle

Tibia

Flexor digitorum
longus muscle

Extensor digitorum
longus muscle

Extensor hallucis
longus muscle

Peroneus longus
muscle

Peroneus brevis
muscle

Fibula

Peroneal artery
and veins

Flexor hallucis
longus muscle

Soleus muscle

Gastrocnemius
muscle

Posterior tibial
artery and veins

Figure 3.84. Medial approach to the peroneal artery in the mid-and lower leg, cross-section view. The posterior tibial vessels are retracted posteriorly. Dissection along the intermuscular septum toward the fibula will lead to the peroneal vessels.

Lateral Exposure of the Peroneal Artery

The lateral approach to the peroneal artery provides a more superficial access to the artery than the medial approach (Fig. 3.85). This access could facilitate the exposure and the construction of an anastomosis to the peroneal artery. An 8- to 10-cm longitudinal skin incision is made over the lateral aspect of the fibula and centered over the segment to be exposed (Fig. 3.86). If the proximal part of the peroneal artery is to be exposed, care should be taken to avoid injury to the common peroneal nerve as it crosses the neck of the fibula.

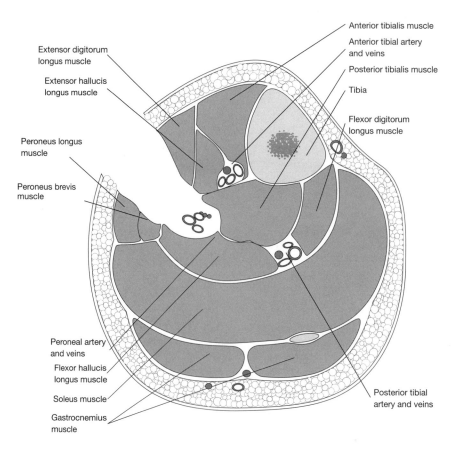

Figure 3.85. Lateral approach to the peroneal artery, cross-section view.

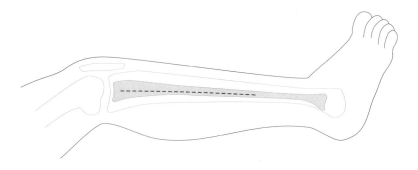

Figure 3.86. A 10- to 12-cm incision is made over the fibula.

The incision is deepened until the fibula is exposed (Fig. 3.87). The periosteum is elevated circumferentially and the fibula is cleared of all tissue attachments. A right-angle clamp is passed underneath the fibula to engage one end of a Gigli saw. The Gigli saw is used to transect the fibula at the proximal and distal end of the incision. (Fig. 3.88). It is important to completely clear the tissues from the fibula before passing the right-angle clamp below it to avoid injury to the underlying peroneal vessels. The exposed segment of fibula is carefully excised. The periosteum of the resected fibula is then incised exposing the peroneal artery and venae comitantes that lie just beneath it (Fig. 3.89). This approach provides an excellent exposure of the peroneal artery down to its terminal branches, especially in redo procedures.

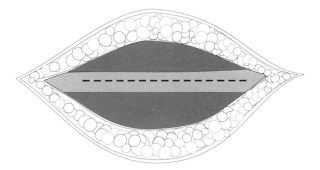

Figure 3.87. The incision is deepened until the periosteum is exposed.

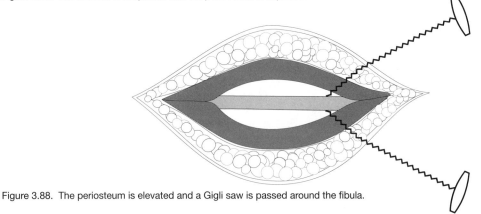

Figure 3.88. The periosteum is elevated and a Gigli saw is passed around the fibula.

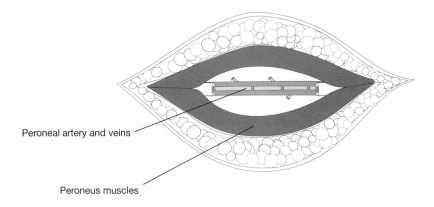

Peroneal artery and veins

Peroneus muscles

Figure 3.89. An 8-cm segment of fibula is resected exposing the peroneal vessels underneath the periosteum.

Exposure of the Anterior Tibial Artery

The anterior tibial artery is usually exposed through a lateral approach (Fig. 3.90). However, the proximal few centimeters of the anterior tibial artery can be exposed from a medial approach by exposing the distal popliteal artery and incising the interosseus membrane. (9) To assist in the exposure of the anterior tibial artery through a medial approach, digital pressure is applied on the anterolateral compartment, displacing the anterior tibial artery medially. Nevertheless, the anterior tibial artery will remain in a deep location, making an anastomosis from this medial approach rather challenging.

Exposure of the Anterior Tibial Artery

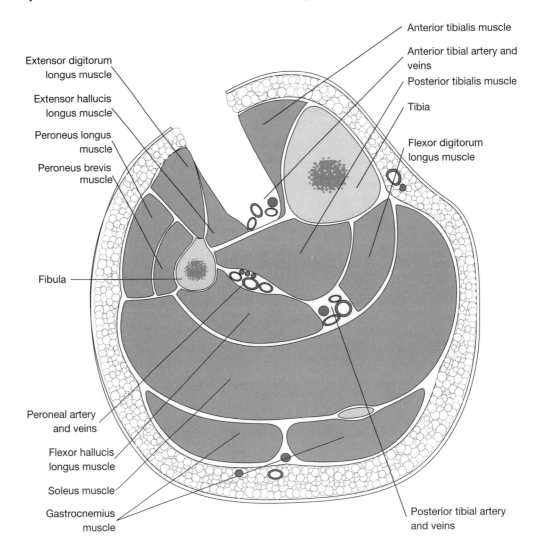

Figure 3.90. Exposure of the anterior tibial artery, cross-section view.

The lateral approach to the anterior tibial artery is achieved through a longitudinal incision performed parallel to the tibia (Fig. 3.91). The incision starts 2 cm inferior to the tibia and extends for 10–12 cm. The skin incision is deepened through the subcutaneous tissue until the fascia is identified (Fig. 3.92). The fascia is incised longitudinally. The first muscle attached to the tibia is the tibialis anterior muscle. The next muscle identified inferior to the tibialis anterior muscle is the extensor hallucis muscle. The longitudinal cleft between these two muscles is entered. Gentle blunt dissection is carried out toward the interosseus membrane (Fig. 3.93). The anterior tibial artery and veins and peroneal nerve will be seen at the deep aspect of the incision (Fig. 3.94). The exposure of the vessels is enhanced by placing the self-retaining retractors deeper in the wound (Fig. 3.95). Due to the size of the musculature of the leg proximally, the proximal portion of the anterior tibial artery is usually more difficult to expose than the distal anterior tibial artery as it lies in a deeper location.

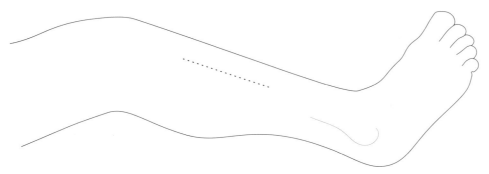

Figure 3.91. A 10- to 12-cm incision is performed 2 cm inferior and parallel to the tibia.

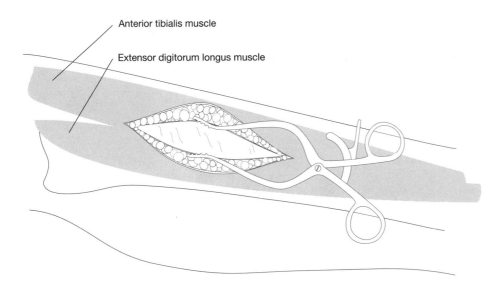

Anterior tibialis muscle

Extensor digitorum longus muscle

Figure 3.92. The incision is deepened through the subcutaneous tissue until the fascia is identified.

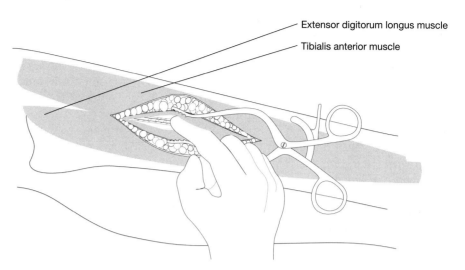

Extensor digitorum longus muscle
Tibialis anterior muscle

Figure 3.93. Using a sweeping motion, the anterior tibialis is separated from the extensor muscles.

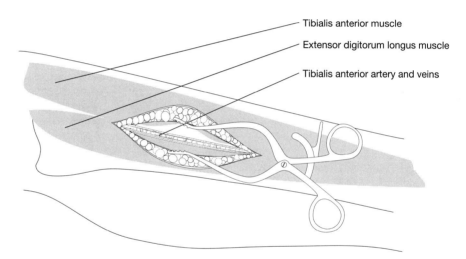

Tibialis anterior muscle
Extensor digitorum longus muscle
Tibialis anterior artery and veins

Figure 3.94. The anterior tibial artery and veins are identified.

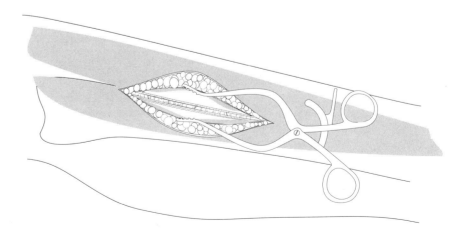

Figure 3.95. The self-retaining retractor is placed in a deeper position to improve the exposure.

Lateral Exposure of the Anterior Tibial Artery in the Lower Leg
In the lower leg, the anterior tibial artery lies between the tendinous portions of
the extensor muscles. A 10- to 12-cm incision is made parallel to the tibia and 2 cm
inferior and lateral to it. The first tendon close to the tibia is the tendon of the
tibialis anterior muscle. On the posterior aspect, the tendon of the extensor hallucis longus muscle is noted. As the anterior tibial artery progresses to become the
dorsalis pedis, it will be seen continuing into the foot and passing underneath
the tendon of the extensor hallucis longus muscle, which crosses from lateral to
medial to attach on the greater toe. More distally, just above the ankle, the anterior tibial artery is exposed by a short longitudinal incision with retraction of the
extensor digitorum longus muscle laterally and the extensor hallucis longus muscle medially (Fig. 3.96). The dorsalis pedis artery is best exposed beyond the
flexor retinaculum in the first metatarsal space (Fig. 3.97). Mapping the dorsalis
pedis artery preoperatively with duplex ultrasonography can guide the placement of the skin incision.

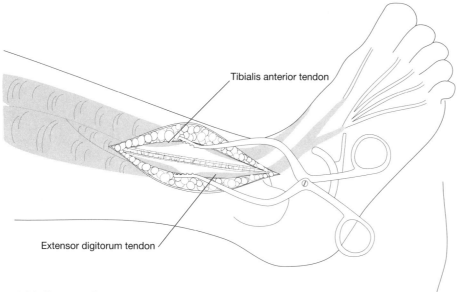

Figure 3.96. Exposure of the anterior tibial artery at the ankle.

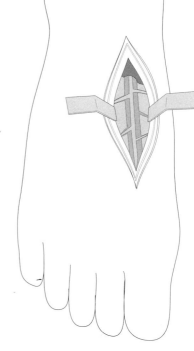

Figure 3.97. Exposure of the dorsalis pedis artery.

VEINS OF THE UPPER AND LOWER EXTREMITIES

ANATOMY OF THE VEINS OF THE UPPER EXTREMITY

The Cephalic Vein

The cephalic vein starts from the volar aspect of the wrist and ascends along the radial aspect of the forearm. In the forearm, the cephalic vein is also referred to as the radial vein. At the level of the elbow, it receives the median cephalic vein and then continues in the upper arm along the lateral border of the biceps brachii muscle (Fig. 3.98). At the level of the shoulder, it continues in the groove between the deltoid and pectoralis major muscles and then starts to move into a deeper plane to join the axillary vein below the clavicle.

The Basilic Vein

The basilic vein starts on the ulnar aspect of the wrist. It ascends along the ulnar aspect of the forearm to join the anterior ulnar and the median antecubital veins at the level of the elbow joint (Fig. 3.98). The basilic vein then ascends along the inner border of the biceps brachii muscle and penetrates the deep fascia at the middle of the arm to run along the brachial artery. It continues onward to become the axillary vein.

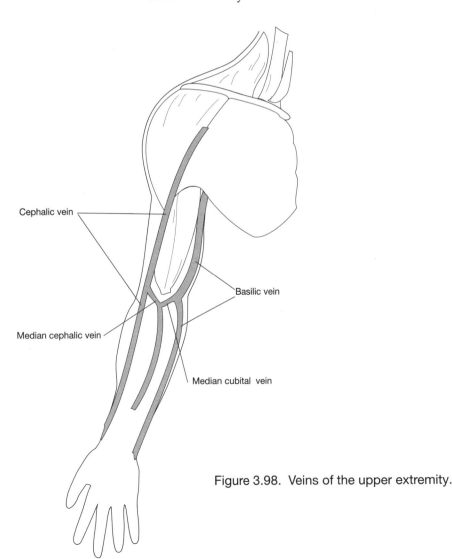

Figure 3.98. Veins of the upper extremity.

EXPOSURE OF THE VEINS OF THE UPPER EXTREMITY

Exposure of the Cephalic Vein

In the upper arm, the cephalic vein can be exposed by starting an incision along the outer border of the biceps femoris muscle. The skin incision is deepened through the subcutaneous tissues and fat. The vein usually lies immediately underneath the skin. The vein can be traced upward until it disappears in the deltopectoral groove. In the forearm the cephalic vein is exposed by a skin incision placed directly over the vein. A tourniquet applied above the elbow joint can help identify the location of the vein before incising the skin.

Exposure of the Basilic Vein

The basilic vein can be accessed by exposing the median antecubital vein at the elbow and then tracing it upward. Alternatively, a longitudinal incision along the medial border of the biceps brachii muscle is performed. The incision is deepened through the subcutaneous tissues and superficial fascia exposing the basilic vein (see Fig. 3.13).

ANATOMY OF THE VEINS OF THE LOWER EXTREMITY

The Greater Saphenous Vein

The greater saphenous vein starts on the medial side of the arch of the dorsum of the foot. It ascends anterior to the tip of the medial malleolus and then over the subcutaneous surface of the lower end of the tibia. The greater saphenous vein continues up to the knee where it moves posterior to the back part of the internal condyle of the femur and then follows the course of the sartorius muscle up to the inguinal region (Fig. 3.99). Below the knee, the greater saphenous vein is accompanied by the great saphenous nerve and lies in a superficial subcutaneous plane. Above the knee, it gradually moves into a deeper subcutaneous plane and penetrates the fascia lata in the upper thigh through the fossa ovale to join the common femoral vein. Frequently a duplicate system can be found in the thigh (35%) or in the leg. The length of the greater saphenous vein in an adult man is estimated to be 60 cm. The vein contains approximately 8–12 valves, with more valves present in the below knee segment.

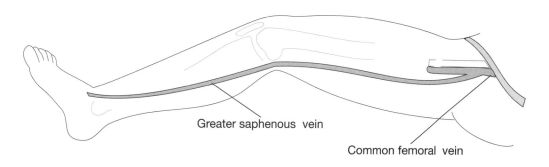

Figure 3.99. Anatomy of the greater saphenous vein.

The Lesser Saphenous Vein

The lesser saphenous vein starts posterior to the lateral malleolus along the lateral border of the Achilles tendon. It crosses above the Achilles tendon and reaches the midline of the posterior aspect of the leg. The lesser saphenous vein continues upward in the subcutaneous tissues and usually penetrates the muscular fascia at the level where the tendon of the gastrocnemius muscle starts. The vein runs just below the fascia to join the popliteal vein between the heads of the gastrocnemius muscle (Fig. 3.100). The lesser saphenous vein is accompanied by the lesser saphenous nerve and measures approximately 30 cm.

The Superficial Femoral Vein

The superficial femoral vein is the continuation of the popliteal vein at the level of the adductor magnus tendon (Fig. 3.100). It ascends in the thigh along the superficial femoral artery receiving several muscular branches. In the inguinal region, it receives the profunda femoris and then the greater saphenous veins and becomes the common femoral vein. In the lower thigh, the superficial femoral vein lies anteromedial to the superficial femoral artery and then moves into a more posterior location running posterior to the artery in the mid- and upper thigh. As it becomes the common femoral vein, it lies medial to the common femoral artery on the same plane.

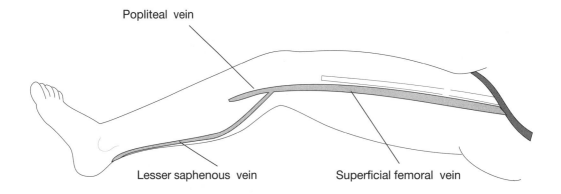

Figure 3.100. Anatomy of the lesser saphenous and superficial femoral-popliteal veins.

Exposure of the Greater Saphenous Vein
Preoperative evaluation of the greater saphenous vein with duplex ultrasonography allows mapping the location of the greater saphenous vein. The skin incision can be carried over the marked skin. Alternatively, the following anatomical landmarks can be used. At the ankle level, a longitudinal incision is placed 1 cm anterior and superior to the medial malleolus. The vein is usually identified directly beneath the skin. At the inguinal region, the incision is started 1.5 cm medial to the femoral pulse and extends at a 30° angle to the vertical axis of the lower extremity. If the femoral pulse is not palpable, the incision is started 1.5 cm medial to a point midway between the pubic tubercle and the anterior superior iliac spine. The incision is deepened through the subcutaneous tissues and Scarpa's fascia to expose the vein (Fig. 3.101). Currently, various methods are available to allow for endoscopic harvesting of the greater saphenous vein through a single small inguinal incision and or additional 1- to 2-cm incisions placed at various locations above or below the knee.

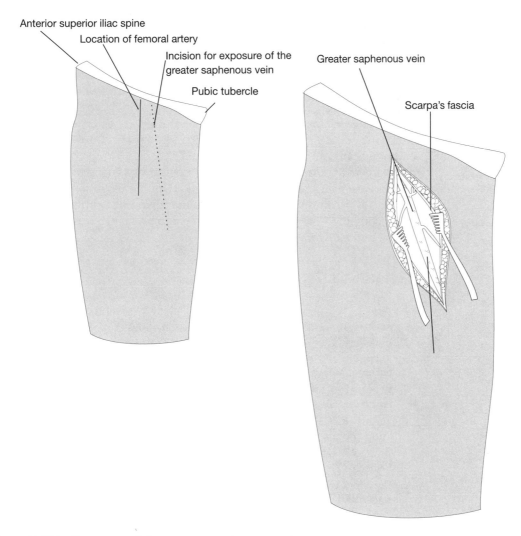

Figure 3.101. Exposure of the greater saphenous vein.

Exposure of the Lesser Saphenous Vein

It is preferable to assess and mark the lesser saphenous vein preoperatively with duplex ultrasonography. If vein mapping is not available, a longitudinal skin incision is started in the middle of the posterior aspect of the calf. The incision is deepened through the subcutaneous tissue until the fascia is identified. The fascia is incised, exposing the saphenous vein directly underneath it. The lesser saphenous vein can be harvested with the patient lying prone or supine. The prone position facilitates the exposure; however, this will usually require turning the patient back to a supine position and reprepping and draping. When the patient is lying supine, external rotation of the leg and the gastrocnemius muscle allows access to the lesser saphenous vein. However, the junction to the popliteal vein remains challenging to expose from this approach. The lesser saphenous vein can also be approached through a medial skin incision, but this requires the creation of large skin flaps and allows access to only a short segment of the vein.

Exposure of the Superficial Femoral Vein

The exposure of the superficial femoral vein is similar to that of the superficial femoral artery. A longitudinal skin incision is performed along the outer border of the sartorius muscle. The incision is deepened through the subcutaneous tissues and fat, exposing the muscular fascia. The muscular fascia is incised and the entire sartorius muscle is mobilized and retracted inferiorly and medially, preserving its segmental blood supply. This procedure will expose the vascular pedicle in the upper thigh and the adductor canal in the lower thigh.

The superficial femoral vein is separated from the artery in the upper thigh and encircled with a silastic vessel loop and then traced toward the knee. The tendinous portion of the adductor canal is incised to expose the superficial femoral vein at that level. When harvesting the superficial femoral vein, multiple large branches are usually identified. Double or suture ligation of these branches is recommended. At the inguinal region, it is important to preserve the junction with the profunda femoris vein to prevent excessive venous hypertension in the lower extremity. (36)

REFERENCES

1. Ascer E, Veith F, Gupta S: Bypasses to plantar arteries and other tibial branches: An extended approach to limb salvage. J Vasc Surg 1985;8:434.
2. Berguer R, Kieffer E. The aortic arch and its branches: Anatomy and blood flow. In Berguer R, Kieffer E (ed): Surgery of the Arteries to the Head. New York: Springer-Verlag, 1992;5–31.
3. Berguer R, Kieffer E. Special surgical problems. In Berguer R, Kieffer E (ed): Surgery of the Arteries to the Head. New York: Springer-Verlag, 1992;167–205.
4 Berguer R, Kieffer E. Repair of the supraaortic trunks. In Berguer R, Kieffer E (ed): Surgery of the Arteries to the Head. New York: Springer-Verlag, 1992;84–108.
5 Bridges R, Gewertz BL. Lateral incision for exposure of femoral vessels. Surg Gynecol Obstet 1980;150:733.
6. Crawford ES, Morris GC, Myhre HO, Roehm JO. Celiac axis, superior mesenteric artery, and inferior mesenteric artery occlusion: surgical considerations. Surgery (St. Louis) 1977;82:856–866.
7. Danese CA, Singer A. Lateral approach to the trifurcation popliteal artery. Surgery (St. Louis) 1968;63:588–590.
8. Dardik H, Dardik I, Veith FJ. Exposure of the tibioperoneal arteries by a single lateral approach. Surgery (St. Louis) 1974;75:377–382.
9. Dardik H, Elias S, Miller N, et al. Medial approach to the anterior tibial artery. J Vasc Surg 1985;2:743.

10. Dardik H, Ibrahim IM, Dardik II. The role of the peroneal artery for limb salvage. Ann Surg 1979;189:189–198.

11. Dean RH, Hansen KJ. Renal revascularization: how to make a difficult operation easier. In: Veith FJ (ed): Current Critical Problems in Vascular Surgery. St. Louis: Quality Medical, 1989:306–308.

12. Dear RH, Foster JH. Surgery of the renal arteries. In: Haimovici H (ed): Vascular Surgery: Principles and Techniques. Norwalk, CT: Appleton-Century-Crofts, 1984:827–840.

13. DeBakey ME, Crawford ES, Garrett HE, et al. Surgical considerations in the treatment of aneurysms of the thoracic and thoracoabdominal aorta. Ann Surg 1965;162:650–662.

14. Demetriades D, Chahwan S, Gomez H, et al: Penetrating injuries to the subclavian and axillary vessels. J Am Coll Surg 1999;188:290–295.

15 DePalma RG. Sexual function and vascular surgery. In: Wilson SE, Veith FJ, Hobson RW, William RA (eds): Vascular Surgery: Principles and Practice. New York: McGraw-Hill, 1987:942–951.

16 Dossa C, Shepard AD, Wolford DG, Reddy DJ, Ernst CB: Distal internal carotid exposure: A simplified technique for temporary mandibular subluxation. J Vasc Surg 1990;12:319.

17. Effeney DJ, Stoney RJ. Extracranial vascular disease. In: Effeney DT, Stoney RJ (eds): Wylie's Atlas of Vascular Surgery. Philadelphia: Lippincott, 1992:18–57.

18. Fisher DF Jr, Fry WJ. Collateral mesenteric circulation. Surg Gynecol Obstet 1987;164:487–492.

19. Fry WJ. Occlusive arterial disease: upper aortic branches. In: Nora PF (ed): Operative Surgery: Principles and Techniques. Philadelphia: Lea & Febiger, 1980:763–777.

20. Graham JW, Hanel KC. Vein grafts to the peroneal artery. Surgery 1981;89:254–268.

21. Green RM, Ricotta JJ, Ouriel K, DeWeese JA. Results of supraceliac aortic clamping in the difficult elective resection of infrarenal abdominal aortic aneurysm. J Vasc Surg 1989;9:125–134.

22. Henry AK. Extensile Exposure, 2nd Ed. New York: Churchill Livingstone, 1945:114–63.

23. Hertzer N, Feldman B, Beven E, et al. A prospective study of the incidence of injury to the cranial nerves during carotid endarterectomy. Surg Gynecol Obstet 1980;151:781.

24. Hoballah JJ, Chalmers RT, Sharp WJ, et al. Lateral approach to the popliteal and crural vessels for limb salvage. Cardiovasc Surg 1996;4:165–168.

25. Imparato AM, Kim GE, Chu DS. Surgical exposure for reconstruction of the proximal part of the tibial artery. Surg Gynecol Obstet 1973;136:453–455.

26. Mattox KL. Approaches to trauma involving the major vessels of the thorax. Surg Clin North Am 1989;69:77–91.

27. Mattox KL. Thoracic great vessel injury. Surg Clin North Am 1988;68:693–703.

28. Minken SL, May AG. Use of the peroneal artery for revascularization of the lower extremity. Arch Surg 1969;99:594–597.

29. Mock CN, Lilly MP, McRae RG, Carney WI Jr. Selection of the approach to the distal internal carotid artery from the second cervical vertebra to the base of the skull. J Vasc Surg 1991;13:846.

30. Naraysingh V, Karmody AM, Leather RP, Corson JD. Lateral approach to the profunda femoris artery. Am J Surg 1984;147:813–814.

31. Nunez AA, Veith FJ, Collier P, Ascer E, Flores SW, Gupta SK. Direct approaches to the distal portions of the deep femoral artery for limb salvage. J Vasc Surg 1988;8:576–581.

32. Padberg FT Jr., Lateral approach to the popliteal artery. Ann Vasc Surg 1998;2:397–401.

33. Rastad J, Almgren B, Bowald S, et al. Renal complications of left renal vein ligation in abdominal aortic surgery. J Cardiovasc Surg 1984;25:432–436.

34. Rob C. Extraperitoneal approach to the abdominal aorta. Surgery 1963;53:87–89.

35. Robbs JV, Reddy E. Management options for penetrating injuries to the great veins of the neck and superior mediastinum. Surg Gynecol Obstet 1987;165:323–326.

36. Schulman ML, Badhey MR, Yatco R. Superficial femoral-popliteal veins and reversed veins as primary femoropopliteal bypass grafts: A randomized comparative study. J Vasc. Surg 1987;6:1–10.

37. Shepard A, Scott G, Mackey W, et al: Retroperitoneal approach to high-risk abdominal aortic aneurysms. Arch Surg 1986;121:444.

38. Sicard GA, Freeman MB, VanderWoude JC, Anderson CB. Comparison between the transabdominal and retroperitoneal approach for reconstruction of the infrarenal abdominal aorta. J Vasc Surg 1987;5:19–27.

39. Stanley JC, Messina LM, Wakefield TW, Zelenock GB. Renal artery reconstruction. In: Bergan JJ, Yao JST (eds): Techniques in Arterial Surgery. Philadelphia: Saunders, 1990:247–263.

40. Stoney R, Wylie E: Surgical management of arterial lesions of the thoracolumbar aorta. Am J Surg 126:157, 1973.

41. Stoney RJ, Schneider PA. Technical aspects of visceral artery revascularization. In: Bergan JJ, Yao JST (eds): Techniques in Arterial Surgery. Philadelphia: W.B. Saunders, 1990:271–283.

42. Usatoff V, Grigg M. Letter to the Editor: A lateral approach to the below-knee popliteal artery without resection of the fibula. J Vasc Surg 1997;26:168–170.

43. Veith FJ, Ascer E, Gupta SK, Wengerter KR. Lateral approach to the popliteal artery. J Vasc Surg 1987;6:119–123.

44. Veith FJ, Gupta S, Daly V. Technique for occluding the supraceliac aorta through the abdomen. Surg Gynecol Obstet 1980;151:426–428.

45. Wylie EJ, Stoney RJ, Erenfeld WK. Aortic aneurysms. In: Wylie EJ, Stoney RJ, Erenfeld WK (eds): Manual of Vascular Surgery. New York: Springer-Verlag, 1980:159–205.

46. Wind G, Valentine RJ. Vessels of the leg. In Wind G, Valentine RJ (eds): Anatomic Exposures in Vascular Surgery. Maryland, Williams and Wilkins, 1991;411–442.

47. Yao JST, Bergan JJ, Pearce WH, Flinn WR. Operative procedures in visceral ischemia. In: Bergan JJ, Yao JST (eds): Techniques in Arterial Surgery. Philadelphia: Saunders, 1990:284–293.

4

Basic Steps in Vascular Reconstructions

Several basic steps are usually carried out during the performance of a vascular reconstruction:

Blood vessel exposure
Blood vessel dissection
Tunneling
Anticoagulation
Blood vessel control
Creation of a blood vessel incision
Preparation of a patch or a bypass
Construction of the suture line
Securing hemostasis
Evaluating the vascular reconstruction

BLOOD VESSEL EXPOSURE

When exposing a blood vessel, the approach that provides a simple and direct access to the vessel of interest is usually the most desirable. In general, the skin incision is placed along the longitudinal axis of the vessel to be exposed. This will facilitate proximal and distal extension of the exposure. Anatomical landmarks or palpation of the pulse are used to select the site of the skin incision. In patients with scarring due to previous procedures (redo operations), or in the presence of infection, an alternate approach may be possible. This may provide access to the blood vessels through nonscarred planes. The common and alternate arterial exposures are listed in Table 1. The anatomy and various exposures of these vessels are reviewed in Chapter 3.

BLOOD VESSEL DISSECTION

Blood vessels are usually dissected sharply using a blunt-tipped scissors. A 15 blade can also be used for the dissection and is especially valuable when dealing with scarred tissues in redo procedures. An inadvertent vascular incision caused by a knife may be easier to repair than a tear produced by a scissors. As the vessel is being exposed, self-retaining retractors are usually placed at progressively deeper levels, applying traction on the tissues to be divided. Retractors should be carefully applied to avoid injury to neighboring vessels or nerves. Once the vessel is adequately exposed, the adventitia on its anterior surface is carefully grasped with a Debakey forceps. While applying gentle traction on the adventitia and countertraction on the surrounding tissues, sharp dissection along the sidewall of the vessel will identify an avascular plane between the vessel and its surrounding

107

Table 1 Vessel anatomy and exposure

Artery	Common exposure	Alternate
Proximal common carotid	Median sternotomy	
Distal common carotid and carotid bifurcation	Anterior border of sternocleidomastoid	Transverse neck
Vertebral	Supraclavicular incision	Anterior neck
Subclavian		
Origin Rt	Median sternotomy	
Origin Lt	Anterior thoracotomy (3rd intercostal space)	Trapdoor
First part	Supraclavicular incision	
Second part	Supraclavicular incision	
Third part	Supraclavicular incision	
Axillary	Infraclavicular incision	Axillary
Brachial	Medial incision	
Suprarenal aorta	Transabdominal Medial visceral rotation (MVR)	Retroperitoneal Thoracoabdominal, (TA)
Celiac	Transabdominal, MVR	Retroperitoneal, (TA)
Superior mesenteric	Transabdominal, MVR	Retroperitoneal, (TA)
Infrarenal aorta	Transabdominal	Retroperitoneal
Common and external iliac	Transabdominal	Retroperitoneal
Internal iliac	Transabdominal	Retroperitoneal
Common femoral	Medial incision	Lateral incision
Profunda	Medial incision	Lateral to sartorius
Superficial femoral	Medial incision	Lateral to sartorius
Popliteal	Medial incision	Lateral incision, Posterior approach
Popliteal, below knee	Medial incision	Lateral incision with resection of fibula
Peroneal	Medial incision	Lateral incision with resection of fibula
Posterior tibial	Medial incision	Lateral incision with resection of fibula
Anterior tibial	Lateral approach	Medial approach

tissues. This plane is developed on each side of the vessel and followed posteriorly to achieve circumferential dissection of the vessel. Although circumferential dissection may be appealing, it is not always necessary. For example, when exposing the infrarenal aorta during an aortic reconstruction, dissection on each side of the aorta down to the spine without circumferential dissection may be sufficient for achieving vascular control. Anterior exposure of the tibial vessels may be all that is needed when a pneumatic external tourniquet or an internal vessel occluder is used for vascular control. Similarly, circumferential dissection is not required when a partially occluding clamp is used to achieve vascular control.

Blood vessels can be traced proximally and distally, anticipating their cylindrical shape and adjacent vascular structures. Throughout the dissection, the vessels should be handled gently; only the adventitia should be grasped with the forceps. Grasping the full thickness of the vessel wall can cause intimal damage. Silastic vessel loops may be passed around a vessel and used for vessel retraction. However, only gentle traction on the vessel loop should be used to avoid damage to the vessel wall. The sites of major vascular branches can be anticipated from knowledge of surgical anatomy. Dividing arterial branches should be avoided as they may represent important collateral channels.

TUNNELING

Bypasses can be tunneled along the vessel being bypassed (anatomically) or extraanatomically. When the tunnel is of a short distance, it can be created with the Metzenbaum scissors alone or in conjunction with blunt finger dissection. Tunneling devices can also be used to pass the graft from one location to another and are essential when the tunnel is of a long distance. Two different types of tunneling devices exist. In one type, the tunneling device is made of an outer tube and an inner obturator. Once the tunnel is created, the obturator is removed and a passer is used to grab the graft and pass it through the outer part of the tunneling device. In the other type, the tunneling device is made of one part with interchangeable heads of different dimensions. After creating the tunnel with the tunneling device, the graft is tied to the tunneler. By withdrawing the tunneler, the graft is pulled into the desired location.

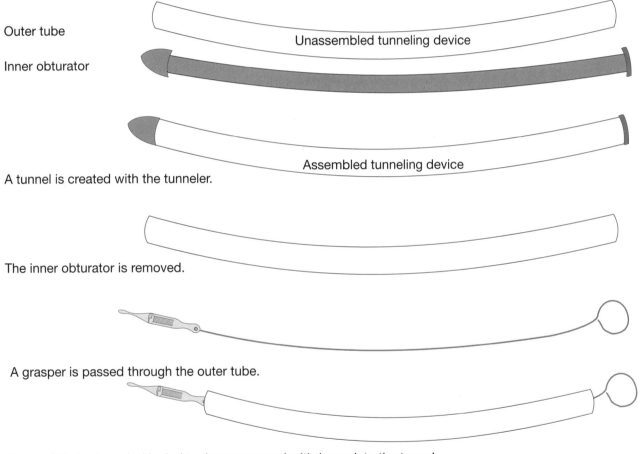

Outer tube

Inner obturator

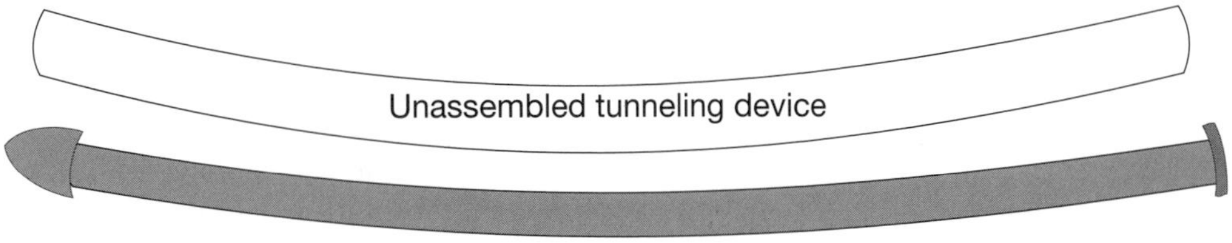
Unassembled tunneling device

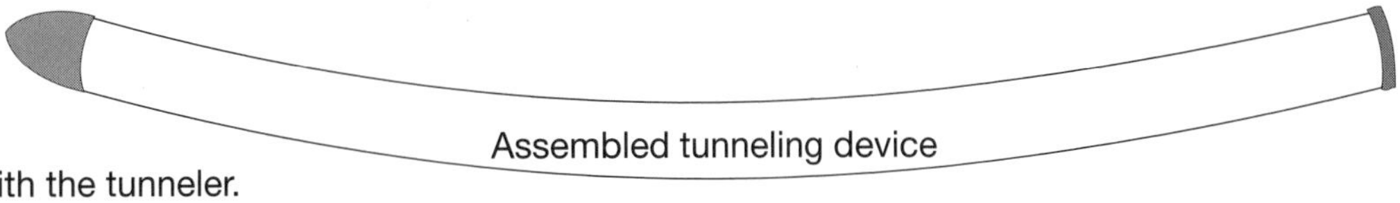
Assembled tunneling device

A tunnel is created with the tunneler.

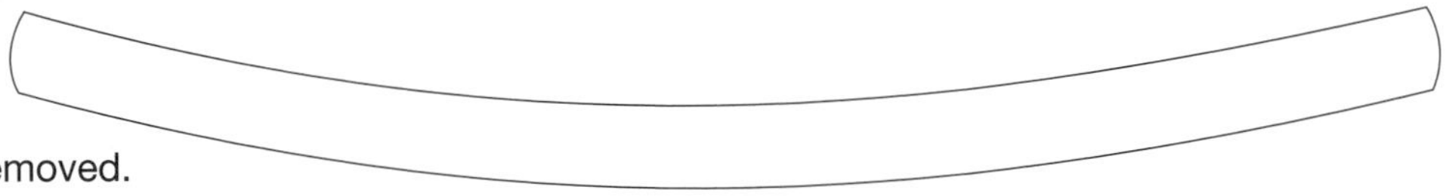

The inner obturator is removed.

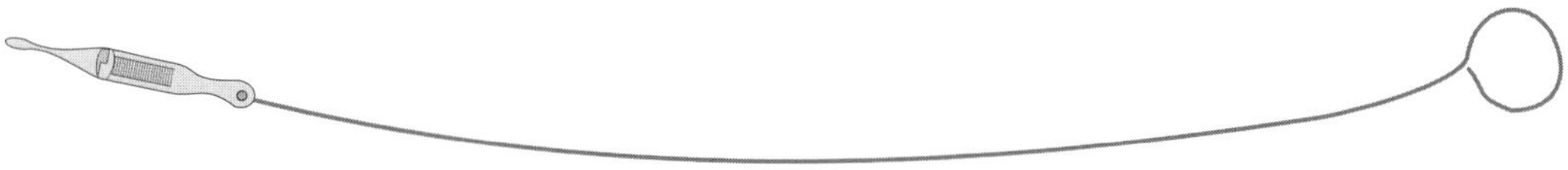

A grasper is passed through the outer tube.

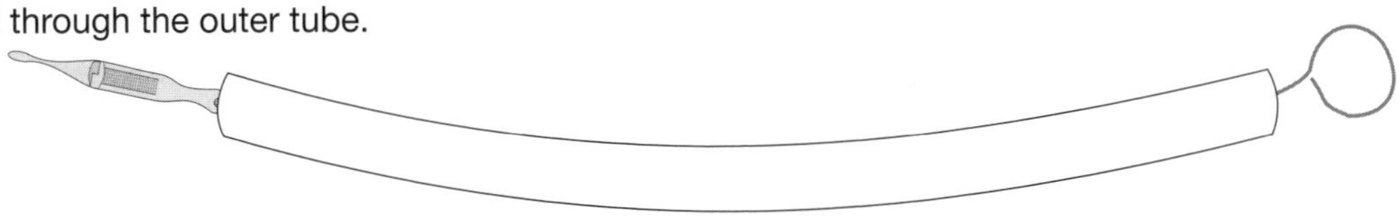

The graft to be tunneled is tied to the passer and withdrawn into the tunnel.

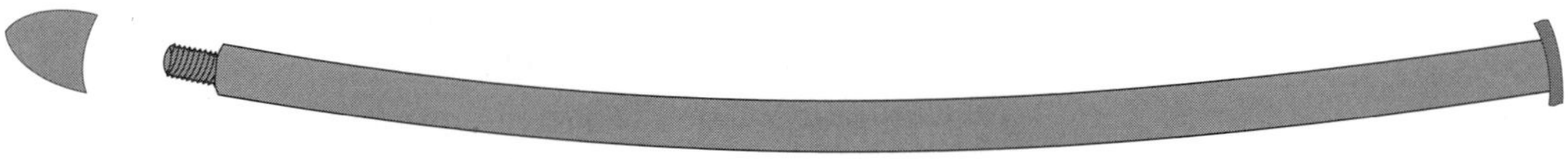

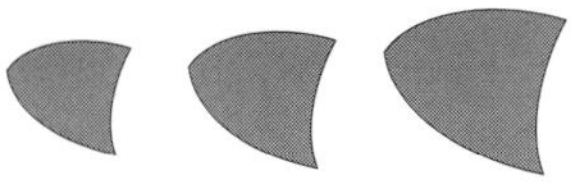

Alternatively a tunneler with interchangeable heads of different sizes can be used.

Tunneling

Tunneling is preferably done before systemic anticoagulation with heparin. The graft should be carefully passed through the tunnel to avoid any twists. In addition, especially when using an autogenous conduit, the graft should be checked very carefully for hemostasis before tunneling to avoid bleeding in the tunnel. The anatomical location of various tunnels created in commonly performed vascular procedures are listed below.

Axillofemoral bypass: In the chest, the tunnel is created to pass anterior to the rib cage and posterior to the pectoralis major muscle. The graft is usually tunneled along the midaxillary line. The graft continues subcutaneously and crosses over the inguinal ligament medial to the anterior superior iliac spine. Adequate length should be available to avoid excessive tension on the proximal anastomosis to the axillary artery. Otherwise, a Y-deformity or very rarely disruption of the axillary anastomosis could occur. A counterincision may be required especially in large individuals. The counterincision is usually made halfway between the inguinal and the infraclavicular incision.

Femorofemoral bypass: The tunnel in a femorofemoral bypass is subcutaneous. It can be started with the Metzenbaum scissors and further developed by blunt finger dissection or with the use of a C-shaped tunneler. A gentle C-curve is important to avoid kinking of the femorofemoral graft at the level of the femoral anastomosis. It is also important to tunnel just anterior to the fascia of the external oblique muscle and to avoid tunneling in a very superficial plane.

Aortobifemoral bypass: Tunneling for the limbs of the aortobifemoral bypass is usually accomplished with blunt finger dissection. One finger is introduced below the inguinal ligament over the external iliac artery. Another finger is introduced over the common iliac artery and advanced toward the inguinal ligament until both fingers meet. Care is taken to keep the tunnel posterior to the ureter. Otherwise, fibrosis and stricture of the ureter can develop in the future where the ureter is sandwiched between the iliac arteries and the graft limb. An aortic DeBakey clamp can be introduced in the tunnel from the inguinal region toward the aorta to grasp and pull the graft limb through the tunnel.

Infrainguinal bypass: Except for an in situ bypass, infrainguinal grafts usually need to be tunneled. The tunnel can be subcutaneous, subfascial, or subsartorial. An advantage of a subcutaneous tunnel is the easy access to the graft should a revision become necessary. If skin flaps were developed during the dissection or vein harvesting, placing the bypass in a deeper subfascial or subsartorial location may be preferred, especially when the wound appears to be at increased risk for infection or nonhealing. The adductor canal is not usually used as a tunnel. Prosthetic grafts are infrequently placed subcutaneously.

Above-knee femoropopliteal bypass: A prosthetic graft is usually placed in a subsartorial or subfascial tunnel. An autogenous vein bypass is placed in a subcutaneous, subfascial, or subsartorial tunnel.

Below-knee femoropopliteal bypass: A prosthetic graft is usually tunneled subsartorially until the above-knee location. From the suprageniculate to the infrageniculate popliteal artery, tunneling behind the knee joint is usually achieved by blunt finger dissection. It is important to make sure that the tunnel is created between the heads of the gastrocnemius muscle, otherwise an iatrogenic entrapment syndrome can develop. A similar tunnel can be used with an autogenous vein bypass. Alternatively, a subcutaneous or subfascial tunnel can be used.

The bypass to the above-knee popliteal artery is tunneled subsartorially. (A)

The bypass to the below-knee popliteal artery is tunneled subsartorially to the above-knee level and then tunneled anatomically behind the knee between the heads of the gastrocnemius muscle.(B)

The bypass to the posterior tibial artery is tunneled subsartorially and then subfascially or subcutaneously below the knee.(C)

The bypass to the anterior tibial artery is tunneled subsartorially above the knee and then through the interosseus membrane. (D)

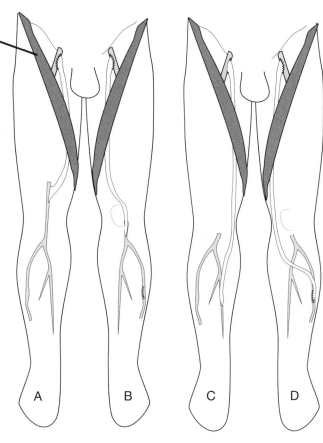

Vein bypasses to the infrapopliteal arteries can also be tunneled subfascially or subcutaneously. (E)

Subcutaneous vein passes to the anterior tibial artery can cross in the leg from medial to lateral anterior to the tibia. (F)

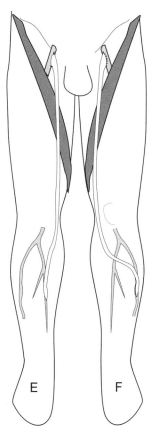

Tunneling

Infrapopliteal bypass: Tunneling to the infrapopliteal level is performed following the same principles used for tunneling a below-knee femoropopliteal bypass. From the infrapopliteal level, autogenous bypasses to the posterior tibial or peroneal artery are usually subcutaneous or subfascial while prosthetic bypasses to the same vessels are placed subfascially. Several options are available for tunneling from the infrapopliteal level to the anterior tibial artery. The bypass can be tunneled from medial to lateral through the interosseus membrane or anterior to the tibia in a subcutaneous tunnel. Bypasses to the anterior tibial artery can also be tunneled on the lateral aspect of the lower extremity. In this situation, the bypass crosses from medial to lateral in the thigh and then continues toward the leg in a lateral subcutaneous tunnel. At the knee level, the bypass is usually tunneled between the lateral tibial condyle and the head of the fibula. This tunneling method can also be used for bypasses to other infrapopliteal vessels exposed through a lateral approach. When using a lateral approach, grafts originating from the proximal common femoral artery are usually tunneled above the sartorius muscle. Grafts originating from the superficial or deep femoral arteries are best tunneled deep to the sartorius muscle to avoid an acute angulation of the proximal conduit.

Subcutaneous bypasses to the anterior tibial artery can also cross from medial to lateral in the thigh and then continue in a lateral tunnel between the head of the fibula and the lateral tibial condyle.

A gentle S-shaped curvature is recommended in the thigh as shown in the right leg (G).

Another route of tunneling is shown in the left leg. This can provide a shorter bypass and is ideal for grafts originating from the common femoral artery (H).

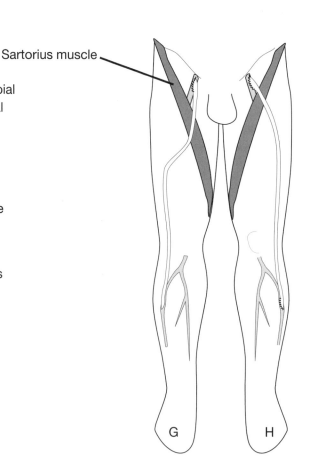

Sartorius muscle

Grafts originating from the superficial femoral or deep femoral arteries are best tunneled deep to the sartorius muscle to avoid acute angulation of the graft in its proximal segment.

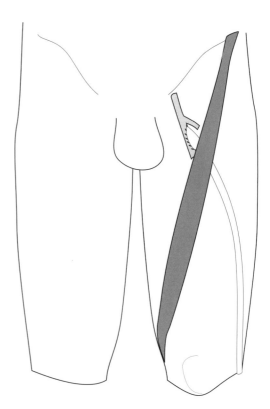

Tunneling is also performed during the creation of arteriovenous fistulae for hemodialysis. Arteriovenous fistulae can be classified into autogenous (primary) or secondary fistulae. In the primary, the vein is anastomosed directly to the artery. In the secondary fistulae, a prosthetic graft is used to connect the artery to the vein. The primary fistulae are constructed using the cephalic or basilic veins. Arteriovenous fistulae to the cephalic vein are constructed at the wrist (radiocephalic) or at the elbow (brachiocephalic) depending on the quality of the cephalic vein. If the cephalic vein is unavailable, arteriovenous fistulae to the basilic vein are constructed at the wrist (radiobasilic) or at the elbow (brachiobasilic) depending on the quality of the basilic vein.

Radiocephalic fistulae: The radiocephalic fistula (Cemino) is usually the fistula of choice if the vein is adequate from the wrist up to the deltopectoral groove. Tunneling is not needed for the creation of this fistula as it is usually done through a transverse incision from the level of the cephalic vein to the radial artery. If longitudinal incisions were used to expose the radial artery and the cephalic veins, a subcutaneous skin flap is usually created. The cephalic vein is transected and passed under the skin flap to reach the artery in a gentle curve.
Brachiocephalic fistulae: The brachiocephalic fistula is performed at the elbow by exposing the cephalic vein and brachial artery through a transverse elbow crease incision. The cephalic vein is dissected distally and transected and then sutured to the brachial artery in an end-to-side fashion. This fistula does not require any tunneling.
Radiobasilic fistulae: The primary fistulae created with the basilic vein require tunneling. Below the elbow, the basilic vein lies on the ulnar aspect of the forearm, which places the fistula in an undesirable position for

Tunneling

dialysis. The vein can then be mobilized through a longitudinal incision placed over the course of the vein. The vein is transected at the wrist and then freed all the way up to the elbow. A tunnel is then created from the level of the radial artery to the antecubital fossa. The basilic vein is then passed through the tunnel and is now placed on the palmar aspect of the forearm in an easily accessible location. The tunnel is created subcutaneously to allow easy access to the vein.

Brachiobasilic fistulae: The basilic vein in the upper arm can also be used for dialysis; however, because of its deep location and being adjacent to the artery, puncture of this vein in its anatomical position is challenging and uncomfortable for the patient. To achieve an autogenous primary fistula, the basilic vein can be completely mobilized from the elbow to the axilla. All communicating branches are ligated and divided. The basilic vein is then transected at the elbow and freed completely up to the axilla. A tunnel is then created from the level of the brachial artery and then along the anterior border of the biceps brachii muscle in a subcutaneous plane. This will allow easy access to the fistula for venipuncture.

Prosthetic arteriovenous (AV) fistulae can be placed in the forearm or upper arm. The alternatives in the forearm include a straight or a loop fistula.

Straight forearm arteriovenous grafts: The straight fistula connects the radial artery to the best available vein at the level of the elbow. The tunnel is created subcutaneously. It is important to avoid creating the tunnel in a subdermal plane as this could compromise the overlying skin. It is also important to avoid tunneling the graft too deep or subfascially as this will make puncturing the graft more difficult.

Loop forearm arteriovenous grafts: In the loop forearm fistula, one end of the graft is connected to the brachial artery just distal to the elbow joint. The other one is connected to the best available vein in the antecubital area. During the tunneling of the forearm loop fistula, it is important to avoid an acute angle in the distal part of the forearm as this could result in kinking of the graft and thrombosis of the fistula. A 3-cm skin incision at the level of the distal forearm is performed and and a small pocket is created between the muscular fascia and the subcutaneous tissue. A subcutaneous tunnel is then created on the ulnar side of the forearm from the brachial incision to the distal forearm counterincision. The graft is then passed in the tunnel. Another similar tunnel is then created along the radial aspect of the forearm. The other end of the graft is then pulled through the tunnel. The graft is inspected through the counterincision to ensure the presence of a gentle curve. In general, the forearm loop configuration is more desirable than the straight, because of a lower rate of thrombosis that can be related to the small size of the radial artery at the wrist.

Straight upper arm arteriovenous grafts: In the upper arm, a prosthetic graft can be placed from the brachial artery to the basilic vein. It is important to tunnel this graft in an anterior location to allow it to facilitate venipuncture. The tunnel is created similar to that of the primary basilic fistula along the anterior border of the biceps brachii muscle.

Loop upper arm arteriovenous grafts: Loop upper arm arteriovenous grafts are created by connecting the brachial artery in the upper arm to the basilic vein in the proximal upper arm. This graft is created when the brachial artery at the elbow cannot be used as an inflow source. The tunneling is similar to that performed for the forearm loop arteriovenous grafts. The counterincision is usually 2 cm proximal to the elbow joint.

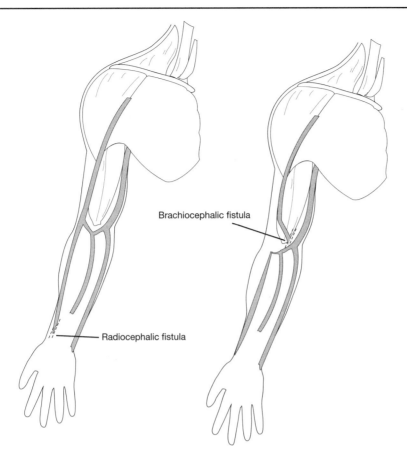

Brachiocephalic fistula

Radiocephalic fistula

Tunneling is not usually necessary for the creation of arteriovenous fistulae to the cephalic vein.

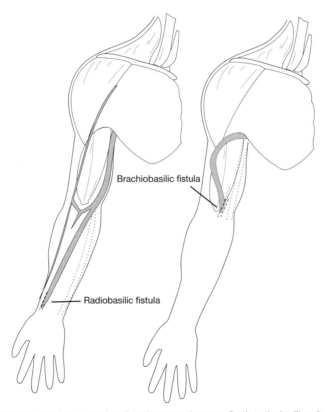

Brachiobasilic fistula

Radiobasilic fistula

Tunneling is necessary for the creation of a primary arteriovenous fistula to the basilic vein to make the vein accessible for venipuncture.

Tunneling

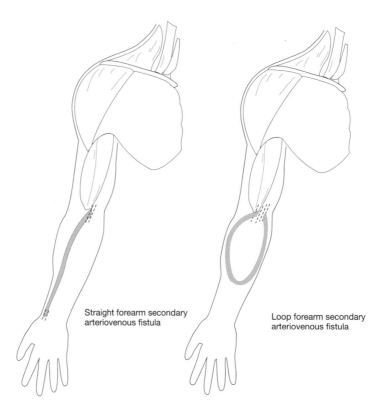

Straight forearm secondary
arteriovenous fistula

Loop forearm secondary
arteriovenous fistula

A gentle smooth curve is necessary when tunneling for a loop forearm fistula.

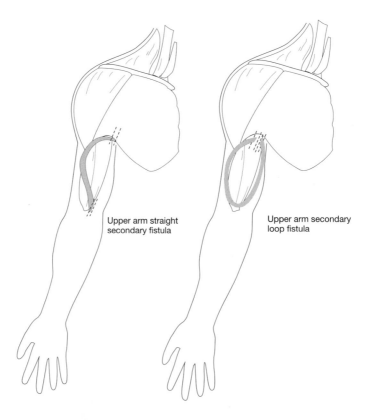

Upper arm straight
secondary fistula

Upper arm secondary
loop fistula

A gentle curve is necessary when creating a straight or loop upper arm fistula.

ANTICOAGULATION

Before occluding the blood vessels to perform a vascular reconstruction, systemic anticoagulation is usually necessary to prevent thrombosis in the distal circulation during the period of cross-clamping. Systemic anticoagulation is usually achieved by the administration of heparin intravenously. A loading dose of 75–100 international units/kg is often used in vascular procedures. Most surgeons will wait 3–5 minutes after the heparin administration before cross-clamping. The effect of a single dose will last approximately 3–4 hours. Supplemental doses of heparin may be necessary if the duration of the cross-clamping is extended beyond 2 hours. Intraoperative dosing of heparin can be guided by measuring the activated clotting times during the procedure.

Antiplatelet therapy is commonly used in conjunction with carotid surgery or infrainguinal reconstructions. Aspirin is usually started preoperatively. Low-dose aspirin irreversibly acetylates cyclooxygenase in platelets, which then prevents platelet synthesis of thromboxane A2. Enteric-coated aspirin, 325 mg daily, is usually continued indefinitely. Aspirin may be used in conjunction with warfarin but with caution as the patients can become more prone to develop bleeding complications.

Dextran is also used as an antiplatelet agent. It is started intraoperatively and continued as an intravenous infusion usually over the ensuing 24 hours. Dextran is a polysaccharide, which decreases platelet adhesiveness and aggregation. It is available in two forms, dextran 40 and dextran 70. Dextran 40 is the form generally used during vascular procedures as an antiplatelet agent while dextran 70 is more commonly used as an intravascular volume expander. Anaphylactic and allergic reactions can be reduced by infusion of dextran 1, a solution of short-chain dextrans, before starting dextran 40. The dosage of dextran used during vascular reconstructions is 500 mL intravenously followed by 500 to 1000 mL over the following 24 hours, given as a continuous infusion. The major complications with dextran use are bleeding and fluid overload.

BLOOD VESSEL CONTROL

Before occluding the vessels to create the vascular incision, the vessels are assessed for presence of atherosclerotic plaque. The dissected artery can be gently palpated with the index finger or pinched between the index finger and the thumb to check for the presence of atheromatous plaque. However, assessment with finger palpation alone may not be adequate. A useful method is to compress the blood vessel with the index finger against a right-angle clamp. This will allow a good evaluation of the vessel with respect to the presence and location of atherosclerotic plaque. Palpation of an artery should be carried out gently and cautiously, as rough manipulation could result in distal embolization and breakage of atheromatous debris into the distal circulation. This could be catastrophic when handling the carotid artery where a "no-touch" technique should be followed when dissecting around the carotid bulb.

Several methods are available for controlling blood vessels. These methods include the use of atraumatic vascular clamps, tapes with Rumel tourniquet, silastic vessel loops, internal occluders, or external pneumatic tourniquet.

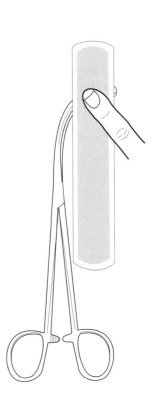

VASCULAR CLAMPS

In the absence of plaque, the vascular clamp is applied in the simplest manner that would not obscure the incision or exposure. In a diseased artery, the presence and location of an atheromatous plaque will dictate the method of clamp

Blood Vessel Control
Vascular Clamps
Rumel Tourniquet

application. The vascular clamp should be applied in a manner that would oppose the soft wall of the artery against the hard plaque without breaking the plaque or tearing the artery.

Before applying a vascular clamp, it is a good habit to check the number of notches needed for complete apposition of the clamp jaws. Excessive clamping may result in injury at the clamp application site even with the use of an "atraumatic" vascular clamp.

When dealing with smaller arteries, such as the profunda femoris or external carotid artery, self-compressing clamps such as the bulldog clamps or aneurysm clips can be very useful. The aneurysm clips (Heifitz clips or Yasargil clips) require a special applicator for placing them, which facilitates their delivery and removal in deep locations.

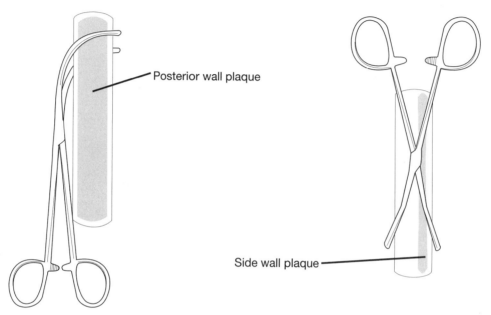

Posterior wall plaque

Side wall plaque

In the presence of posterior plaque, the vascular clamp is applied to appose the anterior and posterior walls together.

In the presence of a plaque on the sidewall, the vascular clamp is applied to appose the lateral and medial walls against each other.

A Rumel tourniquet can be used to achieve vascular control in medium-sized arteries such as the common femoral or common carotid arteries.

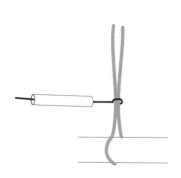

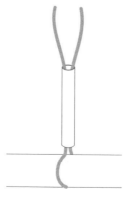

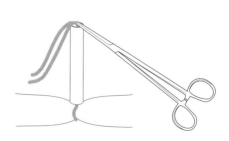

An umbilical tape is placed around the blood vessel.

The umbilical tape is introduced through a segment of the rubber catheter using a snare.

The rubber catheter is pushed against the artery and stabilized by clamping the umbilical tape.

SILASTIC VESSEL LOOPS

Silastic vessel loops are often used to encircle blood vessels. Gentle tension on the vessel loop can help in providing traction on a blood vessel and facilitating the exposure. When double looped, tension on the vessel loop usually results in blood flow interruption. However, excessive tension on the vessel loops can damage the vessel wall. Thus, the least amount of tension capable of interrupting blood flow should be applied. When dealing with very small branches, the vessel loops can be bulky to use and may be replaced by a double loop of 4-0 silk.

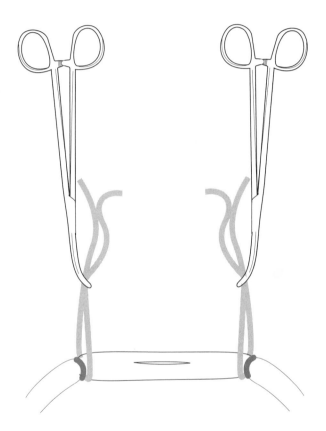

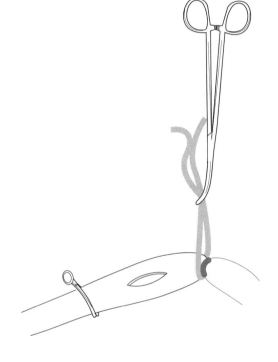

Vessel loops may fail to interrupt the blood flow if used with prosthetic grafts or diseased vessels of the size of the common femoral artery. In addition, if two vessel loops are used for proximal and distal control, the blood vessel segment between the loops may be placed in undue tension and the process of placing the sutures in the arterial wall could be made unnecessarily difficult.

This problem could be avoided by replacing the distal vessel loop with an aneurysm clip.

Blood Vessel Control
Silastic Vessel Loops

Vessel loops can be used to control side branches without having to dissect them circumferentially. This can be particularly helpful when obtaining control of the profunda femoris artery in scarred tissue planes. In this situation, only the common femoral and superficial femoral arteries are dissected. As shown below, the vessel loop is passed underneath the common femoral artery and then underneath the superficial femoral artery.

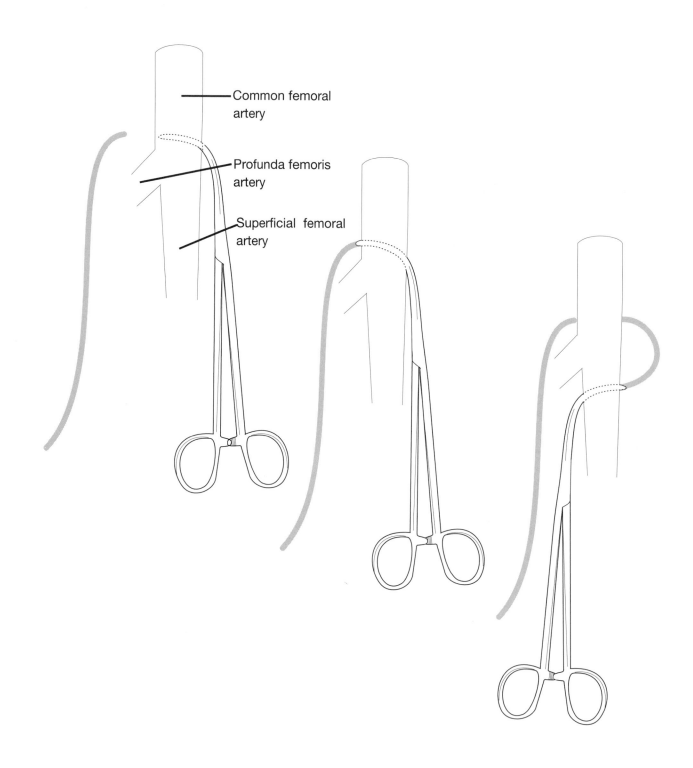

Common femoral artery

Profunda femoris artery

Superficial femoral artery

This process is repeated, which results in placing a double loop around the profunda femoris artery. This double loop can also control branches originating from the posterior aspect of the common or deep femoral arteries.

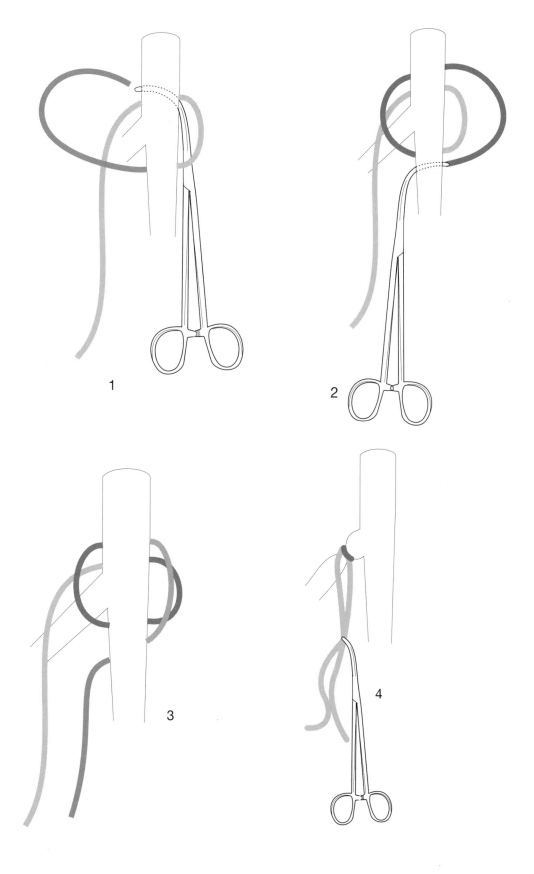

1

2

3

4

Blood Vessel Control
Internal Occluders

INTERNAL OCCLUDERS

Internal occluders are dumbbell-shaped devices that are available in different sizes. They are particularly useful in controlling infrapopliteal vessels. They are inserted through the arteriotomy, and they interrupt the blood flow from within the lumen. Thus, only exposure of the anterior surface of the vessel is required and circumferential dissection becomes unnecessary. This method eliminates the need for external occlusion of the tibial vessels, which could result in arterial spasm or vessel injury, especially in calcified vessels.

The appropriate size of internal occluder should be chosen. A small size could result in bleeding around the occluder. A large size could damage the intima if forced into the lumen. Occasionally, the presence of branches at the site of the arteriotomy or adjacent to the beginning or end of the arteriotomy may result in persistent bleeding. These branches will need to be controlled with silk loops to achieve a dry field.

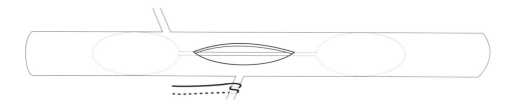

In the presence of heavy calcification, the arteriotomy may not allow the insertion of the internal occluders. Vascular control can be obtained by occluding the vessels from within using two balloon catheters, each attached to a three-way stopcock.

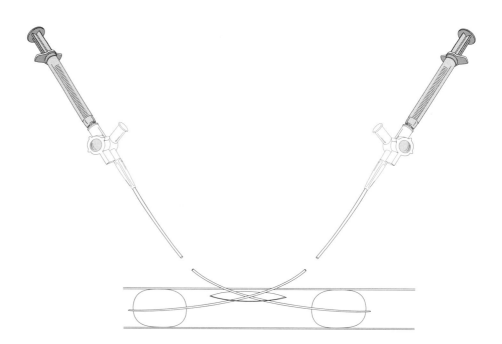

EXTERNAL PNEUMATIC TOURNIQUET

The external pneumatic tourniquet is another method of controlling the infrageniculate blood vessels. This method interrupts the blood flow without placing any intraluminal objects or any clamps that could hinder the exposure or potentially injure the vessel. The tourniquet is particularly helpful in the presence of heavily calcified blood vessels. A sterile tourniquet is applied, usually around the midthigh over a cotton roll. The leg is elevated and drained of the venous blood with the use of an Esmarc bandage. The tourniquet is inflated to a pressure of 250 mmHg and the arteriotomy is created. If the field is not adequately dry, the inflation pressure can be increased to 350 mmHg. If bleeding persists, occluding the profunda femoris artery may provide the desired hemostasis. The alignment of the graft should be well established and double checked before inflating the tourniquet to avoid any twists or unpleasant surprises when the tourniquet is deflated.

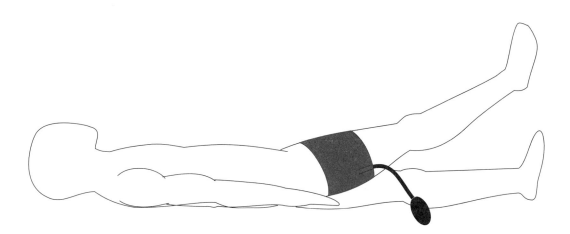

A similar concept to the external pneumatic tourniquet is the "Boazul Roll-On Cuff" (Boazul Medical AB). These cuffs are made of Latex and are available in four different sizes. After choosing the appropriate size, the cuff is inflated to 120 mm Hg, rolled on to the extremity proximal to the site where vascular control is desired and then secured in place using a wedge. These cuffs can be autoclaved and re-used. Furthermore, they eliminate the need for an Esmarc bandage as venous drainage is accomplished during the rolling of the cuff.

**Creation of Blood
Vessel Incision**

CREATION OF A BLOOD VESSEL INCISION

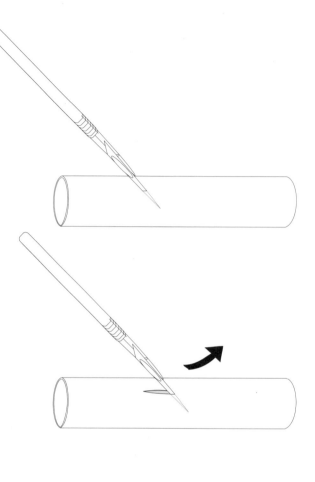

An 11 blade is usually used to start the incision in the blood vessel. The blade is introduced at a 45° angle and then advanced in a forward movement simulating an airplane during takeoff. This will create an opening large enough to easily accommodate the blade of a Potts scissors. The Potts scissors is used to extend the incision to the desired length.

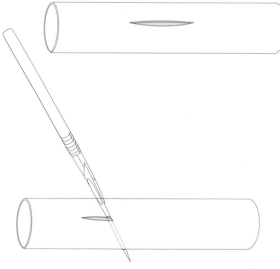

Introducing the blade too deeply can result in an injury to the back wall.

Introducing the blade without a forward movement can result in a very small arteriotomy and a struggle in introducing the blade of the Potts scissors.

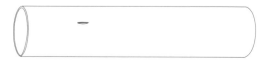

Prosthetic or autogenous patches can be used. Vein patches are usually prepared by harvesting a segment of vein and incising it along its longitudinal axis.

Alternatively, a segment of an occluded superficial femoral artery is harvested. The artery is incised along its longitudinal axis.

The patch is created by performing an endarterectomy of the harvested segment.

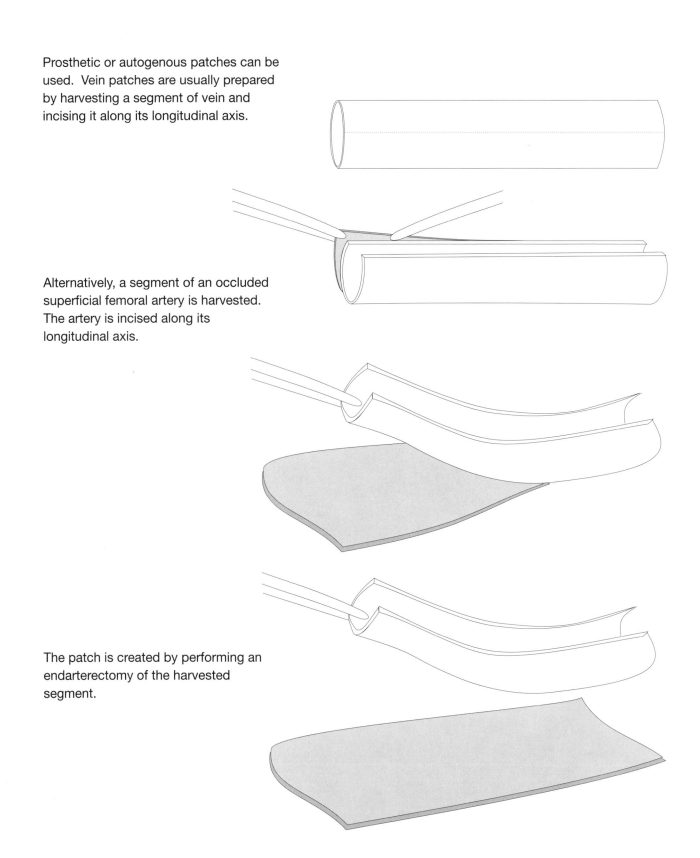

Preparation of a Patch

The patch is prepared for the reconstruction. The edges of the patch are usually trimmed to match the incision in the vessel. Several shapes can be created.

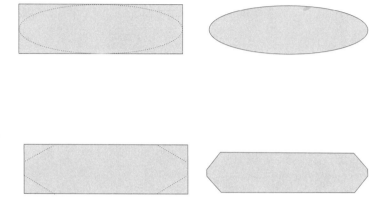

If the edges of the patch are trimmed leaving an acute angle, the placement of the apical sutures can be technically demanding.

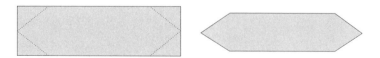

PREPARATION OF A BYPASS

"Measure twice, cut once." When preparing an autogenous vessel for an anastomosis, the vessel is often transected at a right angle and then slit on its posterior aspect, resulting in spatulating the vessel end. Alternatively, the edges of the graft are trimmed to various degrees. The same method can be used with prosthetic grafts.

Incise the vessel along the posterior aspect.

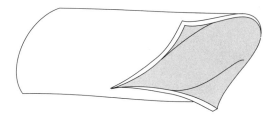

You may cut a wedge of the graft on one side.

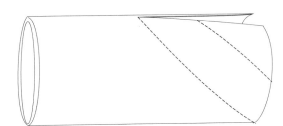
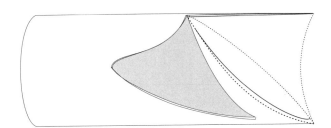

Cut the remaining wedge on the other side.

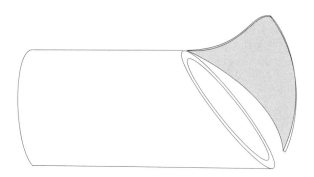
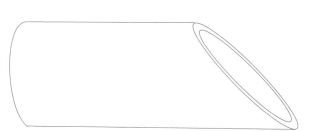

Preparation of a Bypass

Another alternative would be to clamp the graft and then transect it using a new blade along the inner aspect of the clamp.

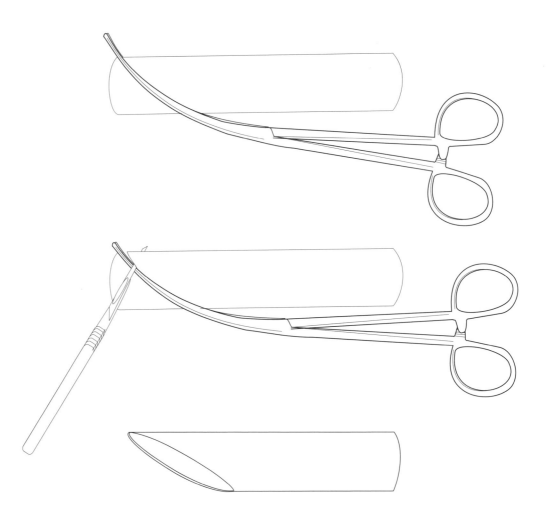

Before starting the suture line, the size of the opening in the bypass should be checked to match appropriately the length of incision in the blood vessel. If after starting the anastomosis the opening in the bypass is found to be larger than the vascular incision, the conduit can be trimmed or the arteriotomy can be lengthened. However, if the length of the arteriotomy is found to exceed the length of the opening in the graft, accommodating for the size discrepancy is more demanding.

CONSTRUCTION OF THE SUTURE LINE

The use of magnifying loupes is recommended especially during the reconstruction of small vessels such as in infrainguinal bypass procedures. Most surgeons will use 2.5–3.5 power loupe magnification. Illumination is as important as magnification. A headlamp may prove to be worth the headache it may cause.

INTRODUCTION OF THE NEEDLE

The needle should be passed through the vessel wall with minimal damage to the wall. In the presence of a plaque, introducing the needle from the adventitial side of the wall can result in separation of the plaque from the arterial wall. Creating a flap or a dissection can be avoided in calcified arteries by always introducing the needle from the intimal side of the arterial wall.

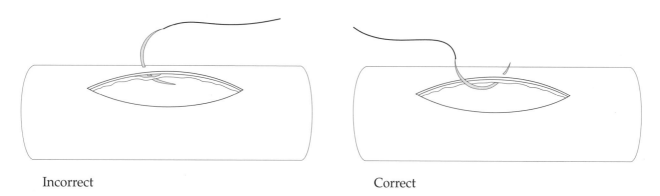

Incorrect   Correct

In soft nondiseased arteries, the needle can be safely placed from the adventitial side of the wall. When placing sutures in veins or prosthetic grafts, the needles should be introduced in the simplest fashion that provides a forehand placement of the suture.

The needle should be introduced at a right angle to the vessel wall. The needle should be passed through the wall while following the curvature with minimal movements to avoid creating large needle holes.

Before pushing the needle through the wall, releasing the needle holder while maintaining control of the needle (unclick before you stick) will result in minimizing the amount of lateral movement of the needle while in the arterial wall. This maneuver will allow passage of the needle without creating large needle holes.

The temptation of holding the tip of the needle should be avoided, as this will result in blunting of the needle tip. Pushing the needle too far in the arterial wall also should be avoided, as it may result in pushing the tip of the needle holder into the arterial wall.

Construction of the Suture Line

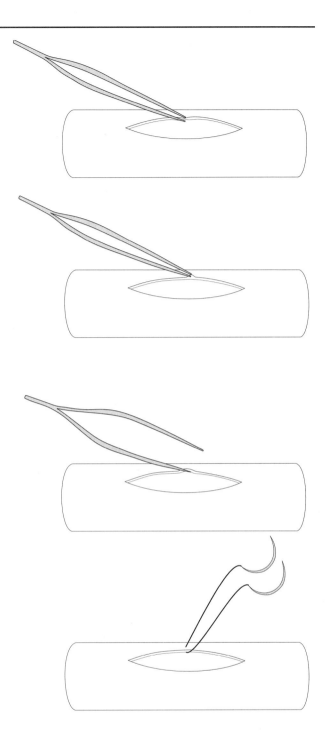

When placing sutures in autogenous vessels, the temptation of holding the entire thickness of the vessel wall with the forceps should be avoided.

It is preferable to hold only the adventitia with the forceps, especially in small vessels. Even the softest "atraumatic" vascular forceps can cause intimal damage. The adventitia should be held carefully to avoid separating it from the rest of the vessel wall.

One option is to retract the vessel wall with one side of the forceps.

Another option is to place stay sutures to retract the vessel wall.

SIZE OF THE BITE

The size of the bite varies depending on the blood vessel being reconstructed. With aortic reconstructions, the bites are usually 3–4 mm deep and 2–3 mm apart. However, larger double-layer bites are recommended for the posterior wall of the aorta, especially when dealing with aneurysmal disease.

With infrainguinal reconstructions, the bites in the common femoral artery are usually 1–2 mm deep and 1 mm apart. In the popliteal artery, the bites are usually placed 1 mm deep while in the infrapopliteal vessels the bites are usually 0.5–1 mm deep. Too few sutures with large advancement could result in bleeding between the sutures. Too many sutures are also not ideal.

The bites should result in intimal apposition, which is usually obtained when the suture line is everting. Adventitial strings should not be allowed to slip in the suture line, as they can be very thrombogenic.

The assistant should follow the surgeon by maintaining tension on the suture line while the surgeon is reloading the needle in the needle holder. Tension on the suture line is briefly released when the surgeon is ready to pull the suture through the vessel wall. The suture is pulled to appropriate tension by the surgeon and the assistant regrasps the suture. When a continuous suture line is being used, the forceps can be used to guide the placement of the suture loop. The location of the suture loop is as important as the placement of the bites.

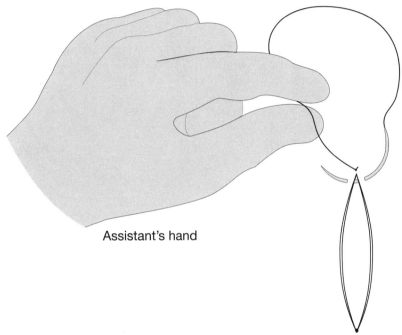

Assistant's hand

It is preferable to place the bites with a forehand rather than a backhand rotation of the needle. However, the surgeon should be comfortable with both forehand and backhand suturing techniques. When suturing away from the surgeon, the surgeon may follow himself/herself and grasps the suture line.

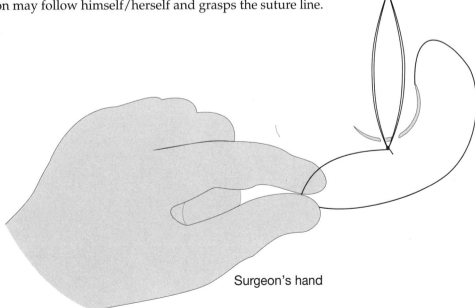

Surgeon's hand

Construction of the Suture Line

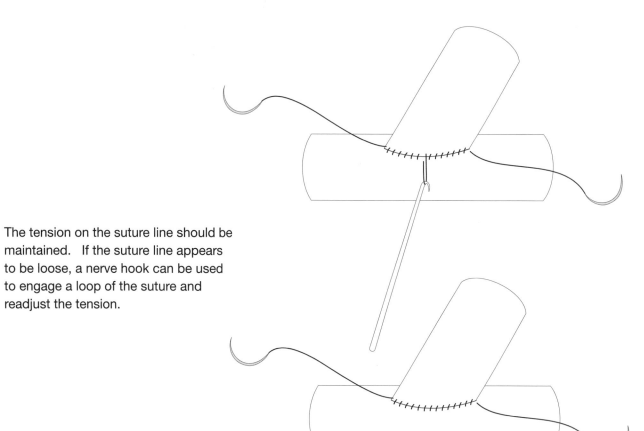

The tension on the suture line should be maintained.   If the suture line appears to be loose, a nerve hook can be used to engage a loop of the suture and readjust the tension.

Excessive tension should be avoided as it can cause a pursestring effect or puckering of the anastomosis.

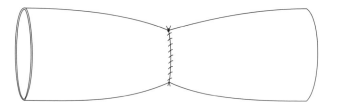

TYING GUIDELINES

Surgeons should use the method with which they feel most comfortable. Crossing the hands while tying is necessary to achieve a square knot. A sliding knot can be helpful in reaching the desired amount of tension. A sliding knot can be created by placing two throws in the same direction without crossing the hands. Even if the first throw was flat, so long as the hands do not cross with the second throw, the knot will slide. Crossing the hands with the third and following throws is necessary to achieve square knots and prevent unraveling of the suture.

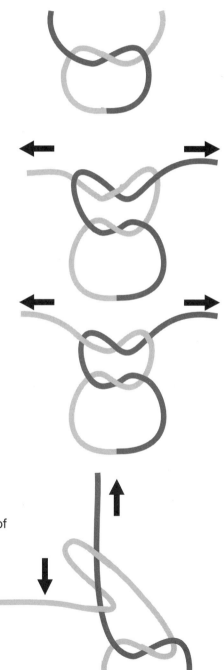

A square knot is started with a flat throw.

Crossing the hands with the second throw will result in a square knot.

When both throws are placed in the same direction, a granny knot is formed. This knot is not secure and can slip.

A slip knot can also be achieved by changing the direction of the tension applied on the strings while tying. This slip knot can be secured by adding multiple square knots.

SECURING HEMOSTASIS

Before tying the suture line, the vessel lumen is irrigated with heparinized saline to flush out any debris. Forward and backward bleeding should also be rechecked before completing the suture line. The distal clamps are released first. The proximal clamps are then partially released to identify obvious leaks. In that situation, the clamps are reapplied and the defect repaired. In the presence of multiple outflow vessels, the circulation is usually first reestablished into the least critical outflow vessel such as the external carotid artery during a carotid endarterectomy. This will allow any debris to travel into the nonvital circulation. After constructing the suture line, hemostasis is secured. In addition, the wound should be carefully checked for lymph leak. Hemostasis is reviewed in Chapter 5.

EVALUATING THE VASCULAR RECONSTRUCTION

After securing hemostasis, the vascular reconstruction is evaluated for patency or the presence of any technical abnormalities. Although the presence of a pulse distal to the reconstruction is very reassuring, most vascular surgeons rely on other methods to assess a newly completed vascular anastomosis. Noninvasive evaluation can be performed using a sterile handheld doppler or duplex ultrasonography. The handheld doppler is usually marched over the vascular reconstruction as well as proximal and distal to the reconstruction site. The doppler signal distal to an anastomosis should diminish with pinching the newly implanted bypass and reaugment with reestablishment of the blood flow. A high-pitched signal is suggestive of a stenotic pathology. Insonation over freshly implanted prosthetic grafts is usually unsuccessful. Duplex ultrasonography has also been used to evaluate vascular reconstruction intraoperatively. This method has been particularly useful for evaluating the carotid arteries following endarterectomy procedures. It has also been valuable following renal artery revascularization. However, its role in evaluating infrainguinal revascularization intraoperatively has not gained wide acceptance as angiography continues to be the method of choice. This can be attributed to the superiority of the images obtained by angiography.

Intraoperative angiography is usually performed by inserting a 20-gauge angiocath or butterfly into the conduit and injecting 10–15 mL of contrast. A side branch can be used as the entry site for the angiocath when a vein conduit is being used. After the angiogram is obtained, the angiocath is withdrawn and the side branch is ligated. This avoids the need for placing a suture to control bleeding for the angiocath insertion site. Angioscopy has also been used for intraoperative assessment of infrainguinal revascularization. Although angioscopy has been successfully used to monitor valvular disruption and the patency of vascular reconstructions, it remains infrequently performed. This can be attributed to concerns related to cost, fluid overload and potential intimal injury to the conduit. Furthermore, angioscopy does not provide any information regarding the outflow vessel distal to the reconstruction.

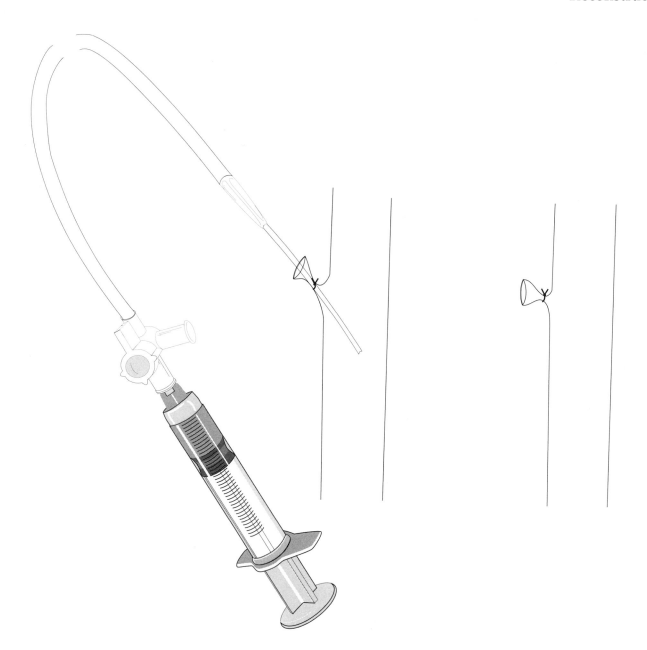

5

Hemostasis

During a vascular reconstruction, standard surgical techniques are used for soft tissue hemostasis. The use of electrocautery should be limited near blood vessels to avoid inadvertent injury to the vessel wall or adjacent nerves. To achieve a desired vascular exposure, some blood vessels may need to be divided. Small vessels are usually double ligated in continuity and then transected.

SUTURE LIGATION

Suture ligation may be required when the transected vessel is expected to have a short stump. Examples include the facial vein during the exposure of the carotid bifurcation or the lateral circumflex vein during the exposure of the profunda femoris artery. Suture ligation may also be needed to control bleeding from vascular orifices such as the backbleeding from the lumbar or inferior mesenteric arteries during abdominal aortic aneurysm replacement.

CLOSURE OF LARGE TRANSECTED ARTERY

When the transected vessel has a wide base, suture ligation may not be adequate. The edges of the transected end can be oversewn with a simple "over-and-over" continuous suture. This closure method may be adequate when the oversewn vessel has a low intraluminal pressure, such as a vein or the distal end of a transected artery. However, when dealing with the proximal end of a large transected artery, an additional suture line is often used to secure the closure. The first row of sutures is usually constructed with horizontal mattress sutures placed proximal to the edges of the transected artery. The horizontal mattress sutures are placed using an interrupted or continuous technique. The second row of sutures will approximate the edges of the transected artery, usually with an "over-and-over" continuous suture. This method of closure is usually used to oversew the aortic stump after the removal of an infected aortic prosthesis.

REPAIR OF LOOSE SUTURE LINE

After completing the vascular reconstruction, the suture line is inspected to ensure hemostasis. In general, the effect of heparin is allowed to wear off without reversal. Heparin can be reversed with protamine sulfate. The dose of protamine is estimated at 1 mg/100 U heparin, taking into consideration when heparin was administered and the decrease in heparin activity over time. Only one-half of the calculated dose of protamine should be given initially as it can cause hypotension and bradycardia if given too quickly. The maximum rate of administration of protamine is 10 mg/min with a maximum of 50 mg in 10 minutes.

Patience is essential when bleeding is noted from needle holes. Needle-hole bleeding will usually stop when the suture line is gently compressed with a dry gauze sponge. The control of needle-hole bleeding may be expedited by the topical application of hemostatic agents such as oxidized cellulose or gel foam. The topical application of strips of gel foam soaked with thrombin is particularly helpful in controlling needle-hole bleeding from polytetrafluoroethylene (PTFE) grafts or patches. A list of topical hemostatic agents is outlined in table 5.1.

Persistent diffuse bleeding from all the needle holes usually suggests a loose suture line. The tension of the suture line can be checked with a nerve hook by carefully engaging one loop in the suture line. Gentle tension on the loop will usually control the bleeding if it is caused by a loose suture line. In this situation, another suture is placed and tied next to the engaged loop. The loop and the new suture are then tied together.

REPAIR OF LONGITUDINAL TEARS

Occasionally, additional sutures may be required to achieve hemostasis. Bleeding from the suture line may also be caused by longitudinal tears in the vessel wall. This is usually controlled by sutures fortified with pledgets. When repairing a bleeding suture line, it is preferable to clamp the vessel proximally. This will avoid placing and tying sutures in a pulsating vessel with a high intraluminal pressure. Otherwise, additional tears in the vessel wall along the needle holes may occur.

Table 5.1

Name	Manufacturer	Ingredients	How Supplied
Actifoam	Davol; Bard	Collagen	Sponge
Avitene; MCH (Microfibrillar collagen hemostat)	Davol; Bard	Partial hydrochloric acid salt of purified bovine corium collagen	Powder; sheet
Avitene Syringe MCH (Microfibrillar collagen hemostat)	Med Chem Products; Davol; Bard	Partial hydrochloric acid salt of purified bovine corium collagen	Powder in a syringe
Gelfoam	Pharmacia UpJohn	Purified pork skin gelatin	Sponge or powder
Helistat	Integra Life Sciences Corp	Bovine collagen (Achilles tendon)	Sponge
Helitene	Integra Life Sciences Corp	Bovine collagen (Achilles tendon)	Fibrillar
Oxycel	Bectim Dickinson Acute Care	Oxidized cellulose	Cotton-like sponge
Superstat	Superstat Corp	Positively charged collagen based agent	Sheet
Surgicel	Johnson & Johnson	Oxidized regenerated cellulose	Sheet; powder
Thrombin	GenTrac, Inc	Bovine thrombin	Vials, Spray
Tisseel VH (Fibrin Sealant)	Baxter	Human thrombin; Human sealer protein concentrate (Fibrinogen cryoprecipitate); Bovine fibrinolysis inhibitor (Aprotinin)	two syringes with a joining piece

Suture Ligation
Small Vessels

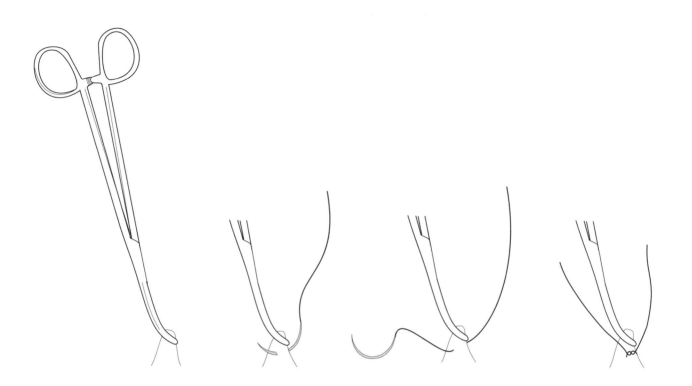

Place a suture in the vascular pedicle. Tie one throw.

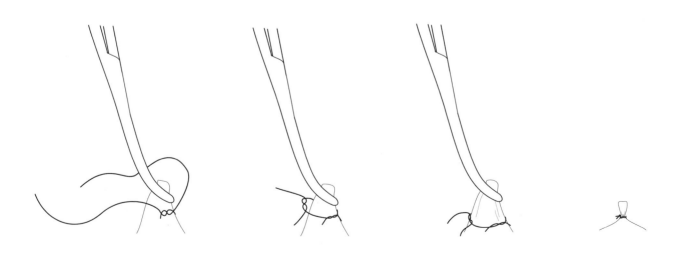

Pass the thread around the clamp and tie the knot.

Suture Ligation
Lumbar Vessels

Bleeding lumbar vessels can be controlled by a simple figure-of-8 suture. In the presence of a calcified plaque, oversewing the orifice of the bleeding vessel will not achieve hemostasis unless preceded by a localized endarterectomy.

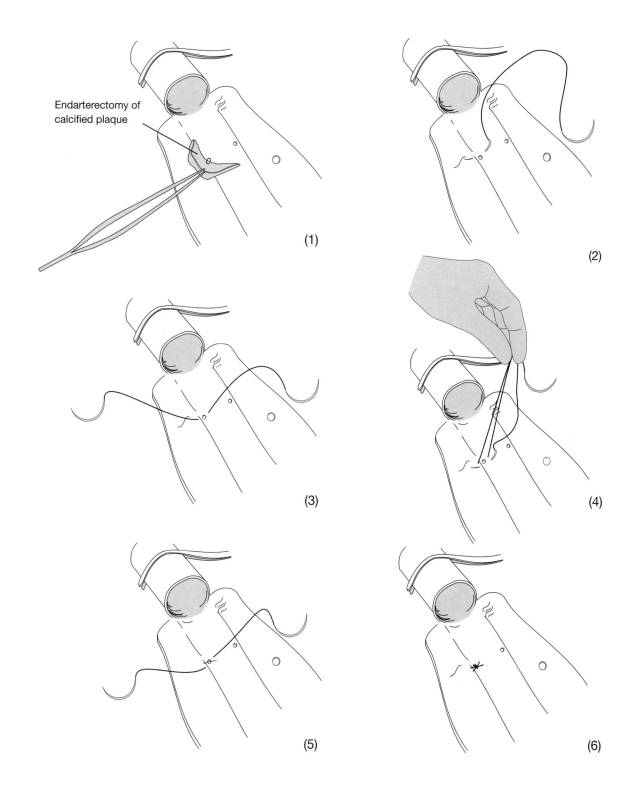

Endarterectomy of calcified plaque

(1)

(2)

(3)

(4)

(5)

(6)

Suture Ligation
Inferior Mesenteric Artery

Blood vessels with large orifices such as the inferior mesenteric artery may need additional bites to secure hemostasis.

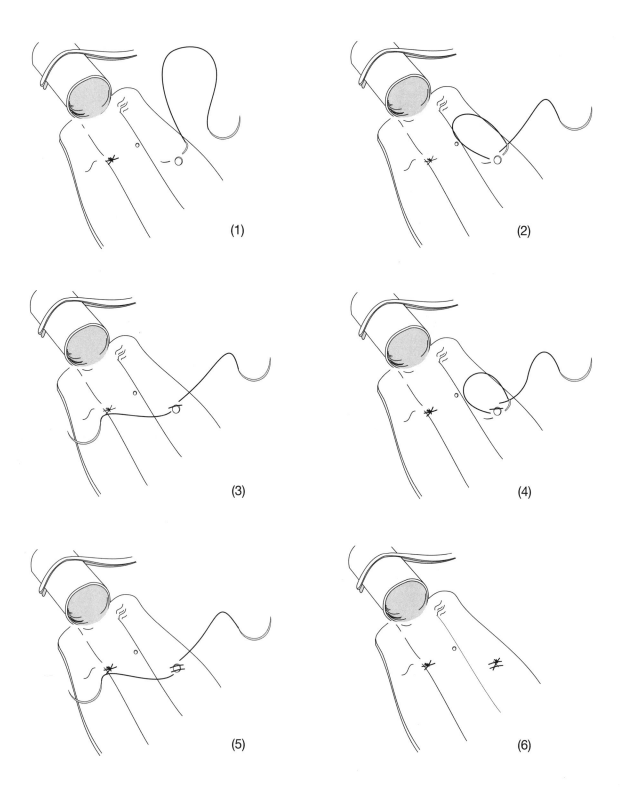

Closure of a Large Transected Artery

Start one suture at one end. Run the suture in a horizontal mattress technique until you reach the opposite end.

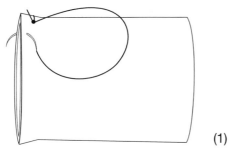

(1)

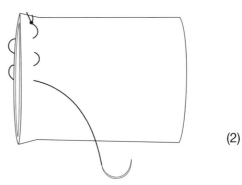

(2)

Tighten the suture line and tie the suture to itself. Start another suture and run it down using a simple continuous closure.

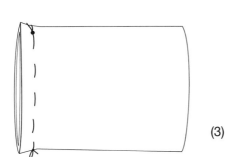

(3)

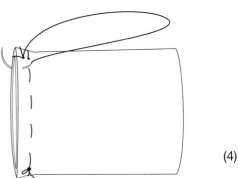

(4)

Place several sutures until you reach the opposite end. Tighten the suture line, and tie the suture to itself.

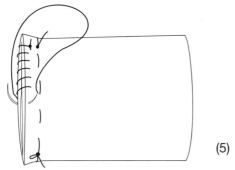

(5)

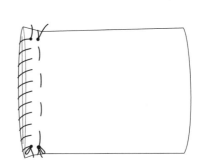

(6)

Alternatively, start by placing a horizontal mattress suture proximal to the edges of the transected end.

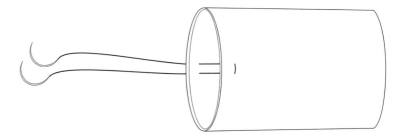

Closure of a Large Transected Artery

Place a row of sutures.

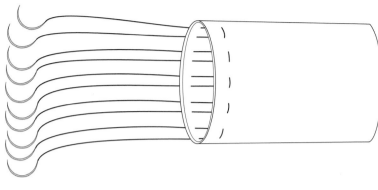

Tie the sutures.

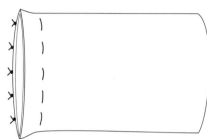

Start another suture at one end. Tie the suture. You may run the suture to the other end using a simple continuous closure.

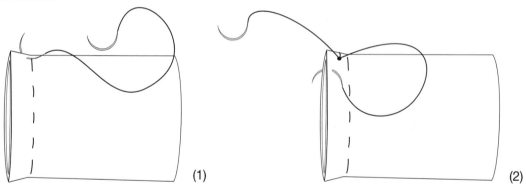

(1)

(2)

Alternatively, you may run the suture using a horizontal mattress technique.

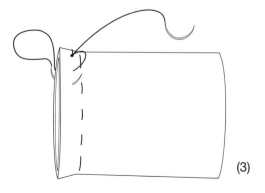

(3)

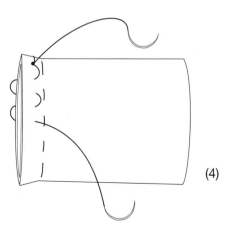

(4)

Closure of a Large Transected Artery

Continue until you reach the opposite end. Tighten the suture.

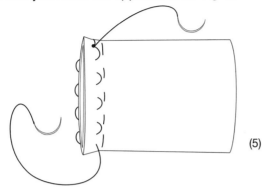

(5)

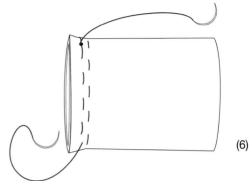

(6)

Run the suture back using a simple continuous closure.

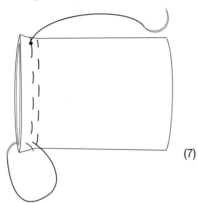

(7)

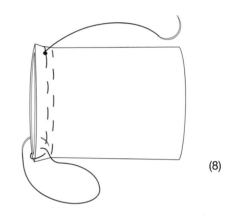

(8)

Place several sutures until you reach the opposite end.

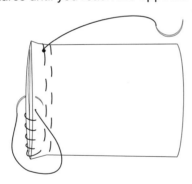

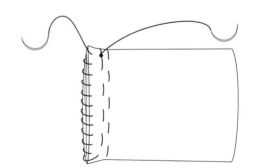

Tighten the suture line and tie both ends together.

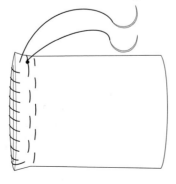

(11)

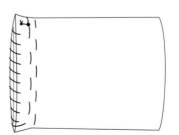

(12)

Repair of Loose Suture Line

Excessive bleeding from the needle holes can occur when the anastomosis has been constructed without maintaining adequate tension on the suture line.

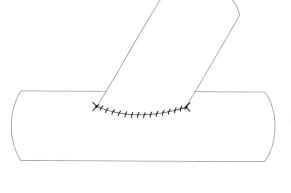

Using a nerve hook, a loop of the suture line is pulled with gentle tension.

A suture of the same type is introduced through the loop. The loop can often be engaged with the needle without the nerve hook.

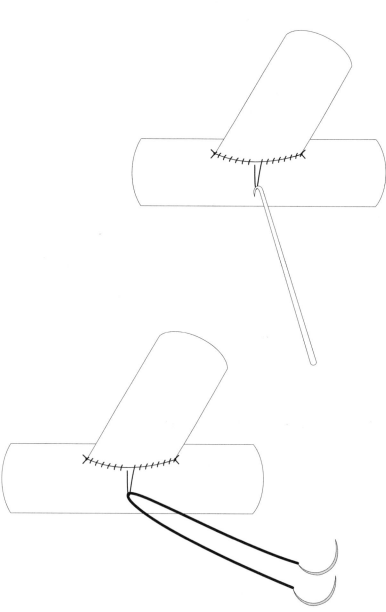

Repair of Loose Suture Line

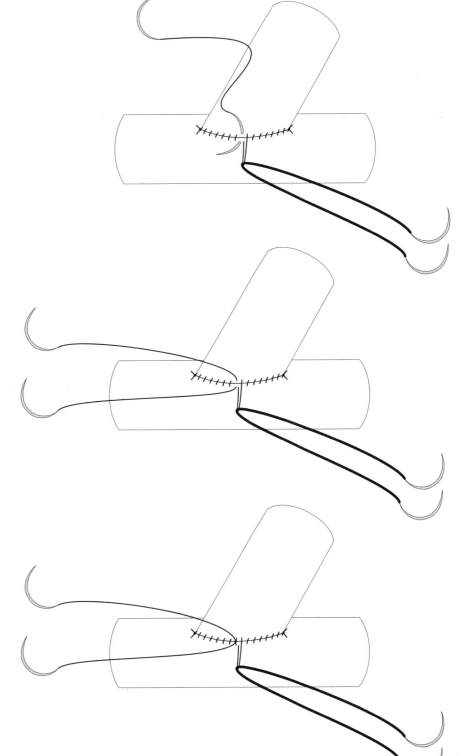

A new suture is then placed
close to the pulled loop.

The new suture is then tied
while maintaining tension on
the loop.

Repair of Loose Suture Line

Tie one end of the suture to
the pulled loop.

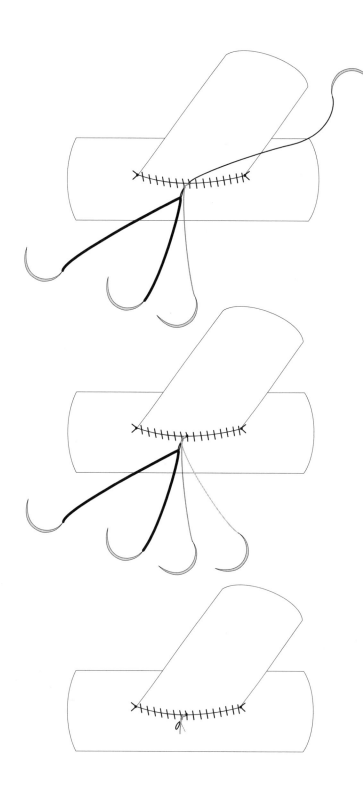

Tie the other end of the
suture to the pulled loop.

Repair of Longitudal Tears

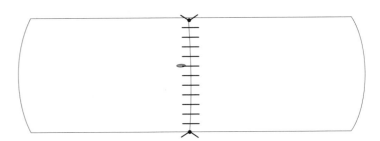

Bleeding from the suture line can be caused by a longitudinal tear along a needle hole.

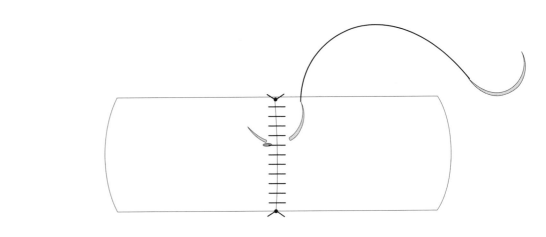

A horizontal mattress suture is placed around the tear.

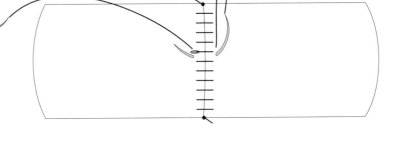

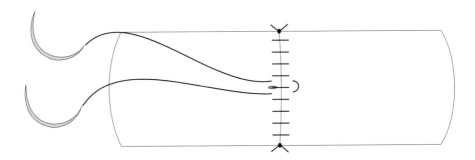

Repair of Longitudal Tears

A pledget is then introduced.

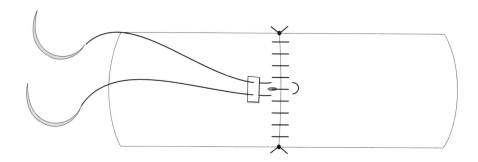

The pledget is advanced to cover the tear.

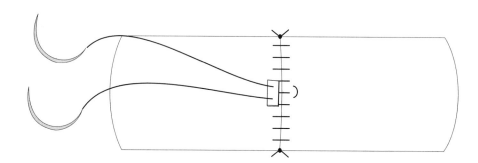

The suture is then tied over the pledget.

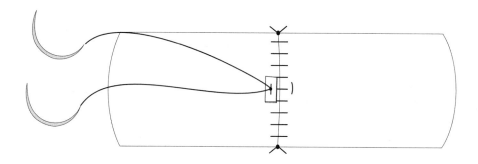

It is preferable to occlude the vessel proximally before placing and tying the suture to avoid additional tears from the repair suture.

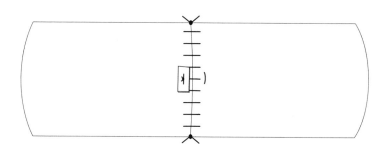

6

Thrombectomy–Embolectomy

THROMBECTOMY–EMBOLECTOMY

Acute arterial occlusion can be caused by embolization or arterial thrombosis. Extractions of the embolus (embolectomy) or thrombus (thrombectomy) are frequently performed vascular procedures. Because thrombosis is very likely to occur distal to an embolization site, an embolectomy is often referred to as thrombo-embolectomy (TE). Several important considerations need to be addressed when performing these procedures. These include the type of blood vessel incision used to remove the thrombi and the methods to minimize blood loss and blood vessel trauma during the procedure. Other important issues relate to the various methods used to achieve retrieval of all offending thrombi in addition to assessing the completeness and effectiveness of the clot extraction. Finally, the examination of the extracted thrombi can be very important, as it can provide insight into the etiology of the occlusive process.

INCISION TYPE

Thrombectomy or embolectomy can be performed through a transverse or a longitudinal incision in the vessel. It is important to ensure that the patient is adequately anticoagulated before occluding the vessels. When the occlusion is suspected to be due to embolization, a transverse incision may be most desirable. In this situation, a transverse incision can be closed primarily with relative ease and without causing any significant narrowing of the lumen. Embolization is usually suspected in a patient with arrythmias and intracardiac thrombi who lacks prior history of chronic arterial insufficiency and presents with acute arterial occlusion. In the presence of significant plaque in the artery or when the occlusion is suspected to be caused by thrombosis secondary to a stenotic pathology, a longitudinal arteriotomy will be most appropriate. Thrombosis secondary to a stenotic pathology is usually suspected when a patient presents with acute ischemia and has prior history of chronic arterial insufficiency in the absence of any cardiac arrythmias. A longitudinal arteriotomy will allow for inspection of the diseased area as well as possible endarterectomy or repair with a patch. In addition, if TE proves to be inadequate and a distal bypass becomes necessary, the incision can serve as the site of the proximal anastomosis of the bypass. The various methods used for closure of vascular incisions are discussed in Chapter 8.

MINIMIZING BLOOD LOSS

Blood loss during a TE can be significant. Most of the blood loss tends to occur when performing TE of the proximal segment of the vessel and reestablishing the arterial inflow. Blood loss may occur while passing the TE catheter beyond the thrombus and while retrieving the thrombus. To minimize blood loss, elastic loops are usually used to encircle and double loop the blood vessel. Gentle tension is then applied on the vessel loop when advancing or withdrawing the catheter. When dealing with a prosthetic graft or a large thickened artery, vessel loops may be inadequate to control bleeding around the TE catheter. In this situation, one option is to use "soft-jaw clamps" such as the Fogarty clamps to occlude the blood vessel. The soft jaws may be able to appose the blood vessel walls just enough to prevent bleeding and still allow the TE catheter to be advanced. The jaws are opened as the inflated TE catheter is being withdrawn. Another useful option is to pinch the vessel between the thumb and the index finger of one hand, while the other hand is manipulating the TE catheter.

AVOIDING VESSEL TRAUMA

Catheter manipulation during a TE can result in significant injury to the blood vessel. (1, 2) Vessel injury can be induced by the tip or the balloon of the TE catheter. The vascular trauma can occur during insertion, advancement, or withdrawal of the TE catheter. One type of injury occurs when the catheter is inadvertently introduced into a subintimal location. Thus, during insertion, it is very important to be sure that the catheter tip is actually going into the lumen of the vessel. If resistance is met and the catheter cannot be advanced any further with gentle manipulation, forceful advancement should be avoided. Forceful advancement can result in vessel perforation or can drive the catheter into a subintimal plane. The latter will result in intimal dissection. Furthermore, upon withdrawal of the inflated TE catheter, part of the intima may be stripped. It is also important to realize that every time an inflated catheter is withdrawn, intimal damage could occur. In fact, this is one of the techniques used in experimental animal models to harvest endothelial cells or to cause endothelial trauma for the evaluation of neointimal hyperplasia. Vessel injury can occur from excessive shear forces on the wall while retrieving the TE catheter, especially if the balloon is overinflated. Balloon overinflation can also result in vessel rupture.

Several steps can be helpful in avoiding vessel trauma during TE. First, it is important to select the appropriate size of the TE catheter. In general, a size 2 Fogarty catheter will be appropriate for vessels less than 2 mm in diameter such as the pedal or hand vessels. A size 3 Fogarty catheter is usually most appropriate for vessels with diameters of 2–4 mm such as the tibial vessels or the infrageniculate popliteal artery. A size 4 Fogarty catheter is usually most appropriate for vessels with diameters of 4–10 mm, such as the above-knee popliteal and superficial femoral arteries, as well as the common femoral artery. A size 4 Fogarty catheter can also be useful for the iliac arteries. A size 5 Fogarty catheter is most appropriate for vessels larger than 10 mm in diameter; it can be useful for TE of some relatively large iliac arteries. Other sizes available include size 6 and 7, which can also be used for thrombectomy of an aortic graft or a saddle aortic embolus. Before inserting the TE catheter, it is imperative to test the balloon and get a visual assessment of its size once fully inflated. It is a good practice to limit the amount of fluid used in the syringe to inflate the balloon to the minimum volume needed for full inflation to avoid overexpansion and rupture of the balloon or the vessel. Another helpful step is to measure the distance from the arteriotomy to the area where the thrombus is expected to be lodged. This will help determine if the catheter has reached far enough to the desired location.

In addition, this may help avoid pushing the catheter beyond the desired location unnecessarily, thus limiting the potential injury to the artery. Once the catheter has reached maximal advancement, gentle inflation while pulling the catheter back will allow feeling the friction between the balloon and the vessel wall. At that point, the balloon should not be inflated any further. The catheter should just be retrieved with that amount of tension. It is very important that the same individual withdrawing the catheter is also controlling the degree of balloon inflation. Similarly, slight deflation of the catheter may be necessary if the catheter is passing across a stenotic area. As the catheter is being pulled back, additional deflation or inflation may be necessary to accommodate for any change in the caliber of the vessel.

ACHIEVING A COMPLETE TE

The ability to retrieve all clots and thrombi depends on getting the catheter into all the desired locations as well as the degree of adherence of the thrombi to the vessel wall. If the TE catheter does not reach the desired location, an angiogram can be very useful to delineate the anatomy. One useful approach is to perform the entire TE under fluoroscopic guidance. Half-strength contrast is used to inflate the balloon. The balloon is first tested under fluoroscopy to appreciate its shape when inflated and deflated. The balloon is then inserted and manipulated based on the prethrombectomy angiogram. This step can be facilitated further if the fluoroscopy machine used has road-mapping capabilities. The fluoroscopy machine will also be used to follow the withdrawal of the catheter. Useful information can be gained from observing the movement of the catheter tip and the inflated balloon under fluoroscopy. First, better insight into the anatomical location of the catheter tip and the vessels that are being catheterized can be obtained. Furthermore, if the inflated catheter is passing across an area of stenosis, the balloon will be seen changing in shape and developing a "waist" at the level of the stenosis.

TE OF THE LOWER EXTREMITY VESSELS

During TE of the lower limb vessels, a Fogarty catheter introduced through the superficial femoral artery will tend to repeatedly travel into the peroneal artery. Thus it is possible to perform a thrombectomy of the peroneal artery alone, leaving behind significant clots in the anterior and posterior tibial arteries. One helpful technique is to bend the tip of the TE catheter with the hope that at the level of the popliteal trifurcation, the bent tip will advance into the anterior or posterior tibial artery. Another helpful technique is to perform the procedure using two TE catheters under fluoroscopic guidance. One TE catheter is placed at the origin of the tibioperoneal trunk and the balloon is then inflated. Another TE catheter with a bent tip is advanced and manipulated under fluoroscopy to proceed into the anterior tibial artery. To catheterize the posterior tibial artery, the balloon of the first TE catheter is inflated at the level of the peroneal artery origin. The second catheter is then advanced after flipping the tip by 180°. Another option is to use special TE catheters that can be introduced over a wire. (Fogarty Thru-Lumen Catheter; Baxter Healthcare Corp., Irvine, CA) The wire will have to be directed first into the desired vessels under fluoroscopic guidance. If despite all these maneuvers the desired vessels cannot be canalized, exposure of the popliteal trifurcation will be necessary. The TE catheter can be introduced into the orifice of each individual tibial vessel under direct vision. Occasionally, exposure of the tibial vessels at a more distal level such as the ankle may be necessary. This allows direct catheterization and TE of the individual tibial vessels.

One of the difficulties encountered with TE of prosthetic grafts is the excessive adherence of the clot to the graft wall. The usual Fogarty catheter may not be able to retrieve the clot, and other catheters can be used. These catheters have been designed specially for the purpose of recovering adherent thrombi. One of these catheters has a mesh over the balloon of the catheter, which theoretically helps in capturing and retrieving adherent clots. (Latis Graft Cleaning Catheter; Applies Medical Resources, Laguana Hills, CA) Other catheters have a curved springy wire at the tip instead of the balloon. The curved wire will serve to strip the adherent thrombus from the vessel wall. (Fogarty Adherent Clot Catheter and Fogarty graft thrombectomy catheter; Baxter Healthcare Corp., Irvine, CA) These special catheters are intended to be used in prosthetic grafts. Their use in native vessels should be avoided.

EVALUATING THE COMPLETION AND RESULT OF THE TE

A thorough irrigation of the lumen with heparinized solution is performed. Angiography or angioscopy can be performed to check for residual clots. If the TE appears to be satisfactory, the arteriotomy is closed. One helpful maneuver is to tighten the suture line without tying of the suture and then allow for reperfusion of the limb. Blood flow distally is then assessed using a doppler probe or angiography. Should additional thrombectomy become necessary, tension is taken off the sutures and the suture line is gently loosened and unraveled. The TE catheter insertion and withdrawal is repeated until no additional clots can be retrieved on two consecutive withdrawals. In the presence of a clot that could not be retrieved, an interoperative injection of a thrombolytic agent (tPA 0.05 mg/kg) into the arterial bed harboring the clot can be helpful. Finally, it is important to check for compartmental hypertension as a possible cause for poor distal doppler signals despite what appears to be an adequate thrombectomy. The normal compartmental pressure should be less than 35 mmHg.

EXAMINATION OF RETRIEVED THROMBI

All retrieved clots and thrombi should be inspected. Inspection of the clots can be helpful in determining the etiology of the occlusion. Clots retrieved when thrombosis develops from low flow secondary to a tight stenosis are similar to coagulated blood. The presence of a grayish granular clot suggests platelet depositions. The presence of a darker or grayish organized clot at the end of the thrombus suggests embolization. An embolus from an atrial myxoma or tumor tends to be gelatinous with a grayish color. In this situation, microscopic examination of the thrombus is essential to delineating the source of the clot and establishing the diagnosis.

REFERENCES

1. Fogarty TJ, Cranley JJ, Krause RJ, et al. A method of extraction of arterial emboli and thrombi. Surg Gynecol Obstet 1963;116:241.
2. Foster JH, Carter JW, Edwards WH, et al. Arterial injuries secondary to the use of the Fogarty catheter. Ann Surg 1970;74:673.

Thrombo–Embolectomy
Minimizing Blood Loss

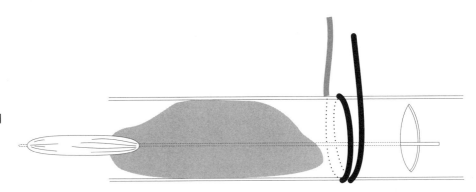

Blood vessel control is achieved using elastic vessel loops. The embolectomy catheter is introduced carefully into the vessel lumen.

The catheter is advanced until it reaches the desired location. Forceful advancement of the catheter is to be avoided.

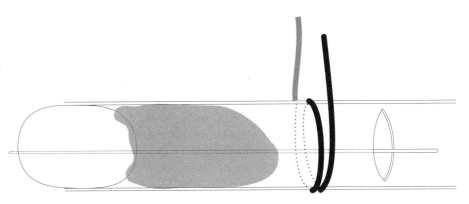

The balloon is gently inflated as the catheter is being pulled back slowly. This allows for feeling the friction between the balloon and the arterial wall. The catheter is withdrawn back while maintaining the least amount of friction and tension.

The vessel loop is kept loose while the thrombus is being extruded out of the vessel.

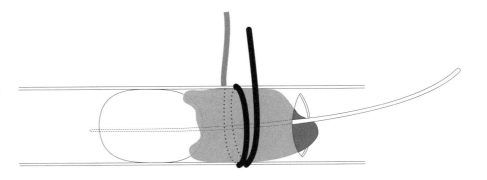

Thrombo–Embolectomy
Minimizing Blood Loss

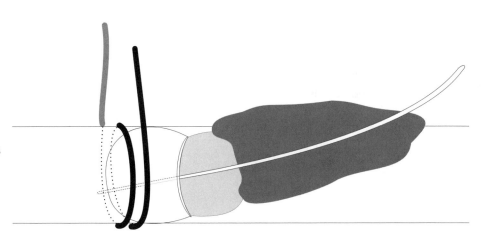

Once the thrombus is
retrieved, a gush of blood is
allowed to flush out any
remaining clot from the
arteriotomy.

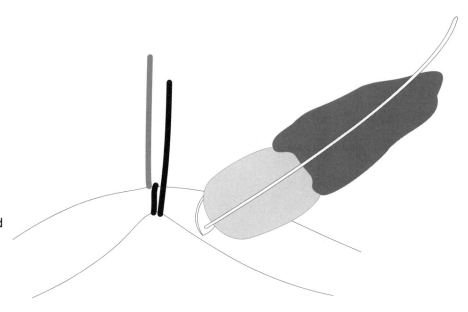

The vessel loop is then pulled
to prevent further blood loss.
The procedure is then
repeated until no further clot
is retrieved.

When performing thrombectomy of a prosthetic conduit, the vessel loop may not be strong enough to compress the graft. Control of the proximal bleeding and the catheter can be achieved using Fogarty vascular clamps. Alternatively, the graft is pinched with the fingers while advancing the embolectomy catheter to prevent excessive blood loss.

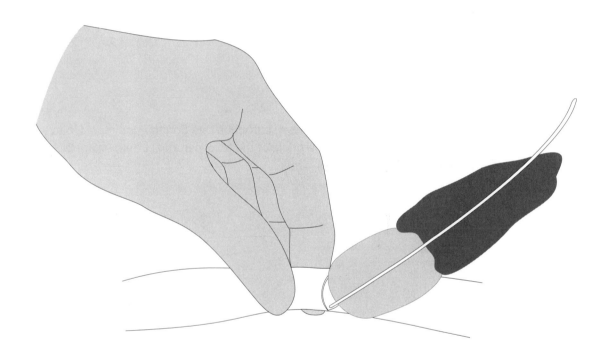

The thrombus is examined. The shape and form of the clot can provide an insight into the etiology of the occlusion. A stasis clot will have the shape of the vessel with the consistency of old clotted blood. A grayish granular thrombus is often seen with excessive platelet deposition. A whitish or darker piece of clot at the distal tip of the thrombus usually suggests an embolic process.

Thrombo–Embolectomy
Thrombo–Embolectomy of Lower Extremity Vessels

When performing a thrombo-embolectomy of the infrapopliteal vessels through a femoral arteriotomy, the catheter tends to repeatedly travel into the peroneal artery.

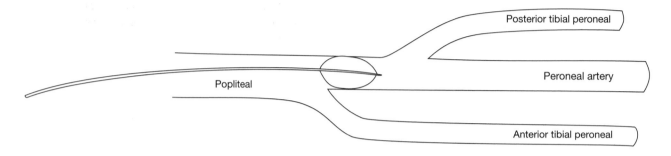

To introduce the catheter into the anterior tibial artery, introduce one Fogarty catheter. Under fluoroscopic guidance, place the catheter at the origin of the tibio-peroneal trunk; inflate the balloon. Introduce another catheter, with the tip slightly bent.

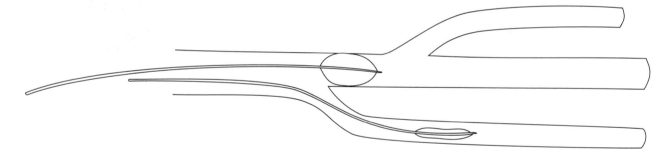

To introduce the catheter into the posterior tibial artery, place the first Fogarty catheter at the suspected origin of the peroneal artery. Introduce the second catheter after rotating it 180°.

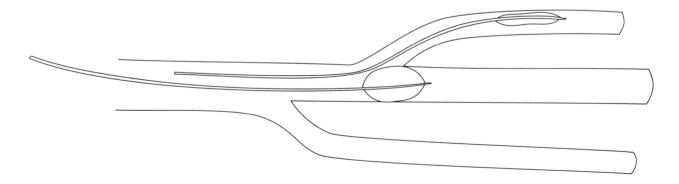

7

Endarterectomy

The histological examination of the cross section of the arterial wall will reveal three layers, the intima, the media, and the adventitia. The innermost layer is the intima, composed of the endothelium and the internal elastic lamina. The endothelium provides a smooth lining and has antithrombotic activity. The media is the inner layer of the arterial wall and is made of layers of smooth muscle cells oriented in longitudinal and circular directions. These layers are surrounded by basal lamina, collagen and elastin fibers. The main role of the media is to regulate blood vessel resistance by constricting and controlling the vessel lumen. The adventitia is the outermost layer and contains the vasovasorum, which provides blood supply to the wall. In addition, it has a collagenous matrix that provides the artery's tensile strength. The purpose of an endarterectomy is to remove an obstructive atherosclerotic plaque from the arterial lumen. This usually results in removing the thickened intima and inner media, leaving behind the outer part of the media and the adventitia. The plaque can be removed by opening the vessel longitudinally and then separating the plaque from the vessel wall (open endarterectomy; Section 1a).

OPEN ENDARTERECTOMY

When performing an open endarterectomy, being in the right plane is very important. Start by holding the edge of the adventitia with a pickup and pulling it away from the plaque. A plane will then develop. Using the Freer elevator, the adventitial wall is pushed away from the plaque. The endarterectomy plane is developed on each side of the vessel wall and advanced posteriorly until it becomes circumferential. On the proximal end, when a normal part of the artery is reached, the plaque is transected flush with the arterial wall without leaving any significant protruding ledge. On the distal end, if a normal segment of the artery is reached, an attempt is made to move the endarterectomy plane to a more superficial level. This usually allows terminating the endarterectomy with a smooth endpoint. Remaining circular fibers of the media can be gently and meticulously peeled off.

TACKING THE ENDARTERECTOMY ENDPOINT

If the disease extends beyond the level where the endarterectomy needs to end, transecting the plaque will create a shelf at the endpoint of the endarterectomy. When prograde flow is resumed, this shelf could lift up and create a dissection

157

or an acute thrombosis. If a smooth transition cannot be achieved at the distal endarterectomy endpoint, the shelf of thickened intima or remaining plaque should be fixed to the vessel wall by "tacking" sutures (Section 1b). This is achieved by placing sutures in the endarterectomized and nonendarterectomized vessel wall segment to prevent separation of the adventitia from the remaining of the arterial wall. Start by placing the suture 0.5–1 mm from the edge of the endarterectomy in the nonendarterectomized segment. This suture should always be placed from the inside of the intima towards the adventitial side to prevent separation of the intima. Place the other suture very close to the edge of the endarterectomy. This suture is also placed from the inside to the outside. Continue by placing several similar sutures almost 3–4 mm apart. Each suture is then tied separately. Great attention should be given to having the appropriate amount of tension on the sutures while tying. Excessive tension can result in tearing of the suture through the intima and media in the nonendarterectomized segment of the wall. Heparinized saline irrigation is then used to test the wall of the artery to check for any area that can still be at risk for lifting up, causing an intimal flap or dissection.

EVERSION ENDARTERECTOMY

When the plaque is removed by everting the vessel wall and pushing the plaque out without opening the vessel longitudinally over the plaque, the procedure is called eversion endarterectomy (Section 2). Semiclosed endarterectomy refers to the procedure where an incision is performed proximally and distally in an artery. The plaque in the vessel segment between the arteriotomies is removed using special instruments known as plaque strippers. Currently, semiclosed endarterectomy is infrequently performed and will not be reviewed in this chapter.

Open Endarterectomy

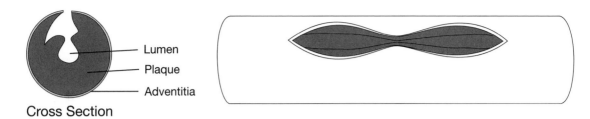

Cross Section

Lumen
Plaque
Adventitia

Incise the artery longitudinally through the plaque until a normal part of the artery is reached.

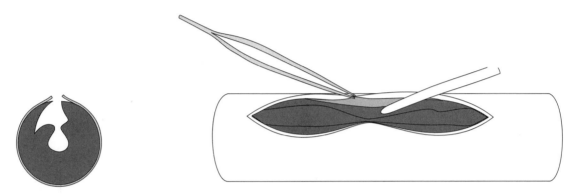

Hold the edge of the adventitia and gently lift it away from the plaque. Use the Freer elevator to identify the correct plane of endarterectomy.

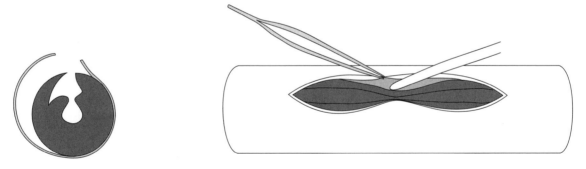

Continue separating the plaque from the adventitia by gently pushing the adventitial wall away from the plaque.

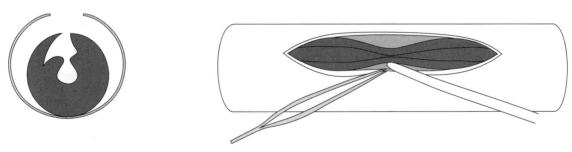

Repeat the same maneuver from the other side of the arteriotomy.

Open Endarterectomy

Pass a right-angle clamp underneath the plaque.

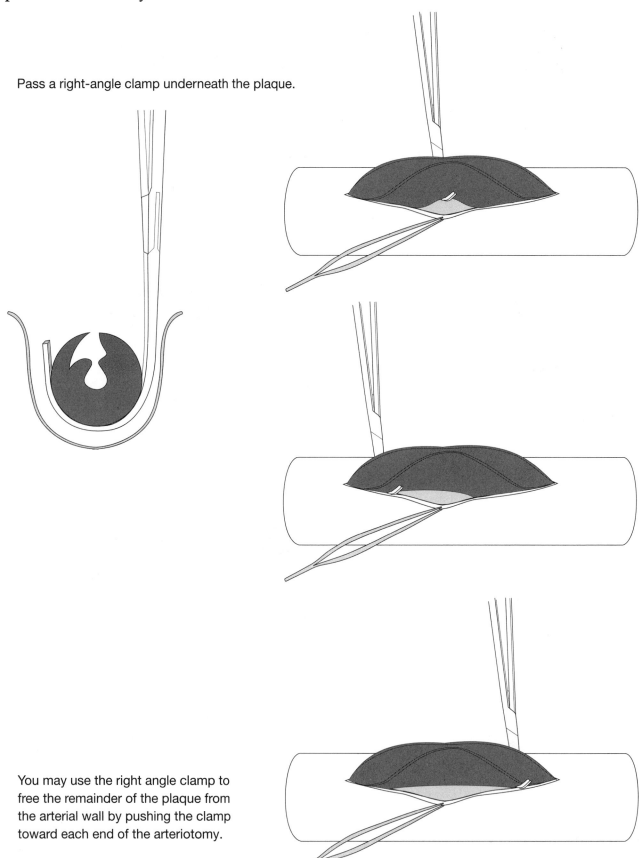

You may use the right angle clamp to free the remainder of the plaque from the arterial wall by pushing the clamp toward each end of the arteriotomy.

Open Endarterectomy
Tacking Sutures

At the level of the distal endpoint, changing the endarterectomy plane into a more superficial one can help in providing a smooth, well-feathered endpoint.

A 15 blade may be used to transect the plaque.

Start by carefully incising the intima at the desired level.

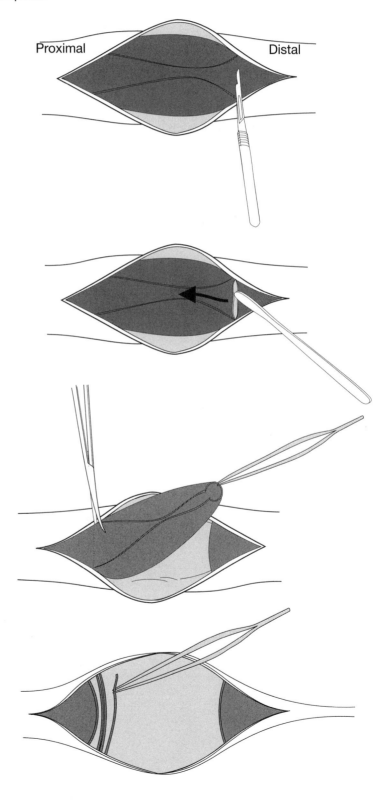

Use the Freer elevator to separate the plaque. Push with the Freer elevator using a sweeping motion toward the proximal endpoint.

Alternatively, you may use the scissors to transect the plaque. Care is taken to avoid leaving an edge of plaque protruding at the endpoint.

Remaining circular fibers are individually peeled off.

Open Endarterectomy
Tacking Sutures

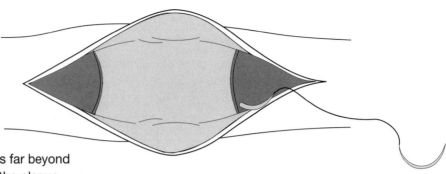

Occasionally, the plaque extends far beyond the arteriotomy. Transection of the plaque may result in an edge that could lift, causing dissection or thrombosis. Tacking the endarterectomy endpoint may be necessary.

Introduce the needle inside out, 1 mm from the edge of the endarterectomy.

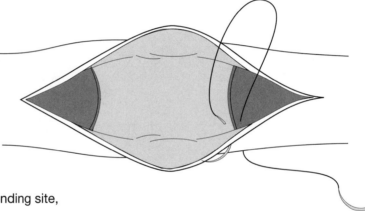

Introduce the needle in a corresponding site, 1 mm from the edge, again inside-out.

Place multiple sutures.

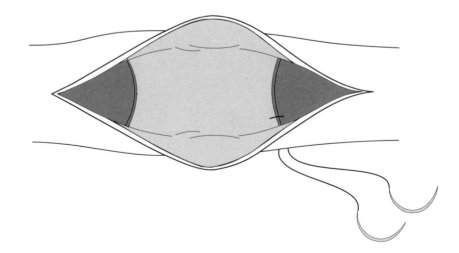

Open Endarterectomy
Tacking Sutures

Tacking of the proximal endpoint is rarely needed.

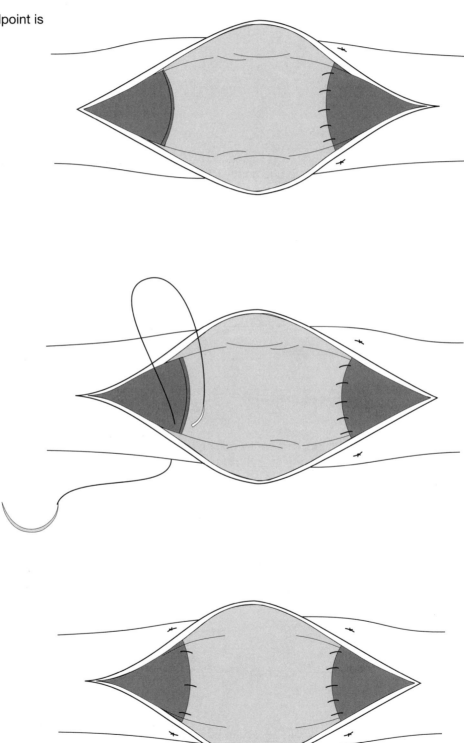

Eversion Endarterectomy

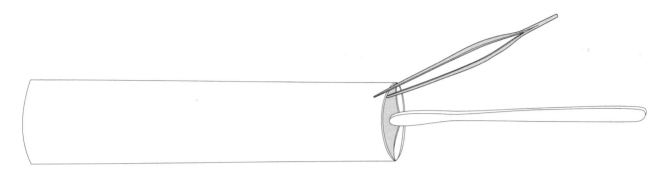

Hold the adventitia with a pickup and gently lift it away from the plaque. Use a Freer elevator to circumferentially dissect the plaque.

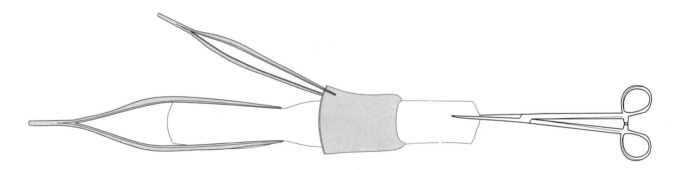

Hold the plaque with a clamp, and gently pull on the plaque while everting the adventitial wall in the opposite direction.

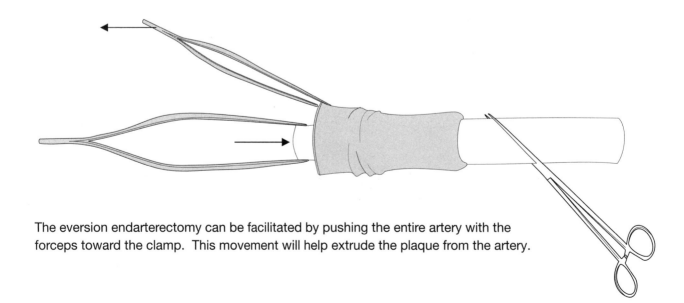

The eversion endarterectomy can be facilitated by pushing the entire artery with the forceps toward the clamp. This movement will help extrude the plaque from the artery.

II

Basic Vascular Reconstructions

8

Closure of an Arteriotomy

An incision in an artery (arteriotomy) can be closed either primarily or with a patch. In a primary closure, the edges of the arterial walls are approximated and sutured directly to each other. In a patch closure, also known as patch angioplasty, a patch is used to bridge the defect between the edges of the incision. The choice of the closure method depends on various factors. These factors include the size of the artery, the direction and the shape of the arteriotomy, and the presence of atherosclerotic plaque at the arteriotomy site.

PRIMARY CLOSURE OF A TRANSVERSE ARTERIOTOMY

Primary closure is a simple and expeditious method of closing an arteriotomy. Most transverse arteriotomies in nondiseased arteries can be closed primarily even in small arteries of 1.5–2.0 mm diameter such as the radial artery or the posterior tibial artery. Similarly, most longitudinal incisions in nondiseased arteries with a diameter greater than 5 mm such as the common carotid artery or the common femoral artery can be closed primarily. However, some degree of narrowing of the lumen is likely to occur with primary closure. Such narrowing could threaten the patency of the reconstruction especially in longitudinal incisions. Thus, whenever there is concern that primary closure will compromise the lumen, patch closure should be considered.

Primary closure is usually performed using a continuous running suture technique (Section 1a). The needle is first introduced from the adventitial surface of one wall and then from the intimal surface of the opposite wall. It is important that the arterial wall at the incision site be free of plaque. Otherwise, as the needle is being passed from the adventitial surface, the needle tip can push the plaque away from the arterial wall and create a nidus for thrombus formation or dissection. Thus, primary closure with continuous sutures is most suitable in normal or minimally diseased arteries. Other applications for primary closure include veins, vein bypasses, prosthetic bypasses, and endarterectomized arteries. The depth and advancement of the bites should be even throughout the length of the suture line. Bites placed inappropriately deep could result in a focal narrowing of the lumen.

Even in the presence of significant plaque at an arteriotomy site, primary closure may still be possible without causing plaque separation from the arterial wall. This may be achieved by using an interrupted suture technique (Section 1b). This technique will allow introducing all the needles from the intimal surface of each wall of the incision, thus pinning the thickened intima to the arterial wall. Placement of deep bites may be necessary to penetrate the arterial wall.

PATCH CLOSURE OF A LONGITUDINAL ARTERIOTOMY

Patch closure is usually utilized in situations where primary closure is likely to cause luminal narrowing or thrombosis. (1) These situations are determined by both technical and nontechnical factors. The technical factors include a jagged incision, a very tortuous artery, a longitudinal incision in an artery smaller than 5 mm in diameter, and the presence of calcified plaque at the arteriotomy site. If the edges of the vessel wall cannot be approximated because of scarring or the presence of a large defect in the vessel wall secondary to trauma or debridement, a patch closure becomes necessary. Furthermore, obstructing pathology that cannot be excised from the vessel wall, such as neointimal hyperplasia or residual plaque, requires closure with a patch. Nontechnical factors suggesting the need for patch closure include uncontrollable risk factors for atherosclerosis such as hyperlipidemia, heavy smoking, female gender, and a history of recurrent stenosis. In patch closure, the needle can be introduced constantly from the adventitial aspect of the patch and then from the intimal aspect of the arterial wall. This avoids the possibility of pushing a plaque fragment into the lumen and precipitating thrombosis or dissection. Patch closure will allow placing good-size bites in the patch and in the artery without compromising the lumen. However, careful bite placement is still required, especially at the apices where improperly placed bites can cause undesirable luminal narrowing. Furthermore, with patch closure, the width of the patch should be well selected. Aneurysmal dilatation at the reconstruction site could occur when the width of the patch significantly exceeds the diameter of the vessel to be repaired.

Patch closure is performed using either an anchor technique or a parachute technique. In the anchor technique, the initial suture is tied down, thus anchoring and stabilizing the patch for the placement of the remaining bites (Section 2a). The simplest method is to start an anchoring suture at one apex, and to place another anchoring suture at the other apex after trimming the patch to the appropriate length. The anchoring suture can be a simple or horizontal mattress suture. The horizontal mattress suture helps to evert the suture line. In small- and medium-size vessels, it is prudent to avoid placing wide horizontal mattress sutures at the apex to avoid narrowing the lumen.

In the parachute technique, several bites are initially placed without pulling down the suture (Section 2b). This technique is particularly helpful when the arteriotomy is in a deep location. The patch is held a few centimeters away from the artery. After placing five or six bites in the patch and in the artery, each end of the suture will be pulled simultaneously while the patch is brought down toward the incision like a parachute. Gentle tension should be applied to each end of the suture because rough handling could result in the suture line cutting through the arterial wall, especially in thin vessels. The starting suture in the parachute technique is usually a horizontal mattress suture. The suture line can be started at the apex, a few bites off the apex, or a combination of both (Section 2b).

REFERENCES

1. De Bakey ME, Crawford ES, Morris GC, Cooley DA. Patch graft angioplasty in vascular surgery. J Cardiovasc Surg 1976;131:452.

Primary Closure of a Transverse Arteriotomy
Continuous Sutures

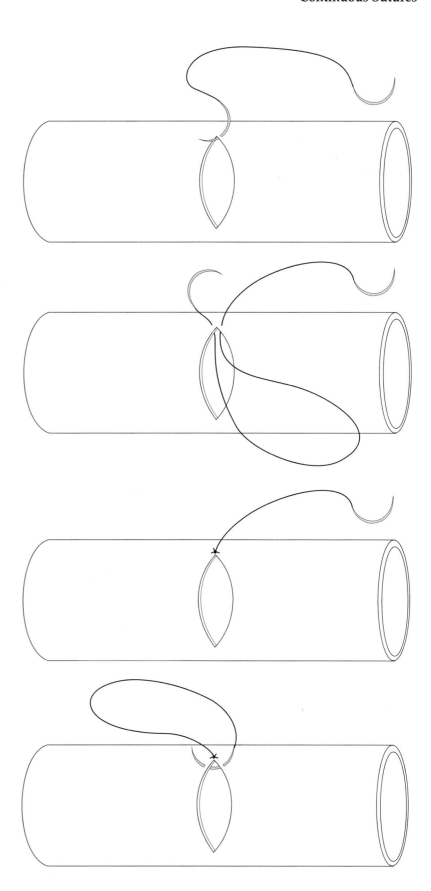

Introduce the needle
from the adventitial side
of the arterial wall.

Introduce the needle
from the intimal side
of the arterial wall.

Tie the suture and cut
one end.

Start running the suture
towards the midpoint of
the arteriotomy.

Primary Closure of a Transverse Arteriotomy
Continuous Sutures

You may continue
running the suture all
the way towards the
end of the arteriotomy.

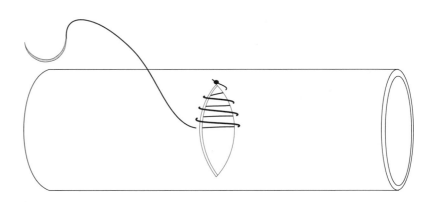

Place the last two
bites closely spaced.

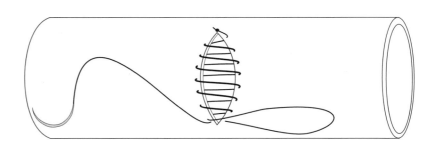

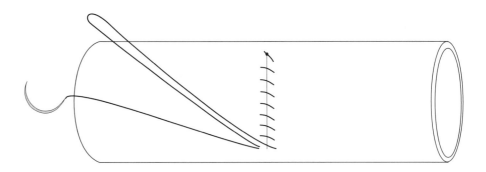

Pull the suture and
tie it to itself.

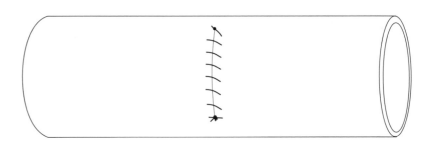

Primary Closure of a Transverse Arteriotomy
Continuous Sutures

Alternatively, you may start another suture at the other end of the arteriotomy to avoid the need to tie the suture to itself.

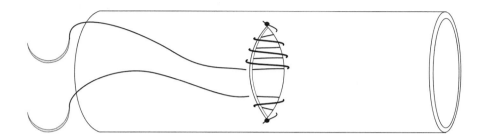

Run the second suture towards the midpoint of the arteriotomy.

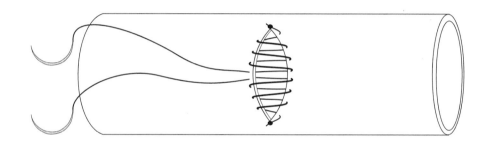

Tie both sutures.

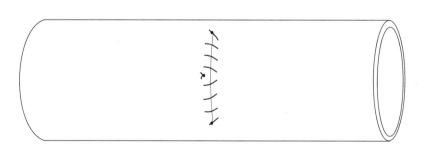

Primary Closure of a Transverse Arteriotomy
Interrupted Sutures

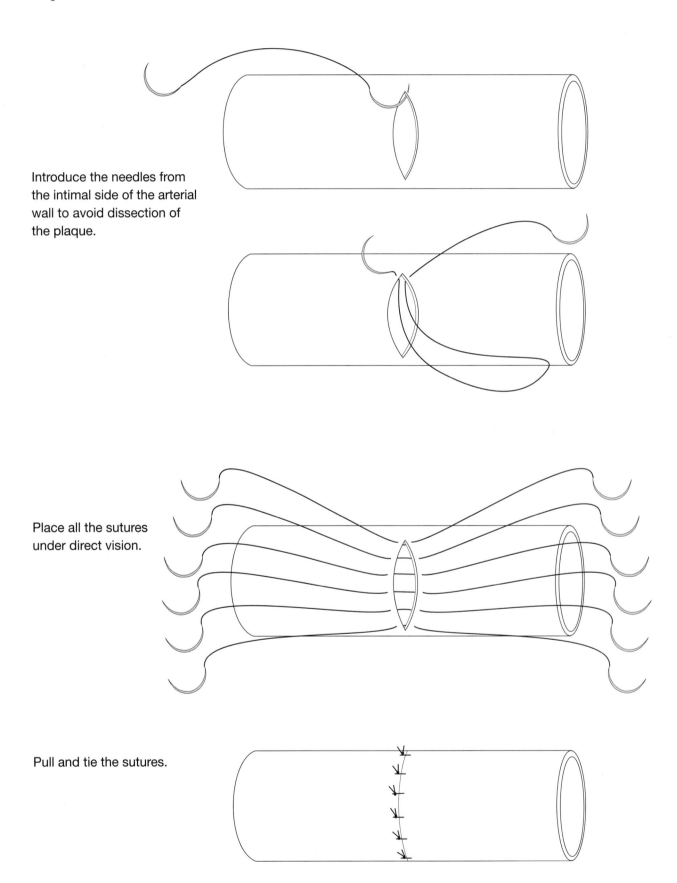

Introduce the needles from the intimal side of the arterial wall to avoid dissection of the plaque.

Place all the sutures under direct vision.

Pull and tie the sutures.

Patch Closure of a Longitudinal Arteriotomy
Anchor Technique

Start by placing a suture at the apex. This suture may be a horizontal mattress or a simple suture as shown here.

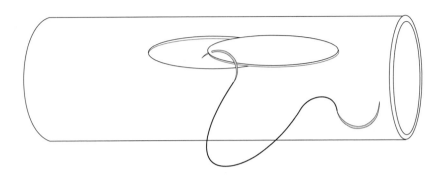

The needle should be introduced from the adventitial side of the patch and from the intimal side of the artery.

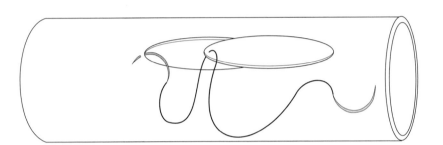

After ensuring that both sides are of equal length, tie the suture. Three throws are usually sufficient.

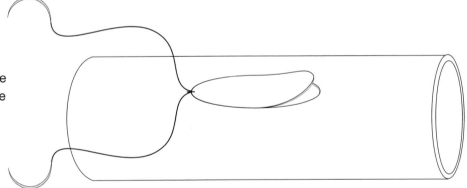

Start suturing with one end. The needle should penetrate from the adventitial side of the patch and then from the intimal side of the artery.

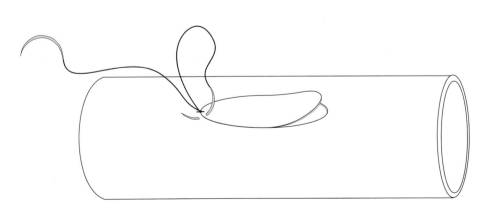

Patch Closure of a Longitudinal Arteriotomy
Anchor Technique

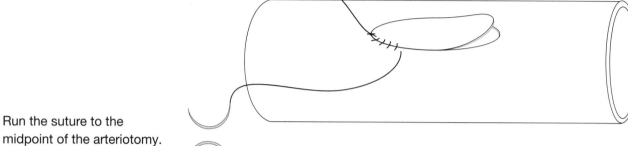

Run the suture to the midpoint of the arteriotomy.

Similarly, run the other end of the suture to the midpoint of the arteriotomy.

Again, the needle should penetrate outside-inside in the patch and inside-outside in the artery.

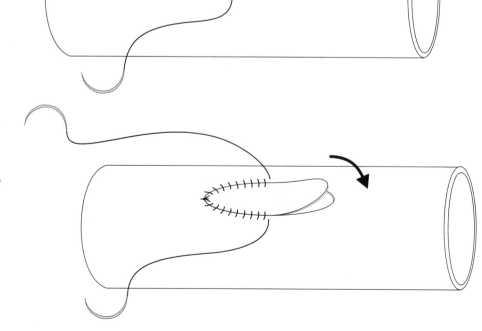

Patch Closure of a Longitudinal Arteriotomy
Anchor Technique

You may continue running this suture until you reach the other end.

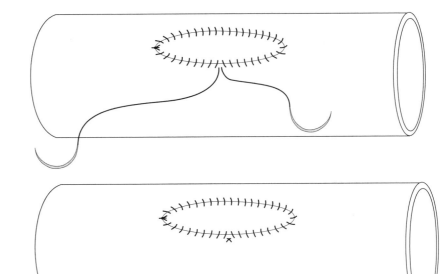

Tie both ends.

Alternatively, after suturing one half of the patch, you may start another suture at the opposite end. This suture may be a simple or a horizontal mattress suture as shown here.

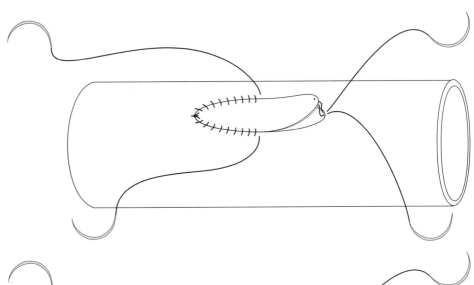

Tie the suture.

In small vessels, it is preferable not to place a wide horizontal mattress suture at the apex to avoid puckering or narrowing the lumen at the apex.

Patch Closure of a Longitudinal Arteriotomy
Anchor Technique

Begin suturing with one end. Again, outside-inside in the patch, inside-outside in the artery.

Run one end of the suture to the midpoint of the patch.

Tie both sutures.

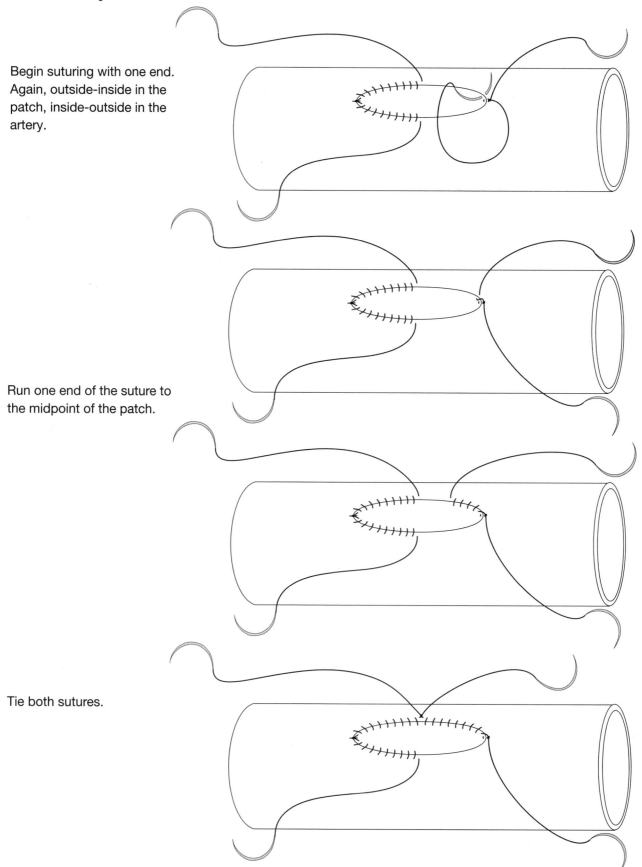

Patch Closure of a Longitudinal Arteriotomy
Anchor Technique

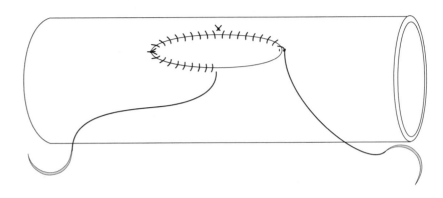

Run the other end of the suture in the other direction to the midpoint of the arteriotomy.

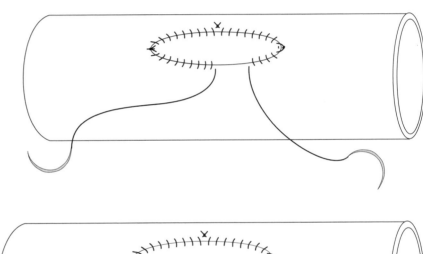

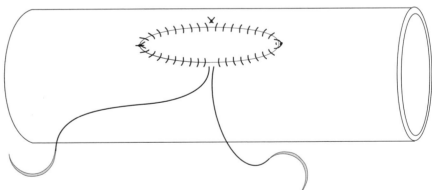

Tie both sutures.

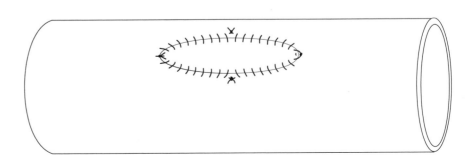

Patch Closure of a Longitudinal Arteriotomy
Parachute Technique

You may start at the apex or a few bites off the apex, as shown here.

Introduce the needle in the patch three bites away from the apex, outside-inside in the patch.

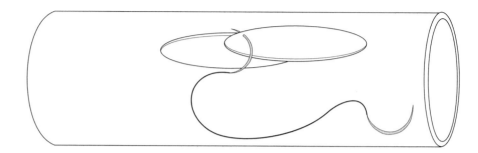

Introduce the needle in a corresponding location inside-outside in the artery.

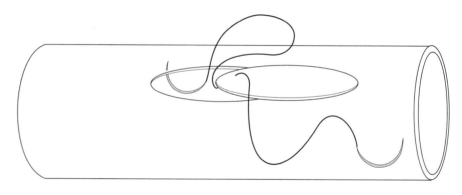

Continue suturing until you have placed three bites past the apex.

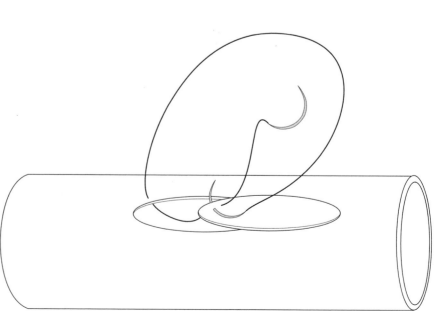

Patch Closure of a Longitudinal Arteriotomy
Parachute Technique

Pull down the suture and the patch.

Placing more than three bites on each side of the apex could create difficulty in pulling and tightening the suture line.

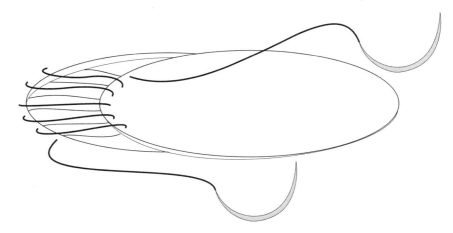

Enlarged view of the suture line before being pulled.

Pulling the loop at the center of the apex with a nerve hook could facilitate tightening the suture line.

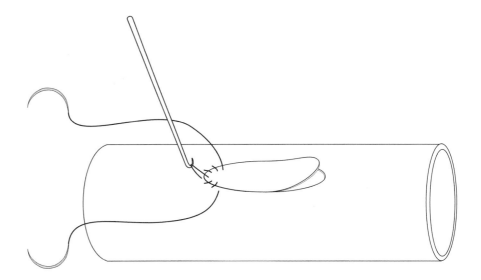

Continue suturing until you reach the middle of the arteriotomy.

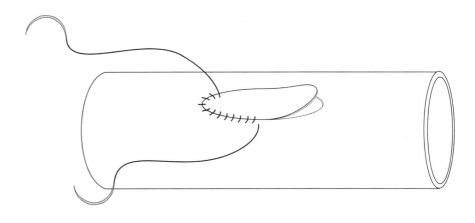

Patch Closure of a Longitudinal Arteriotomy
Parachute Technique

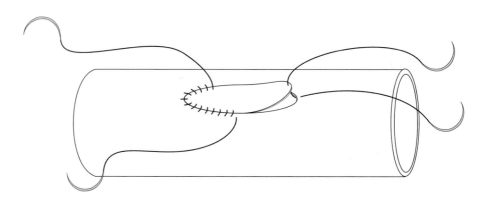

The next suture can be started a few bites off the apex or at the apex as shown here.

Again, introduce the needle outside-inside in the patch, inside-outside in the artery.

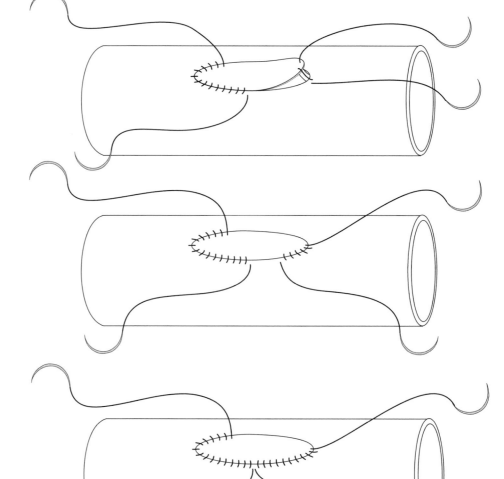

Run the suture on one side until it meets the previous suture.

Tie both sutures.

Patch Closure of a Longitudinal Arteriotomy
Parachute Technique

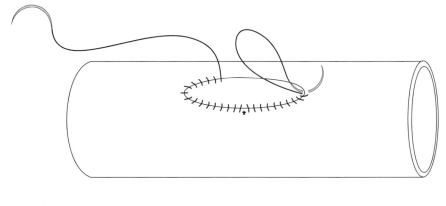

Start suturing with the other end. The needle is first introduced outside-inside in the patch, and then inside-outside in the artery. This first suture should be placed very close to the previous one, as it will become a horizontal mattress suture.

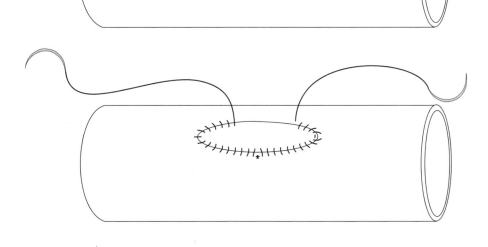

Continue suturing towards the remaining suture.

Tie both sutures.

9

End-to-Side Anastomosis

In most bypasses performed for occlusive disease, the proximal and distal anastomoses are constructed in an end-to-side fashion. Such a configuration allows for constructing the proximal anastomosis in the least diseased area of the inflow vessel while maintaining the original circulation. The distal anastomosis is constructed distal to any occlusive pathology and provides both antegrade and retrograde blood flow. The revascularization provided by the end-to-side configuration protects the limb from ischemia between the proximal and distal anastomoses. This condition, often referred to as "interval ischemia," is more likely to occur when both anastomoses are constructed using an end-to-end configuration.

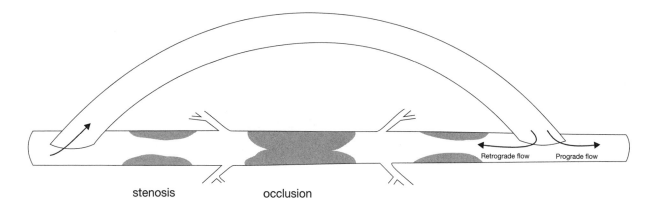

stenosis   occlusion

GEOMETRY OF AN END-TO-SIDE ANASTOMOSIS

The geometry of an end-to-side anastomosis depends on the diameters of the bypass and the artery and the length of the anastomosis, which will influence the angle of transection of the bypass. The ideal dimensions of an end-to-side anastomosis are ill defined as is the optimal length of an anastomosis. Because the diameter of the recipient artery cannot be changed, the geometry of an end-to-side anastomosis depends greatly on the length of the arteriotomy.

The length of the proximal anastomosis of an infrainguinal bypass usually varies from 1 to 2 cm. Some surgeons recommend that the length of the distal anastomosis should be twice the bypass diameter. (3) Others recommend an arteriotomy greater than 2 cm (4) or creation of an arteriotomy 2–4 times the diameter of the recipient popliteal artery and 10–20 times the diameter of the recipient infrapopliteal artery. (5) Other surgeons prefer creating a relatively short arteriotomy 1–1.5 cm in length to avoid having to sew a long anastomotic

suture line, especially in a diseased small-diameter tibial artery. (1) A short arteriotomy 4–6 mm in length is usually recommended for a coronary artery vein
bypass. (2) In a vein bypass, technical imperfections may be more responsible
than the geometry of the anastomosis for the development of distal anastomotic
stenotic pathology. (1) The end-to-side reconstruction can be carried using either
an anchor technique (Section 1) or a parachute technique (Section 2).

END-TO-SIDE ANASTOMOSIS: ANCHOR TECHNIQUE

In the anchor technique, the anastomosis is usually constructed by first placing
a suture at the heel. The suture is tied down, anchoring and stabilizing the bypass. The suture is then run in a continuous manner on either side of the heel.
Frequently, another suture is then started at the apex and tied. The apical suture
is run in a continuous manner on either side of the apex to complete the anastomosis. This technique can be ideal for large vessels, especially if they are not in
deep locations.

An end-to-side anastomosis can have numerous variations. When the anchor
technique is used, the sutures at the apex and the heel can be simple (Section
1a) or horizontal mattress sutures (Section 1b). The horizontal mattress sutures
may help in everting the suture line. However, in small vessels, wide horizontal
mattress sutures at the apex or the heel can cause narrowing of the lumen.

Another variation in the anchor technique relates to the apical part of the
anastomosis where interrupted sutures are used instead of a continuous suture
(Section 1c). This variation may have some theoretical advantages in very small
vessels by allowing the anastomosis to stretch with arterial pulsations and not
be limited by the length of the continuous suture.

Another variation in the anchor technique relates to the location of the initial
anchoring suture, which usually depends on the surgeon's preference. In this
variation, instead of placing the anchoring suture at the center of the heel, the
suture is started mid distance between the apex and the heel (Section 1d). In
this method, suturing around the heel may be technically demanding. In addition, it is important in this variation that the distance from the heel to the anchoring suture is well matched between the bypass and the arteriotomy to
prevent any torsion at the heel of the anastomosis.

Another variation in the anchor technique utilizes staples for constructing
the anastomosis (Section 1e). The role of this evolving technology is yet undetermined. This technique may offer some advantages with respect to expediency and minimizing the bleeding from needle holes, especially with
polytetrafluoroethylene grafts. However, when dealing with small veins and
arteries the precision achieved with suturing cannot yet be duplicated with the
current generation of staples available.

END-TO-SIDE ANASTOMOSIS: PARACHUTE TECHNIQUE

The parachute technique differs from the anchor technique in that the sutures at
the heel and the apex are not pulled down initially. Thus, the bypass is still a
few centimeters away from the arteriotomy and should not obscure the placement of the heel and apical sutures. Several bites are first placed in the bypass
and the arteriotomy. Tension is then gently applied on either end of the suture.
The bypass is advanced toward the arteriotomy as the suture line is tightened
at each end in a seesaw fashion. It is important to note that if more than five
bites are placed before "parachuting" the bypass, pulling on each end of the suture may not result in a tight suture line. A useful maneuver in this situation is
the use of a nerve hook to pull up on the loop at the center of the heel. Tension

on either side of the suture will then successfully tighten the suture line. Excessive tension and rough manipulation of the suture line could result in cutting of the suture line through the vessel wall.

The parachute technique is especially useful if the vessels are small or in a deep location. In such situations, visualization of the first few bites at the apex and the heel may be suboptimal. Better visualization and placement of the sutures at the heel and the apex can be facilitated by the use of the parachute technique. Furthermore, if an autogenous bypass is in spasm following transection, the anastomosis may be initially under slight tension. In this situation and especially in thin small vessels, using a parachute technique could distribute the tension over several bites and prevent the possibility of the suture tearing through the vessel wall.

In the parachute technique, the main variation relates to the site where the suture is started. The suture may be started exactly at the center of the heel or a few bites off the center of the heel. Starting the suture at the center of the heel and the apex (Section 2a) is the simpler method and may allow for a better appreciation of the size match between the arteriotomy and the transected vessel. In addition, it may avoid the possibility of uneven advancement between the different sides of the anastomosis.

Starting a few bites away from the center of the heel (Section 2b) may be more challenging when first learning the technique, with possible entanglement of the suture line. However, once past the learning curve, this technique could facilitate the placement of the difficult heel sutures in a continuous forward movement. Infrequently, the graft is in a location that does not allow flipping the graft around the heel. In this situation, constructing the entire posterior wall of the anastomosis first may be necessary (Section 2c).

Additional variations in the end-to-side anastomosis include using an anchor technique for the heel portion and a parachute technique for the apical portion or vice versa. These variations are usually dictated by individual circumstances. For example, the exposure may be such that the heel portion of the anastomosis is more suitable for reconstruction with a parachute technique while the apical portion of the anastomosis is more amenable to construction with an anchor technique or vice versa.

When constructing an anastomosis to a heavily calcified vessel, the needle tip may become dull from repeated impacts against the calcified plaque. Starting new sutures may be necessary to provide a sharp needle point that can penetrate the calcified plaque without tearing the vessel wall.

REFERENCES

1. Hoballah JJ, Mohan CR, Chalmers RTA, Schueppert MT, Sharp WJ, Kresowik TF, Corson JD. Does the geometry of a distal anastomosis affect patency? Vasc Surg; 1996;30(5):371
2. Kirklin JW, Barratt-Boyes BG. Ischemic heart disease. In: Cardiac Surgery, 2nd Ed. New York: Churchill-Livingstone, 1993:309.
3. Rutherford RB. Atlas of Vascular Surgery: Basic Techniques and Exposures. Philadelphia: Saunders, 1993:48–49.
4. Sotturai VS, Batson RC. Use of nonreversed, translocated saphenous vein graft. In: Bergan JJ, Yao JST (eds): Techniques in Arterial Surgery. Philadelphia: Saunders, 1990:184–191.
5. Taylor LM, Porter JM. Technique of reversed vein bypass to distal leg arteries. In: Bergan JJ, Yao JST (eds): Techniques in Arterial Surgery. Philadelphia: Saunders, 1990:109–121.

Anchor Technique
Simple Anchoring Sutures

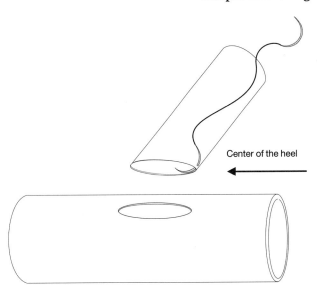

Create an incision in the artery. Transect the graft in a beveled fashion to match the size of the arteriotomy.

Start at the center of the heel. Introduce the needle outside-inside in the graft.

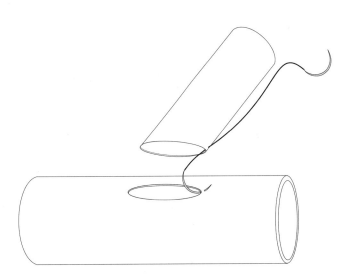

Introduce the needle in a matching location in the artery (inside-outside). This suture may be a horizontal mattress suture or a simple suture as shown here.

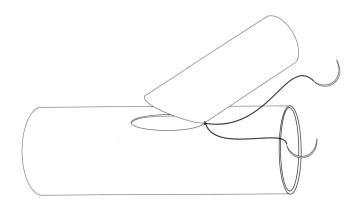

Tie the suture. Three throws are usually sufficient.

Anchor Technique
Simple Anchoring Sutures

Continue with one end of the suture. Introduce the needle in the graft.

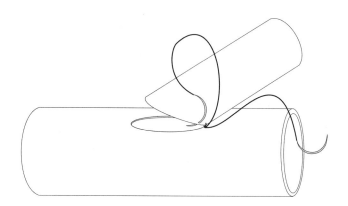

Introduce the needle in the artery. Very often the first few bites after tying down the suture will need to be placed separately in the graft and then in the artery to ensure ideal placement.

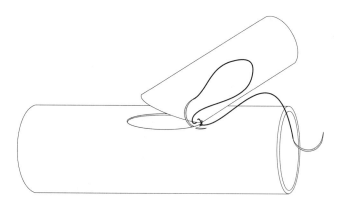

Place several sutures on one side.

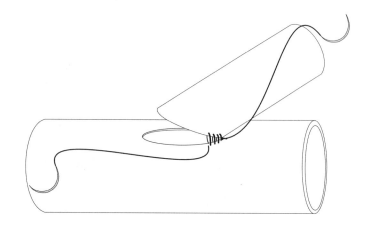

Anchor Technique
Simple Anchoring Sutures

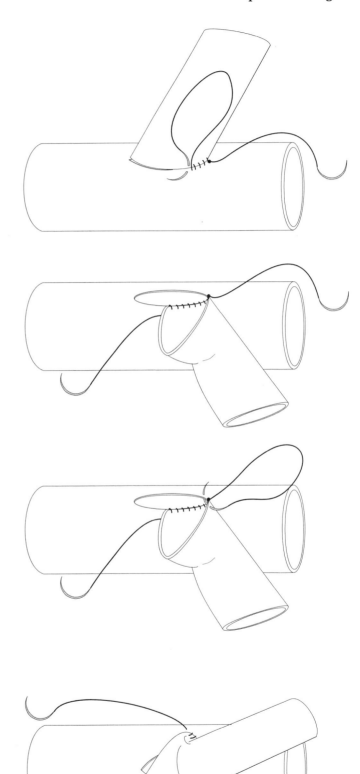

Tighten the sutures. At this stage, you may be able to suture the graft and the artery together in a single bite.

Flip the graft to the other side.

Start suturing on this side. Again, introduce the needle from the adventitial side of the graft and then from the intimal side of the artery.

Place several bites.

Anchor Technique
Simple Anchoring Sutures

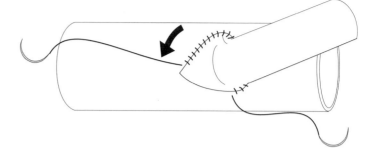

You may continue with the upper
suture and run it around the apex
until it meets the other end.

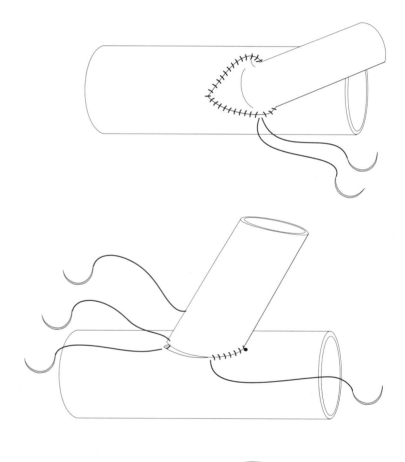

Alternatively, you may start a new
suture at the apex. The new suture
may be a horizontal mattress or a
simple suture as shown here.

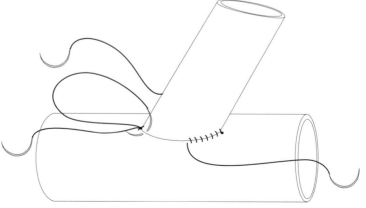

Tie the suture. Introduce the needle
from the adventitial side of the graft
and the intimal side of the artery.

Anchor Technique
Simple Anchoring Sutures

Place several more bites.

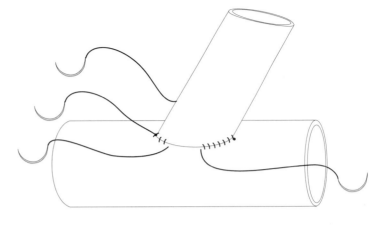

Run the suture line toward the heel until it meets the other suture.

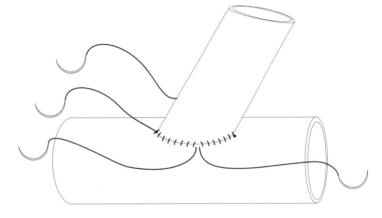

Tie both sutures together.

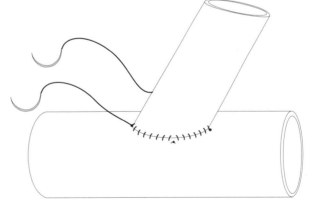

Flip the graft to the other side.

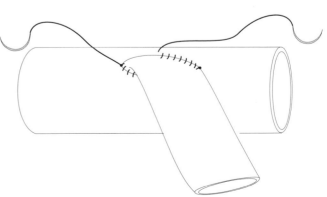

Anchor Technique
Simple Anchoring Sutures

Again, introduce the needle from the
adventitial side of the graft and the
intimal side of the artery.

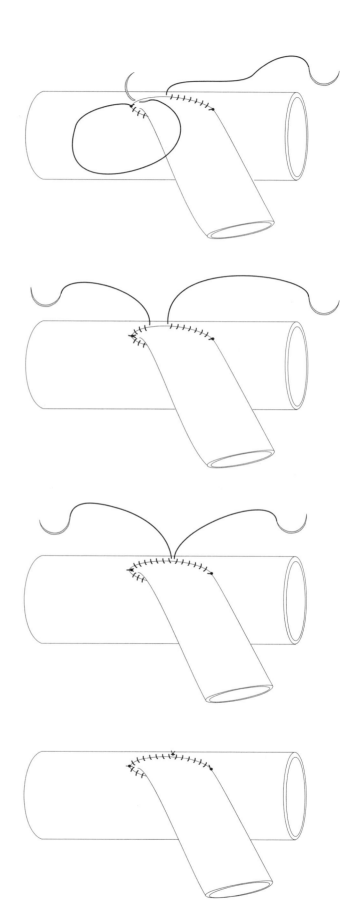

Place several more bites.

Run the suture line toward the heel
until it meets the other suture.

Tie the sutures.

Anchor Technique
Horizontal Mattress Anchoring Sutures

In this variation, the fixing sutures are horizontal mattress sutures.

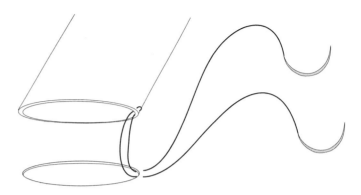

These mattress sutures may help fold the graft and the artery to achieve an everted suture line with an ideal intima-to-intima opposition.

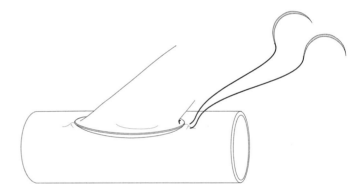

In small vessels, it is important to avoid taking wide horizontal mattress sutures at the toe or the heel, as they may cause puckering or narrowing of the lumen.

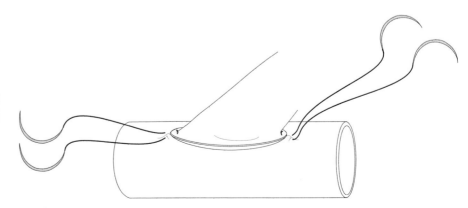

Anchor Technique
Construction of the Apex with Interrupted Sutures

Another variation is the construction of the toe portion of the anastomosis. In very small vessels, interrupted sutures may be used to construct the toe of the anastomosis. The interrupted sutures at the anastomosis may allow for expansion of the anastomosis with arterial pulsations.

Construct the heel as previously described.

Place one suture just proximal to the apex. Again, outside-inside in the graft, inside-outside in the artery.

Place another suture at the apex.

Anchor Technique
Construction of the Apex with Interrupted Sutures

Place a third suture distal to the apex.

Usually, three sutures are sufficient, however, additional interrupted sutures may be placed if deemed necessary.

Tie the sutures.

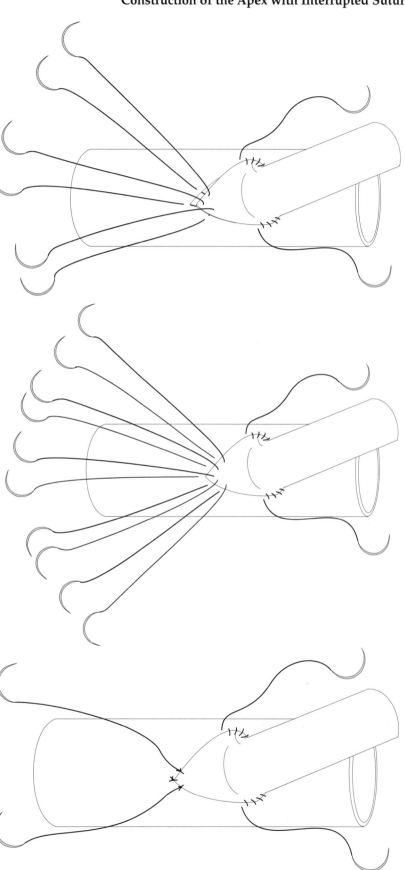

Anchor Technique
Construction of the Apex with Interrupted Sutures

Start suturing with one end.

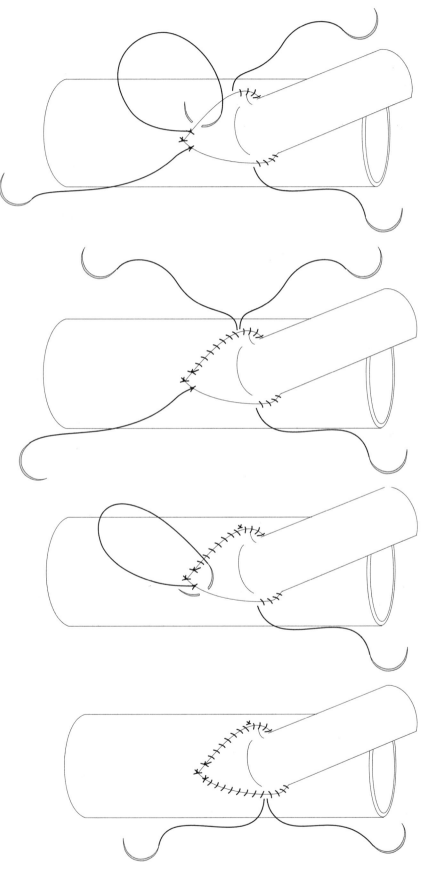

Run the suture until it reaches the heel suture.

Start suturing with the other end.

Run the suture toward the heel.

Anchor Technique
Anchoring Suture Starting Mid Distance Between the Apex and the Heel

Introduce the needle outside-inside in the graft mid distance between the apex and the heel.

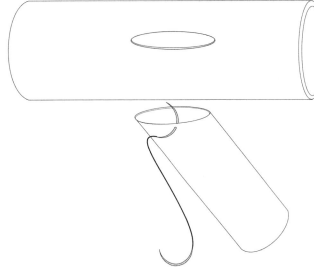

Introduce the needle in a corresponding site inside-outside in the artery.

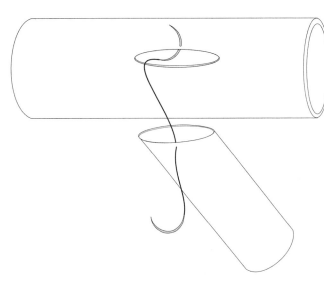

Tie the suture.

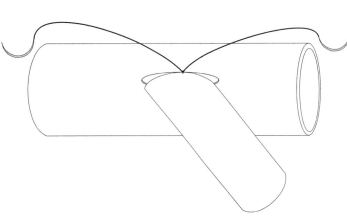

Anchor Technique
Anchoring Suture Starting Mid Distance Between the Apex and the Heel

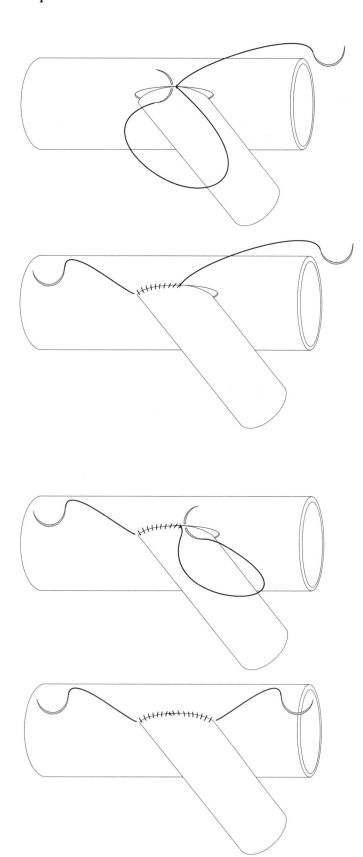

Run one end of the suture toward the apex.

The needle should penetrate from the adventitial side of the graft and the intimal side of the artery.

Run the other end toward the heel.

Anchor Technique
Anchoring Suture Starting Mid Distance Between the Apex and the Heel

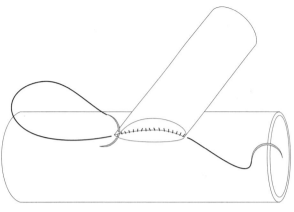

Flip the graft. Continue running the suture from the apex toward the heel.

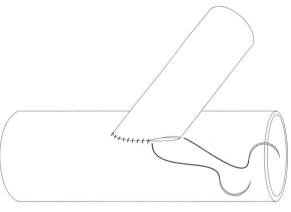

Resume suturing with the other end of the suture from the heel toward the apex.

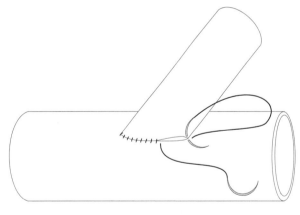

Anchor Technique
Stapled Anastomosis

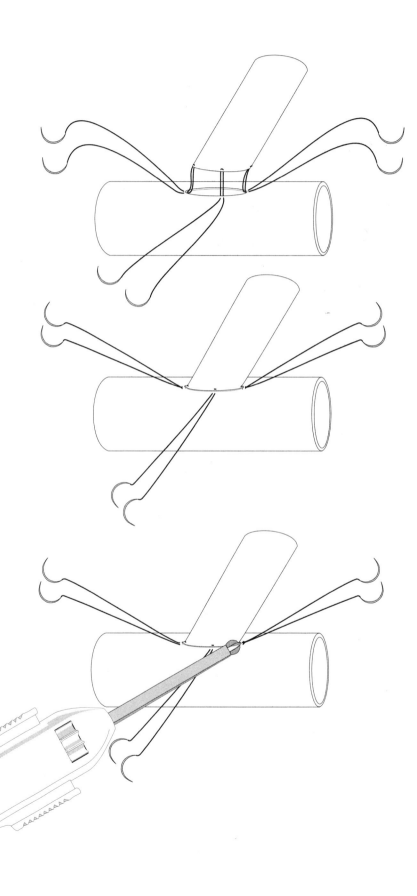

Place horizontal mattress sutures at the apex, heel, and the midpoint between the apex and the heel.

Pull and tie the sutures at the apex and the heel. The mattress sutures will help evert the suture line.

Use the heel suture as a handle. Pull on the suture and start stapling from the heel toward the apex.

Anchor Technique
Stapled Anastomosis

Continue stapling until you reach the middle stay suture. Using an everting forceps could be helpful in applying the staples.

Pull on the apical suture and start stapling at the apex.

Continue stapling toward the heel.

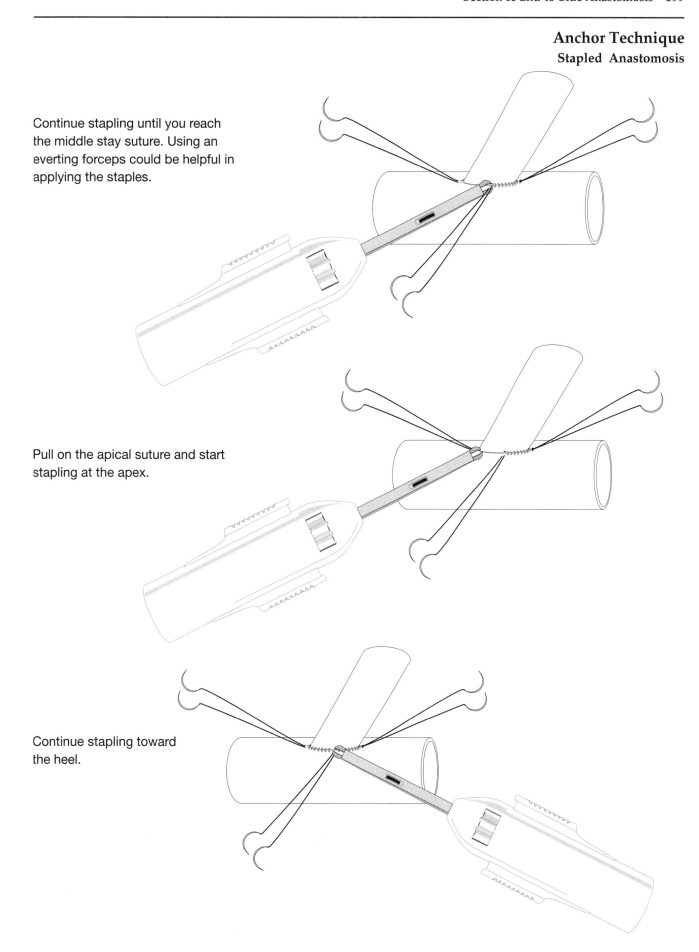

Anchor Technique
Stapled Anastomosis

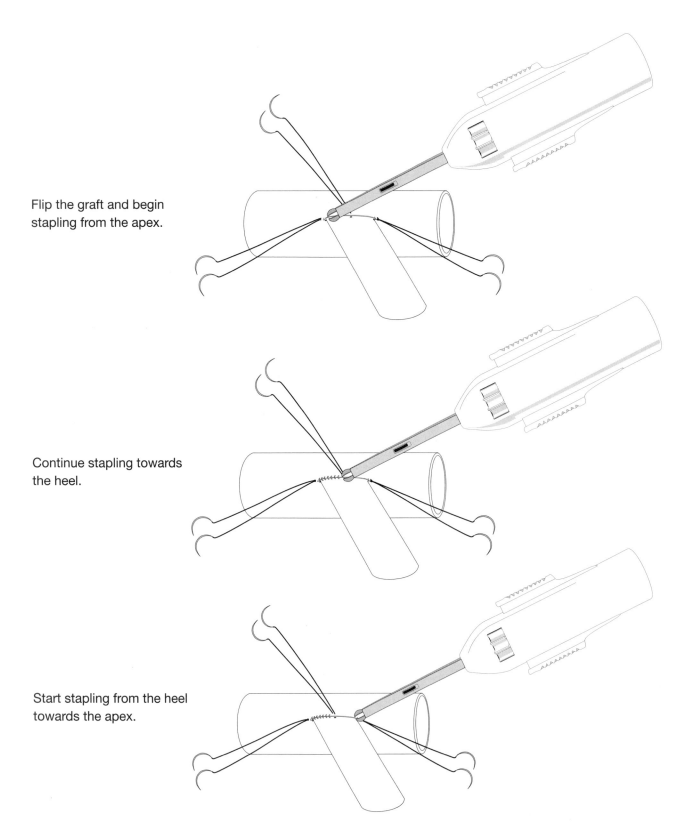

Flip the graft and begin stapling from the apex.

Continue stapling towards the heel.

Start stapling from the heel towards the apex.

Anchor Technique
Stapled Anastomosis

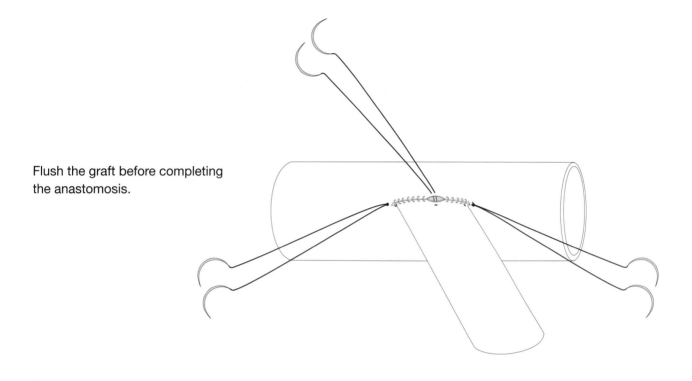

Flush the graft before completing the anastomosis.

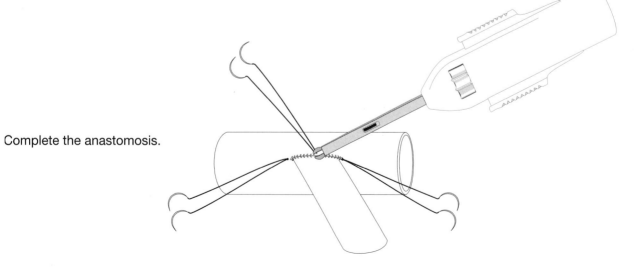

Complete the anastomosis.

Parachute Technique
Starting at the Center of the Heel

Start the suture at the center of the heel. Introduce the needle in the graft (outside-inside).

Introduce the needle in a matching location in the artery (inside-outside).

Progress with the suturing toward the apex.

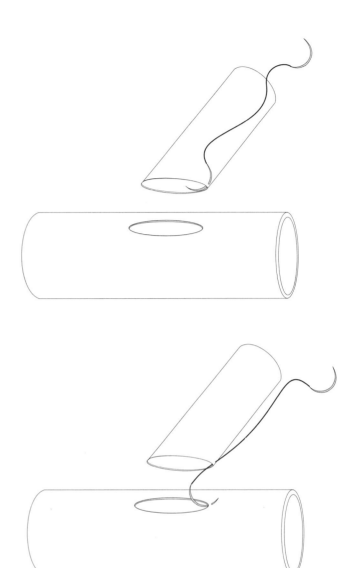
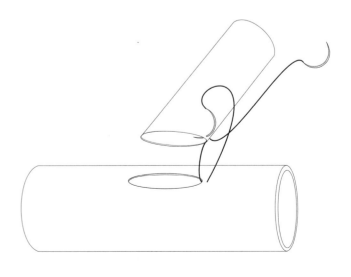

Parachute Technique
Starting at the Center of the Heel

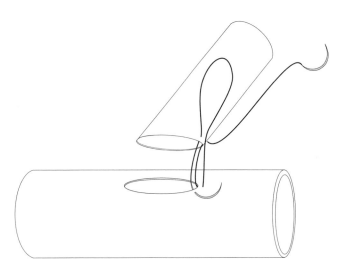

Continue suturing toward the apex
for a few bites.

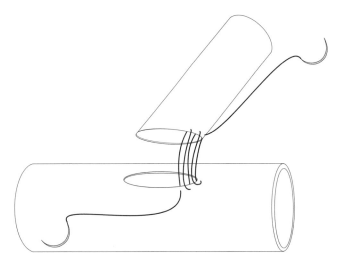

Flip the graft.

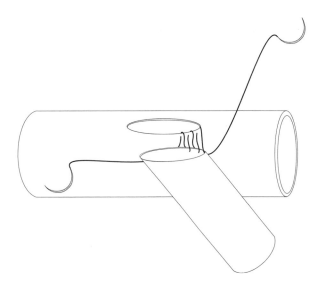

Parachute Technique
Starting at the Center of the Heel

Resume suturing at the center of
the heel. Introduce the needle
(outside-inside) in the graft. This
suture will be a horizontal mattress
suture.

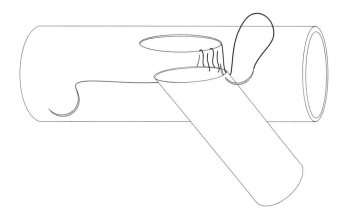

Introduce the needle in a matching
location in the artery.

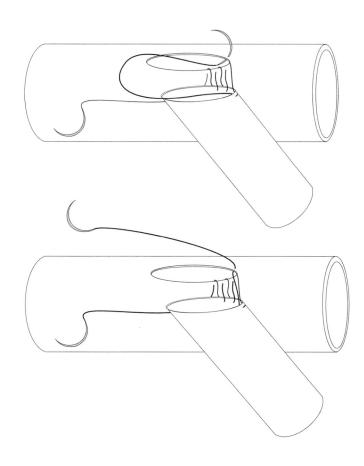

Parachute Technique
Starting at the Center of the Heel

Progress with the suturing forward toward the apex for a few bites.

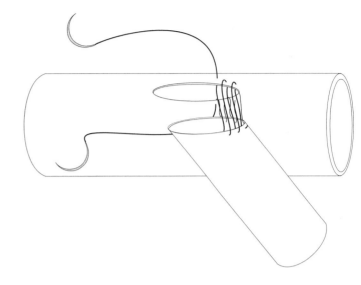

Pull and tighten the suture line.

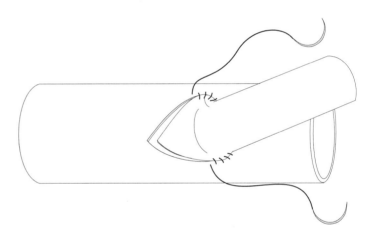

Start another suture at the apex, outside-inside in the graft and inside-outside in the artery.

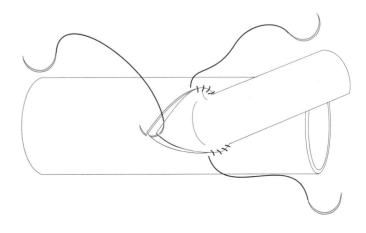

Parachute Technique
Starting at the Center of the Heel

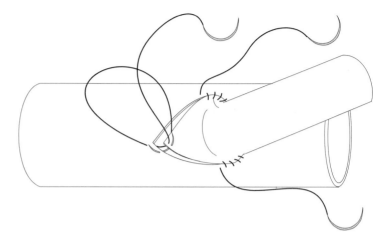

Progress with the suturing toward
the heel for a few bites.

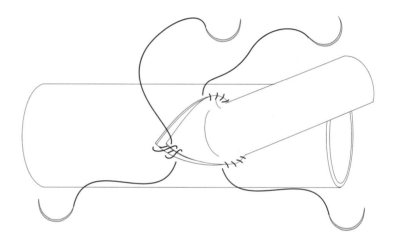

Resume suturing with the other end
of the apical suture. This suture will
become a horizontal mattress
suture.

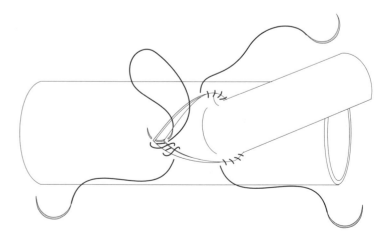

Parachute Technique
Starting at the Center of the Heel

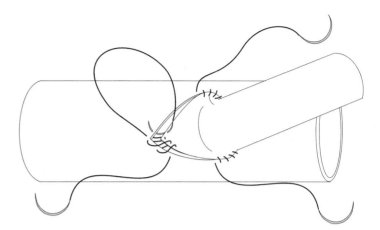

Progress with the suturing toward
the heel for a few bites.

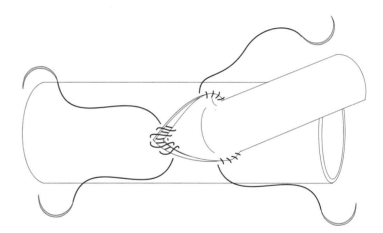

Pull and tighten the suture line.

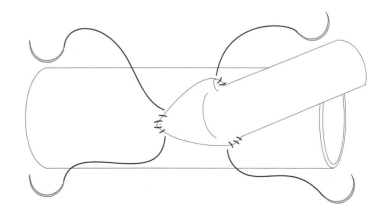

Parachute Technique
Starting at the Center of the Heel

Progress with the suturing toward
the heel.

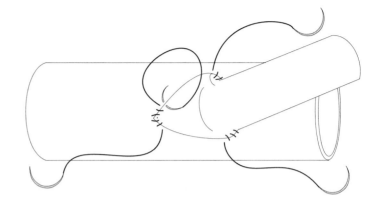

Tie the sutures.

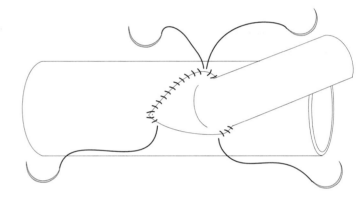

Resume suturing with the other end
of the apical suture toward the heel.

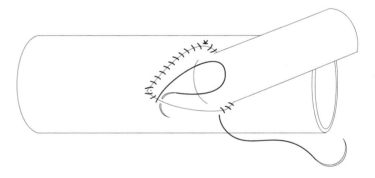

Tie the sutures.

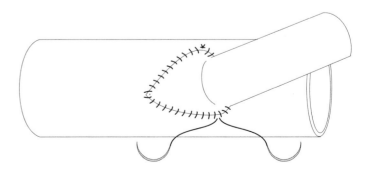

Parachute Technique
Starting a Few Bites from the Center of the Heel

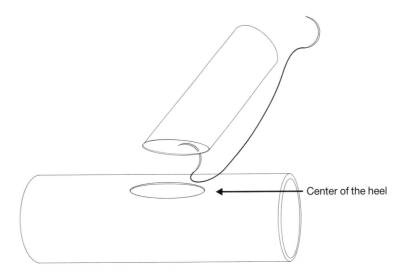

Start by introducing the needle through the adventitial side of the graft a few bites away from the center of the heel.

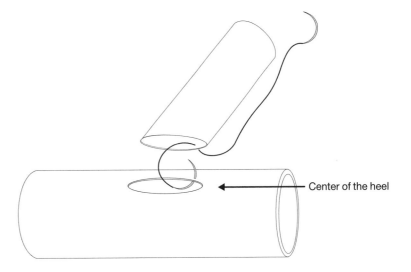

Introduce the needle in a corresponding site through the intimal side of the artery a few bites away from the center of the heel.

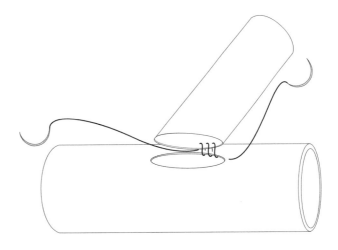

Place several more sutures.

Parachute Technique
Starting a Few Bites from the Center of the Heel

Continue until you have placed a few bites past the center of the heel.

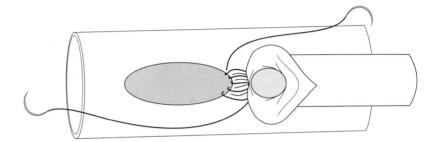

Pull the ends of the sutures and parachute the graft down toward the artery.

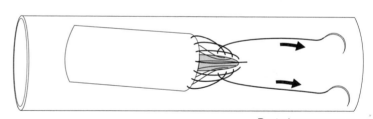

Posterior appearance of the suture line .

Tighten the suture line.

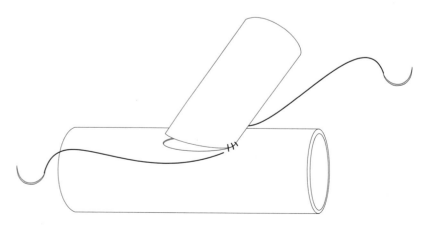

Parachute Technique
Starting a Few Bites from the Center of the Heel

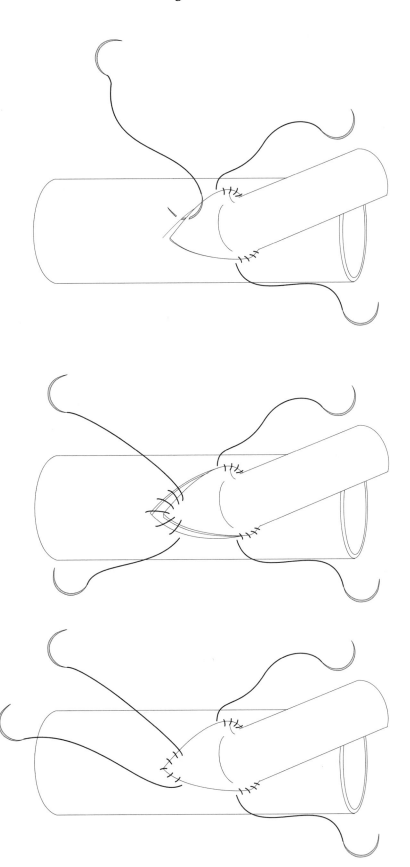

Start another suture a few bites away from the apex.

Introduce the needle from the adventitial side of the graft and the intimal side of the artery.

Continue the suture line until you have placed a few bites past the apex.

Tighten the suture line and pull down the graft.

Parachute Technique
Starting a Few Bites from the Center of the Heel

Continue suturing with one end until the heel suture is met.

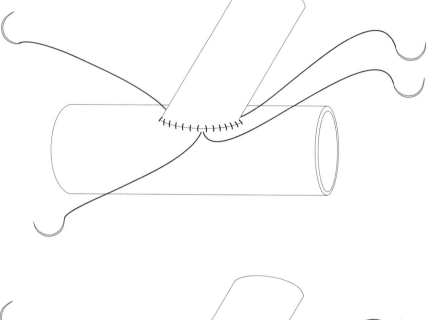

Tie both ends.

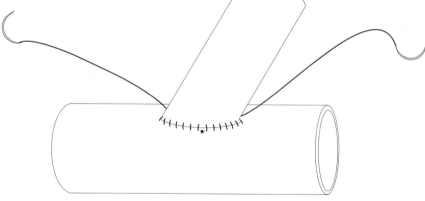

Flip the graft and continue suturing with the other end. Again, start by introducing the needle from the adventitial side of the graft.

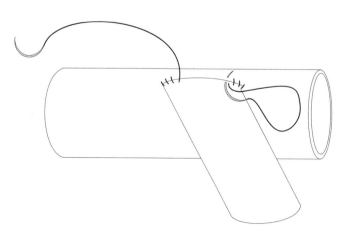

Parachute Technique
Starting a Few Bites from the Center of the Heel

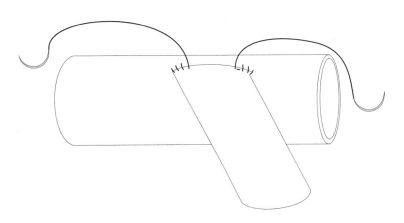

Run the suture toward the
apex until it meets the other
suture.

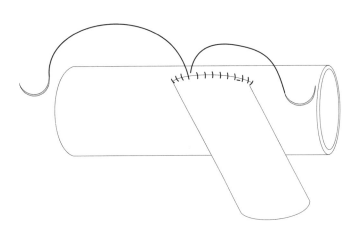

Tie the sutures.

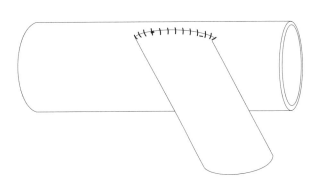

Parachute Technique
Starting at the Center of the Apex
Initial Completion of the Posterior Wall

Start at the center of the apex. Introduce the needle in the graft (outside-inside).

Introduce the needle in a matching location in the artery (inside-outside).

Run the suture along the posterior part of the anastomosis.

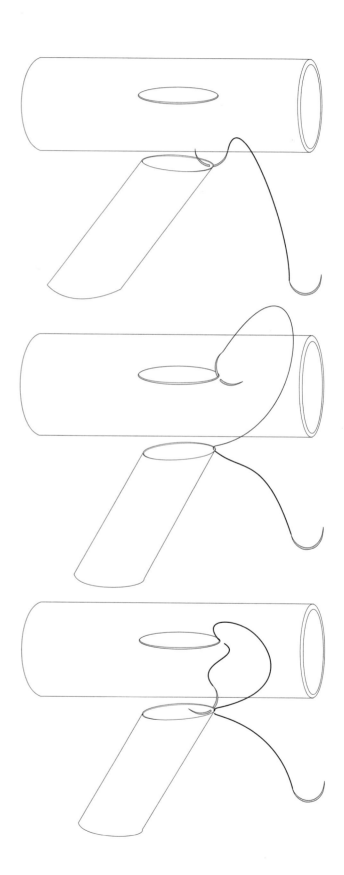

Parachute Technique
Starting at the Center of the Apex
Initial Completion of the Posterior Wall

Continue running the suture along the posterior wall until you reach the heel.

Use a nerve hook to facilitate tightening the suture line.

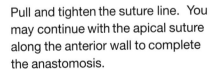

Pull and tighten the suture line. You may continue with the apical suture along the anterior wall to complete the anastomosis.

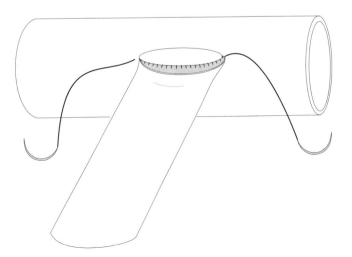

Parachute Technique
Starting at the Center of the Apex
Initial Completion of the Posterior Wall

Alternatively, you may start another suture at the apex as shown here. Start the new suture at the apex very close to the starting point of the previous suture.

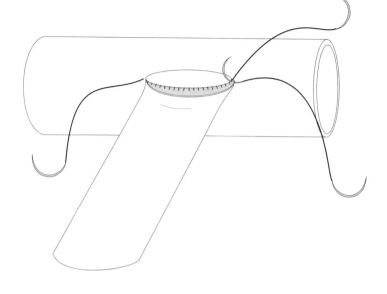

Again, introduce the needle outside-inside in the graft and inside-outside in the artery.

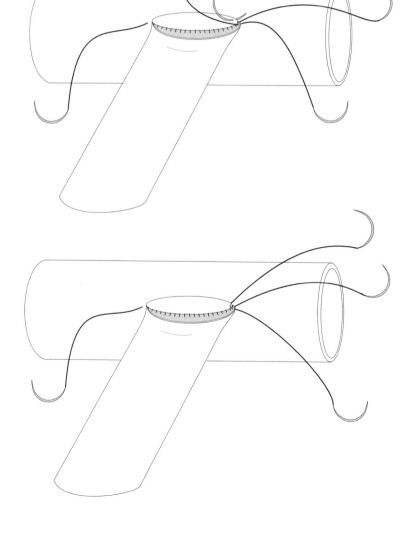

Parachute Technique
Starting at the Center of the Apex
Initial Completion of the Posterior Wall

Tie the new apical suture. Three throws are usually sufficient. Tie one end to the first sutures.

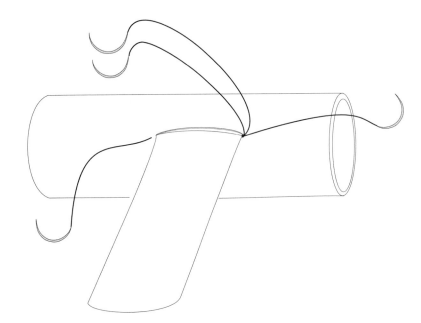

Start suturing the anterior wall. Outside-inside in the graft, inside-outside in the artery.

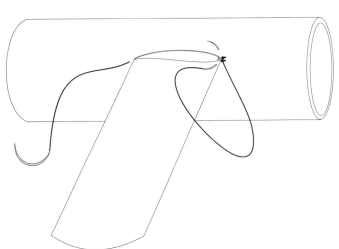

Progress with the suturing until you reach the heel suture.

Pull and tighten the suture line and tie the sutures.

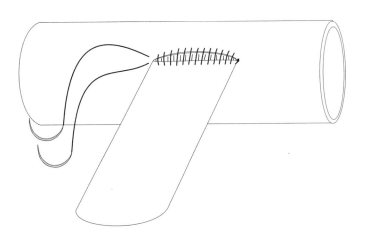

10

End-to-End Anastomosis

An end-to-end anastomosis is usually performed in trauma or for aneurysmal disease to replace an injured or aneurysmal vessel. An end-to-end anastomosis is also used when constructing a composite bypass or when replacing a diseased segment of a bypass. Furthermore, an end-to-end configuration may be chosen when preservation of retrograde flow is not essential, such as in a renal or celiac artery bypass.

Numerous methods are available for constructing an end-to-end anastomosis. The choice of the method will depend on several factors. These factors include the diameter of the vessels to be anastomosed, their mobility, and their ability to be rotated along their long axis. End-to-end anastomoses are usually performed with a continuous running suture technique. A continuous suture line can be started using an anchor technique, a parachute technique, or a combination of both. When a combination of both techniques is used, an anchor technique may be utilized for the posterior part of the anastomosis and a parachute technique for the anterior part or vice versa. In very rare situations, such as in children, the whole anastomosis or a portion of it is constructed with interrupted sutures to accommodate for future growth of the vessel.

END-TO-END ANASTOMOSIS
IN LARGE VESSELS OF COMPARABLE DIAMETER
(8 mm or Greater in Diameter)

When constructing an end-to-end anastomosis between two large vessels of comparable diameters, the vessel transection and the anastomotic suture line are usually in a plane perpendicular to the long axis of the vessels. If both segments are freely movable, one simple technique involves dividing the anastomosis into an anterior and a posterior part by placing two diametrically opposed sutures (Section 1). The sutures are tied and the anterior part of the anastomosis is constructed first. The vessels are then flipped 180° placing the posterior walls in an anterior location for completion of the anastomosis. One modification of this technique is the triangulation method first described by Alexis Carrel (Section 2). In this method, the anastomosis is divided into three parts. The vessels are joined by three individual sutures placed and tied one-third of the circumference of the anastomosis apart. This approach may help to prevent uneven advancements between the sutures on either side of the vessels, especially when dealing with large vessels of comparable but unequal diameters. When the vessel segments are not freely movable and will not allow for rotating the anastomosis 180°, the posterior walls are sutured first. This can be performed using a parachute technique (Section 3) or an anchor technique. In either technique, the suture may be started in the center or at one end of the posterior wall.

END-TO-END ANASTOMOSIS
IN SMALL VESSELS OF COMPARABLE DIAMETER
(6 mm or Smaller in Diameter)

When constructing an end-to-end anastomosis between two small vessels, a beveled or spatulated anastomosis is necessary to avoid compromising the lumen (Section 4). A simple method is to start one anchoring suture at the heel and then progress with the suturing on each side of the heel toward the apex. Another suture is then started at the apex after ensuring that the size of the vessels match appropriately. The anchoring sutures may be simple or horizontal mattress sutures. The anchoring sutures will stabilize the graft for the placement of the remaining bites. Once well apposed, both walls may be sutured together with a single passage of the needle. However, at the apex and the heel, it is preferable to pass the needle separately in each vessel wall to ensure optimal placement of the bites.

Autogenous vessels may contract and shorten transiently after transection. Approximation of the shortened vessels may place the anastomosis under slight tension. If the vessels are thin, the anchoring suture may tear through the vessel wall, especially if a simple suture was used. In this situation, using a parachute technique may be helpful. The parachute technique will spread the tension over several bites in the posterior wall rather than confining the tension to the area of a single anchoring suture. The parachute technique in spatulated vessels is similar to that shown in Section 3.

One useful additional technique that is used infrequently is the end-to-end anastomosis with anterior patch angioplasty. (2) This technique is useful when the debrided ends of an injured artery can only be approximated together if the anastomosis is constructed without beveling or spatulation. In this situation, the length of the arterial segments is not sufficient to allow for spatulation despite maximal mobilization. This technique involves creating an anterior arteriotomy in both vessel segments. The ends of the vessels are sutured together after aligning the anterior arteriotomies. The anastomosis is completed by covering the anterior defect using a vein patch angioplasty (Section 5). The main advantage of this technique is avoiding the placement of a very short interposition graft.

END-TO-END ANASTOMOSIS
BETWEEN VESSELS OF UNEQUAL CALIBER

Several methods have been described to facilitate the construction of an end-to-end anastomosis between two vessels of unequal calibers. In such reconstructions, it is helpful to minimize trimming the smaller caliber vessel and to create a long spatulated anastomosis. This can help in providing a smooth transition between the anastomosed structures and may prevent an acute angulation caused by the diameter mismatch (Section 6).

If an undesirable angulation is likely to develop following an end-to-end anastomosis between unequal-sized vessels, a patch angioplasty may be necessary to correct the deformity. The technique of end-to-end anastomosis with anterior patch angioplasty described in Section 5 can be used to create an anastomosis between two relatively small vessels of unequal calibers. The patch is tailored to accommodate for the diameter mismatch.

When the size discrepancy is so large that an end-to-end anastomosis cannot be constructed, the options available become limited. One alternative involves oversewing the transected end of the larger-diameter vessel. This is followed by connecting the end of the smaller-diameter vessel to the side of the larger-diameter vessel. The resulting configuration is an end-to-side anastomosis, which is a functional end-to-end anastomosis (Section 7).

Another alternative is to consider other reconstructive alternatives. One such example is the composite vein graft, which is usually constructed by joining two vein segments together. If there is a notable size discrepancy, the large end of one segment will need to be anastomosed to the small end of the other segment. This difficult anastomosis can be avoided if one segment of vein is used in a reversed manner (1) while the other is used in a nonreversed manner. The change in the orientation of one vein segment will allow suturing the larger ends of the veins together. The valves in the nonreversed segment are then disrupted after arterializing the graft (Section 8).

REFERENCES

1. Hoballah JJ, Chalmers RTA, Sharp WJ, Corson JD. Composite vein bypass: a simple technique for venovenous anastomosis. Ann Vasc Surg 1994;8(4);400–402.
2. Reiner JAM, Van Dongen MD. End to end anastomosis with anterior patch angioplasty. In: Reconstructive Arterial Surgery. New York: Springer-Verlag, 1970:11.

Large Vessels, Freely Movable; Transection Perpendicular to the Longitudinal Axis
Anchor Technique

Transect the vessels at a right angle to their longitudinal axis.

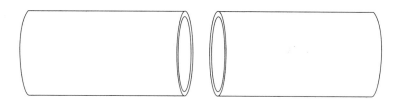

Start by placing one suture at the base of each vessel.

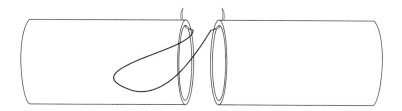

Tie the suture.

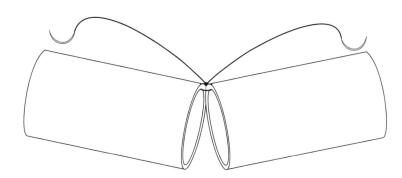

Place an identical suture diametrically opposite to the first suture.

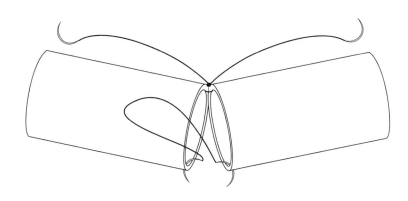

Large Vessels, Freely Movable; Transection Perpendicular to the Longitudinal Axis
Anchor Technique

Start suturing on the anterior wall.

Run the suture along the
anterior wall until it meets the
inferior suture.

Tie the sutures.

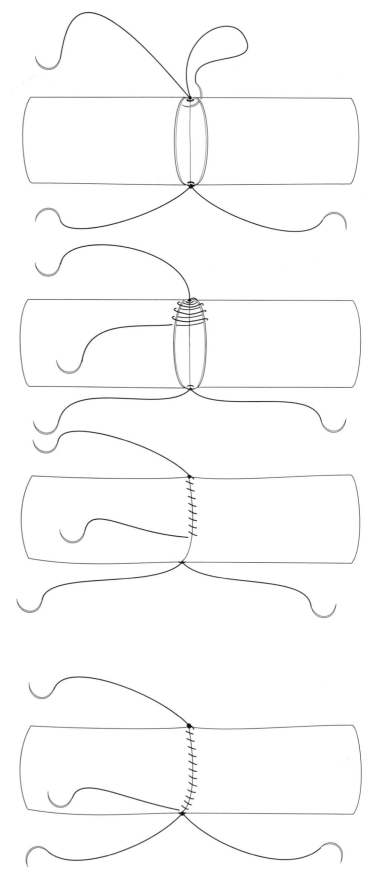

Large Vessels, Freely Movable; Transection Perpendicular to the Longitudinal Axis
Anchor Technique

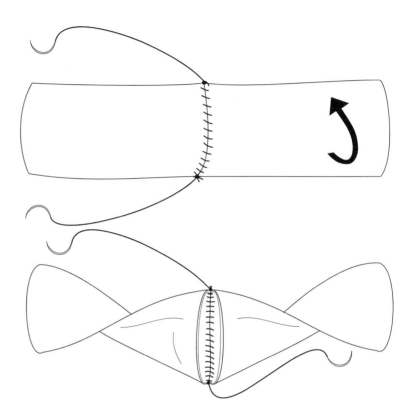

Flip the graft 180°, bringing the posterior wall to an anterior location.

Run the remaining end of the superior suture toward the inferior suture.

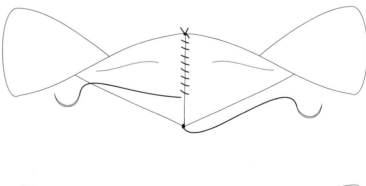

You may continue with the superior suture until it meets the inferior suture.

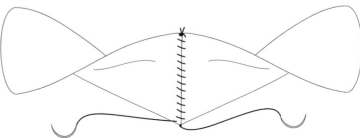

Large Vessels, Freely Movable; Transection Perpendicular to the Longitudinal Axis
Anchor Technique

Alternatively, you may start suturing with the lower suture toward the upper suture.

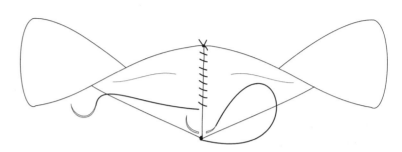

This variation will avoid the need to tie to a suture that already has a knot at its base, which could result in a bulky knot.

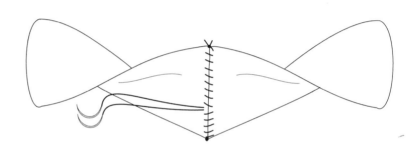

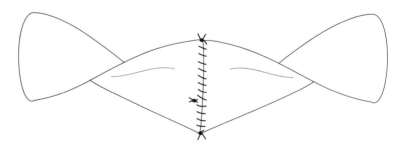

Tie the sutures and flip the graft back to its original position.

Large Vessels, Freely Movable; Transection Perpendicular to the Longitudinal Axis
Triangulation Technique

Place the first suture at the apex.

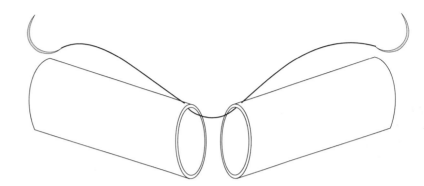

Place the next suture one-third the circumference away from the first suture.

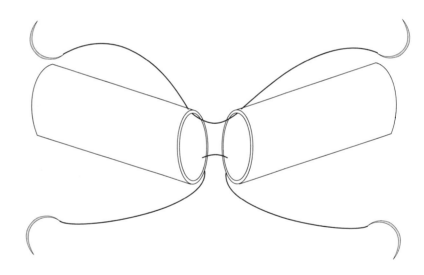

Place the third suture one-third the circumference away from the second suture.

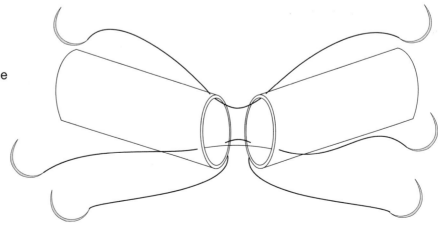

Large Vessels, Freely Movable; Transection Perpendicular to the Longitudinal Axis
Triangulation Technique

Tie all the sutures. The suture
line will now resemble an
equilateral triangle.

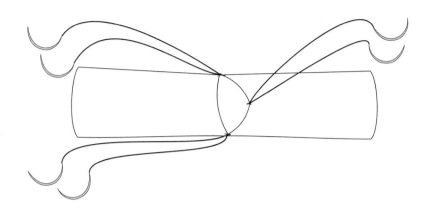

Start running one end of the
apical suture toward the next
suture.

Large Vessels, Freely Movable; Transection Perpendicular to the Longitudinal Axis
Triangulation Technique

Tie the sutures to one end of the middle suture.

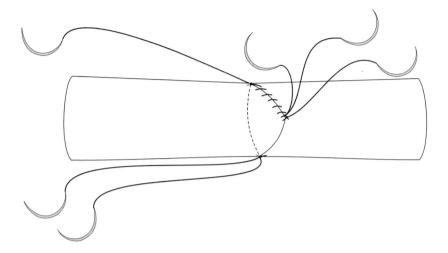

Run the remaining end toward the inferior suture.

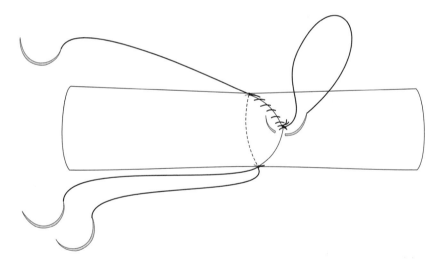

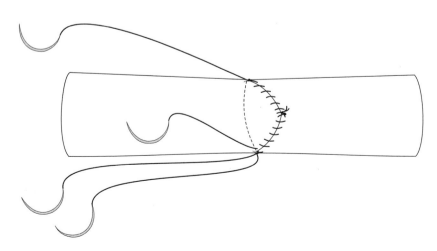

Large Vessels, Freely Movable; Transection Perpendicular to the Longitudinal Axis
Triangulation Technique

Tie the suture to one end of the inferior suture.

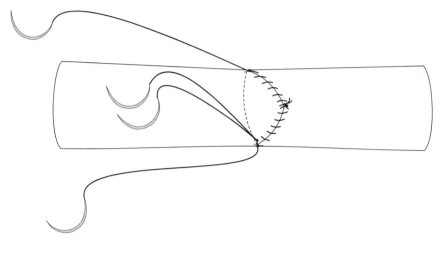

Flip the vessels 180°.

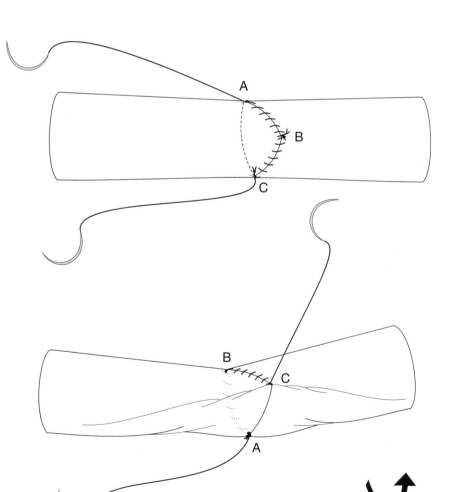

Large Vessels, Freely Movable; Transection Perpendicular to the Longitudinal Axis
Triangulation Technique

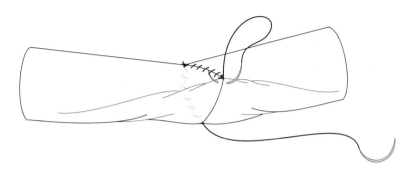

Run the upper suture toward
the lower suture.

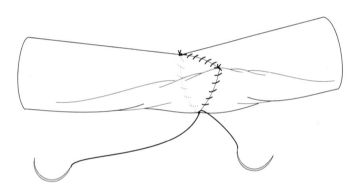

Tie both sutures.

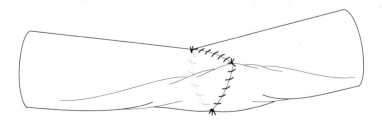

Large Vessels, Fixed; Transection Perpendicular to the Longitudinal Axis
Parachute Technique

When the vessels cannot be rotated 180°, the back wall will have to be sutured first.

Start by placing one suture at the base of each vessel.

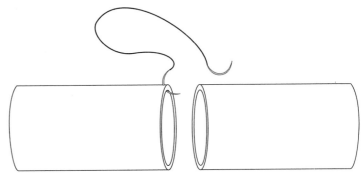

You may tie the suture or continue suturing the back wall without tying, as illustrated here.

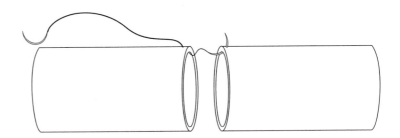

The needle will be introduced from the adventitial side of vessel A and the intimal side of vessel B, thus allowing the suturing to be performed in a forehand manner.

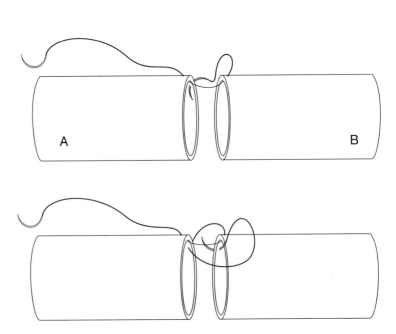

Large Vessels, Fixed; Transection Perpendicular to the Longitudinal Axis
Parachute Technique

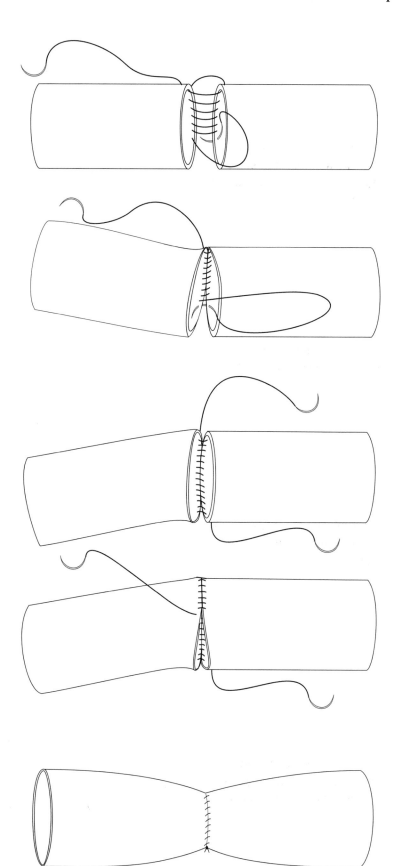

Continue placing the sutures until the posterior suture line is completed.

Tighten the suture line.

You may continue with the upper suture until it meets the other end. Avoid excessive tension on the suture line.

A waist or pursestring effect can occur at the anastomosis if excessive tension is applied to the suture line.

Large Vessels, Fixed; Transection Perpendicular to the Longitudinal Axis
Parachute Technique

Alternatively, you may start another suture. This suture may be a simple or a mattress suture as shown here.

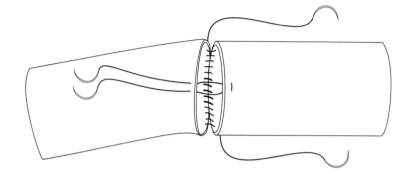

You may tie the suture and continue running the suture line.

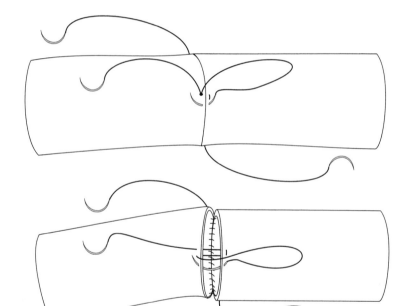

Alternatively, you may continue suturing without tying, as shown here.

Introduce the needle on the adventitial side of vessel B and on the intimal side of vessel A.

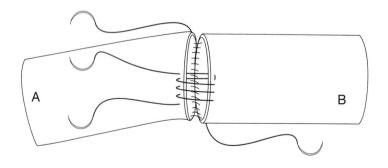
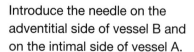

Large Vessels, Fixed; Transection Perpendicular to the Longitudinal Axis
Parachute Technique

Continue suturing until you reach the inferior suture.

Tie the sutures.

Start suturing toward the superior suture.

Tie the sutures.

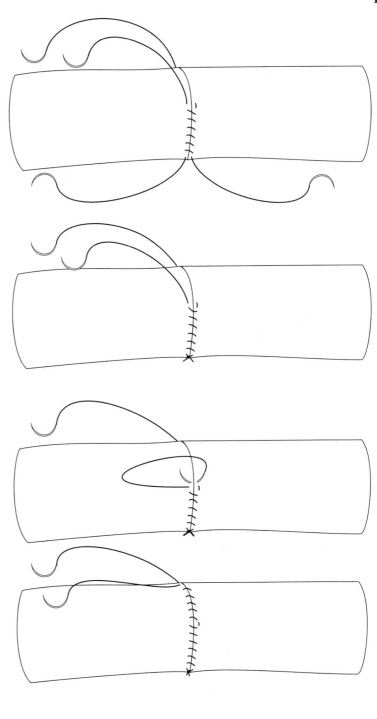

Small Vessels; Beveled Transection
Anchor Technique

This section depicts an end-to-end anastomosis between a graft (A) and an artery (B).

The vessels are beveled as previously described. In small vessels, spatulation may be helpful. The edges can be trimmed as necessary.

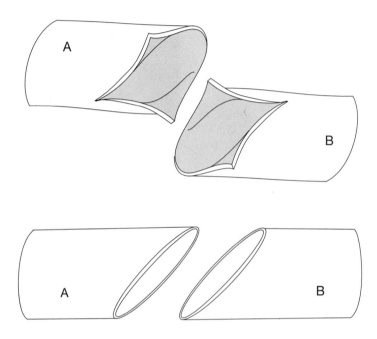

Start the suture at the center of the heel.

Introduce the needle from the adventitial side of the graft and the intimal side of the artery.

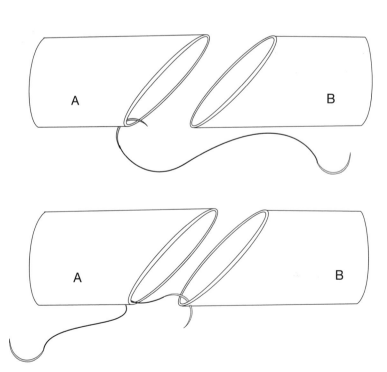

Small Vessels; Beveled Transection
Anchor Technique

This suture may be a horizontal mattress or a simple suture as shown here.

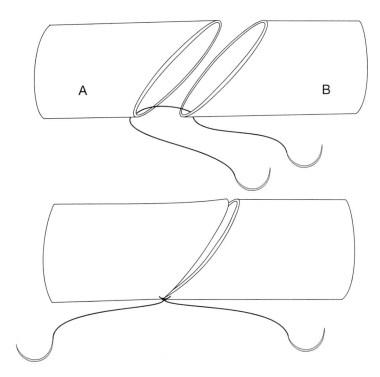

Tie the suture.

Introduce the needle from the adventitial side of the graft.

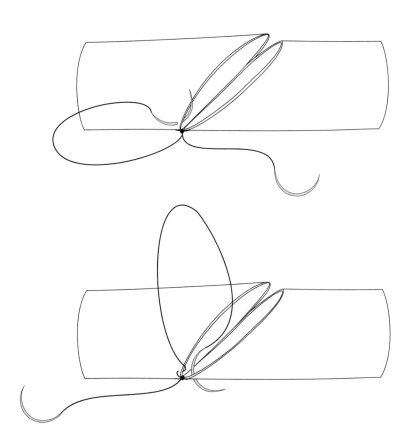

Introduce the needle from the intimal side of the artery.

Small Vessels; Beveled Transection
Anchor Technique

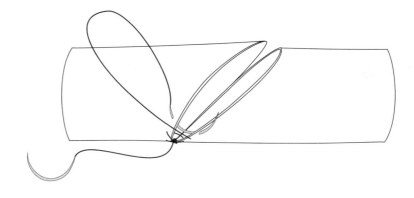

Run the suture toward the apex.

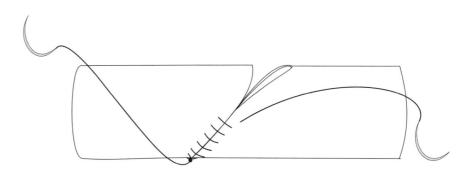

Tighten the suture line.

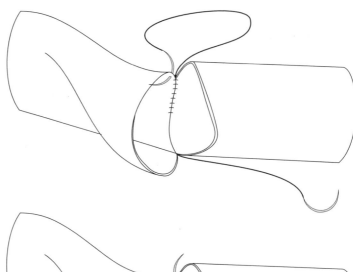

Flip the graft and start suturing with the other end of the suture.

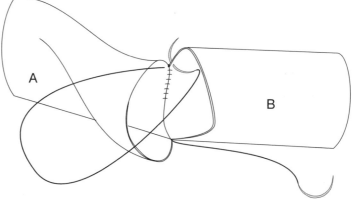

Again, introduce the needle from the adventitial side of the graft (A) and the intimal side of the artery (B).

Small Vessels; Beveled Transection
Anchor Technique

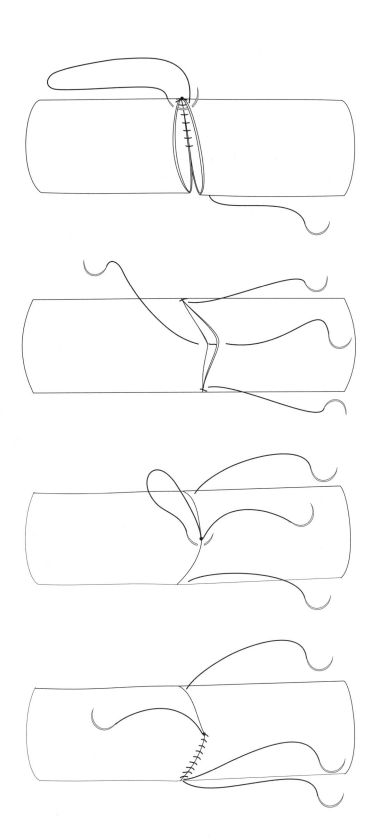

Run the suture until it reaches mid distance to the apex.

Start another suture at the apex. This suture may be a horizontal mattress suture or a simple suture as shown here.

Tie the suture.

Run one end of the suture towards the heel until it meets the other suture.
Tie the sutures.

Small Vessels; Beveled Transection
Anchor Technique

Start suturing toward the
superior suture. Again, outside-
inside in the graft (A), inside-
outside in the artery (B).

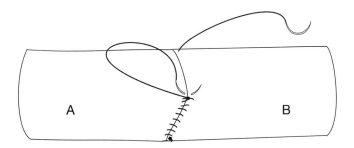

Tie the sutures.

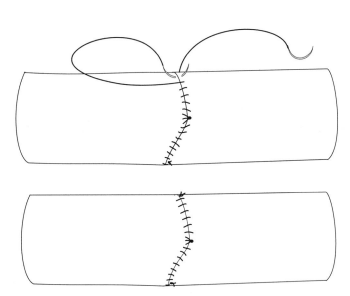

Small Vessels; Transection Perpendicular to the Longitudinal Axis
End-to-End Anastomosis with Anterior Patch Angioplasty

Incise the vessels along the anterior surface.

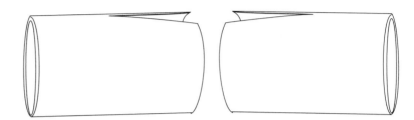

Introduce the needle on one side of the anterior surface.

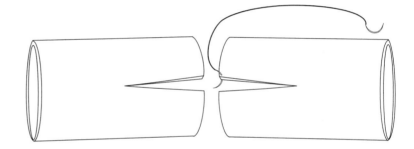

Introduce the needle in a corresponding site in the other vessel.

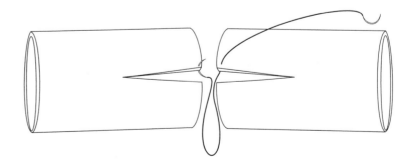

Small Vessels; Transection Perpendicular to the Longitudinal Axis
End-to-End Anastomosis with Anterior Patch Angioplasty

Place an identical suture in the other edge of the anterior incision.

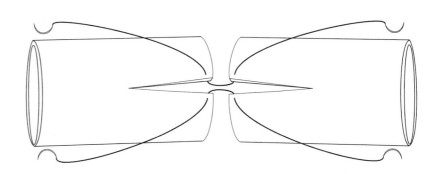

Tie the sutures.

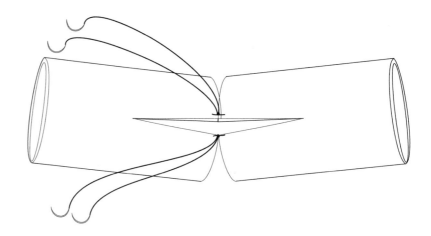

Introduce the needle (outside-inside) closely spaced to the starting point. This will allow suturing the posterior wall from within the lumen.

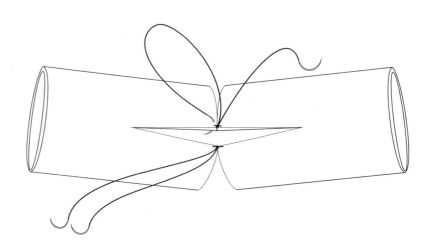

Small Vessels; Transection Perpendicular to the Longitudinal Axis
End-to-End Anastomosis with Anterior Patch Angioplasty

Apply traction on each suture in opposite directions.

Start suturing the posterior wall from within.

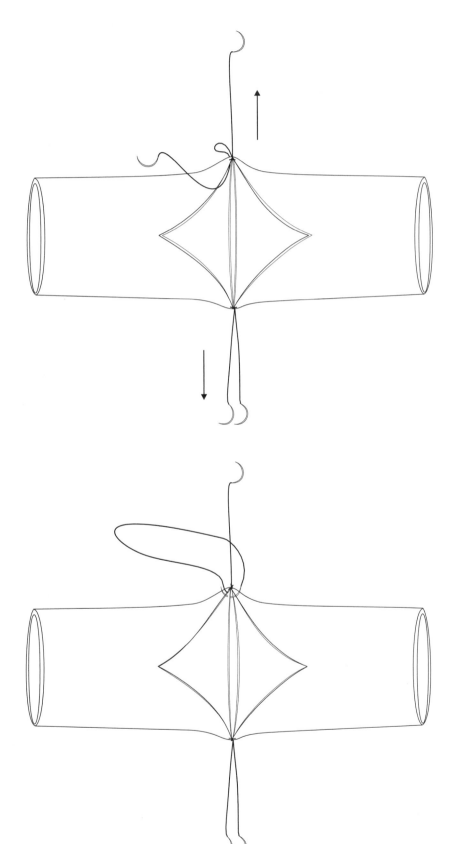

Small Vessels; Transection Perpendicular to the Longitudinal Axis
End-to-End Anastomosis with Anterior Patch Angioplasty

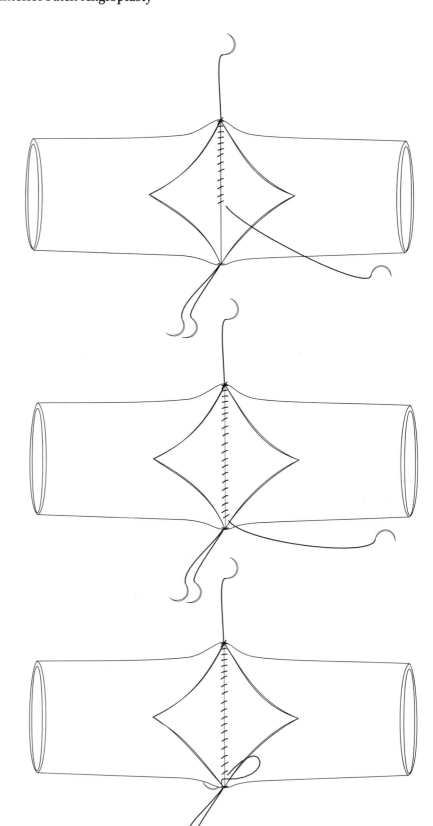

Keep running the superior suture towards the inferior suture.

Introduce the needle (inside-outside) to bring the suture back to the anterior surface.

Small Vessels; Transection Perpendicular to the Longitudinal Axis
End-to-End Anastomosis with Anterior Patch Angioplasty

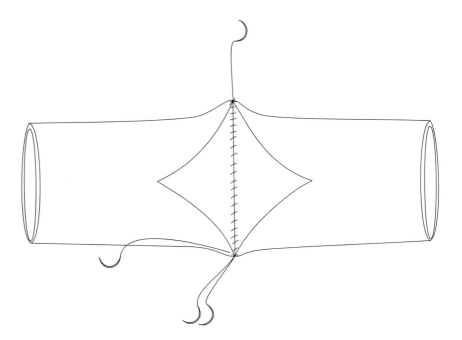

Tie the sutures.

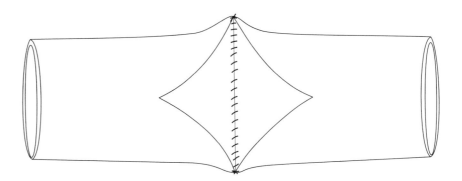

Appearance of the joined
vessels after the tension on the
stay sutures is removed.

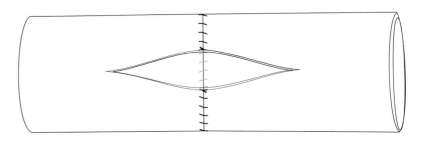

Small Vessels; Transection Perpendicular to the Longitudinal Axis
End-to-End Anastomosis with Anterior Patch Angioplasty

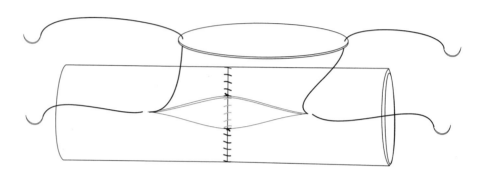

Close the anterior defect in the joined vessels with a patch as previously described.

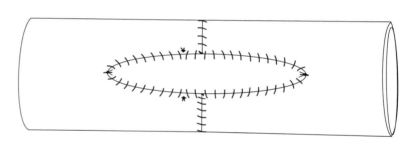

Vessels of Unequal Diameter; Beveled Transection
Combined Technique; Anchor Heel, Parachute Apex

Transect each vessel at a right angle to the longitudinal axis. Make an anterior slit in the larger vessel and a posterior slit in the smaller vessel.

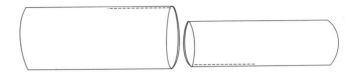

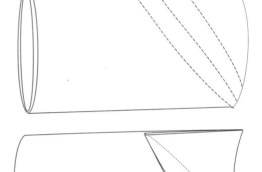

Cut a wedge of the vessel on one side.

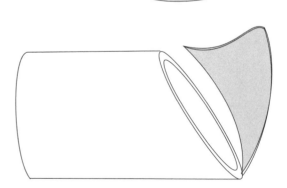

Cut the remaining wedge on the other side.

Use the length of the excised wedge to determine the approximate length to which the smaller vessel should be trimmed.

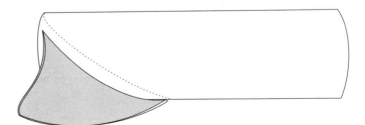

Vessels of Unequal Diameter; Beveled Transection
Combined Technique; Anchor Heel, Parachute Apex

This section describes an end-to-end anastomosis between a small diameter graft and a larger artery. To illustrate the various possible alternatives, the heel suture will be started using an anchor technique. The apical suture will be constructed using a parachute technique.

Start a heel suture penetrating from the adventitial side of the graft and then penetrating from the intimal side of the artery.

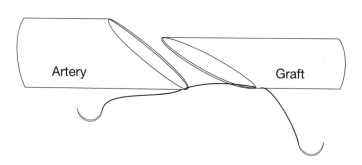

This suture may be a horizontal mattress or a simple suture as shown here. Tie the suture.

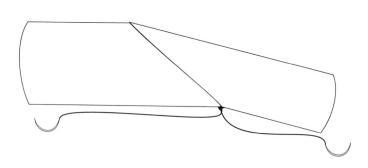

Start running the suture on one side until you have reached mid distance to the apex.

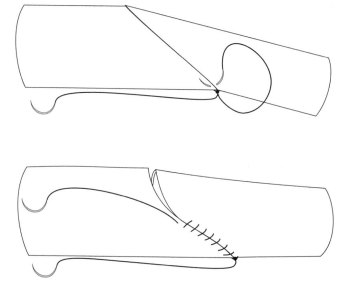

Vessels of Unequal Diameter; Beveled Transection
Combined Technique; Anchor Heel, Parachute Apex

Flip the graft. Introduce the needle from the adventitial side of the graft and through the intimal side of the artery.

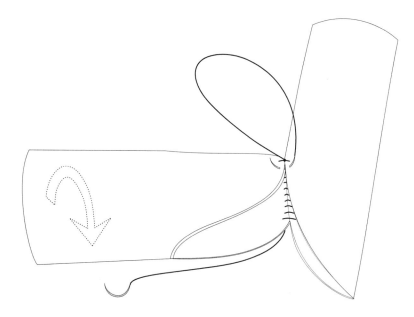

Run the suture until you reach mid-distance to the apex.

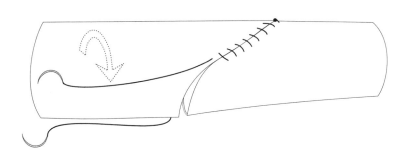

Check that the length of the arteriotomy matches the length of the graft. If the graft is too long for the arteriotomy, you may have to trim the graft or extend the arteriotomy along the dotted line.

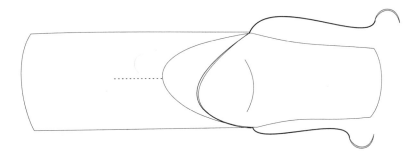

Vessels of Unequal Diameter; Beveled Transection
Combined Technique; Anchor Heel, Parachute Apex

Start the apical suture two bites away from the center of the apex.

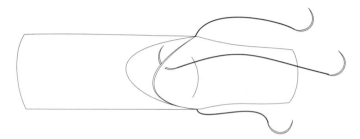

Again, the suture should penetrate on the adventitial side of the graft and then through the intimal side of the artery.

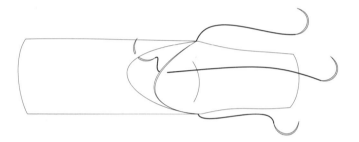

Continue placing the sutures until you have placed two bites past the center of the apex.

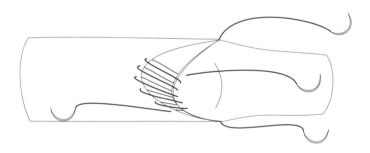

Tighten the suture line and pull down the apex of the graft.

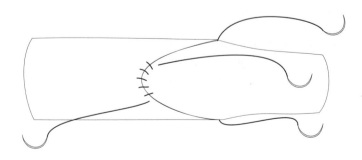

Vessels of Unequal Diameter; Beveled Transection
Combined Technique; Anchor Heel, Parachute Apex

Continue running the suture until it meets the heel suture.

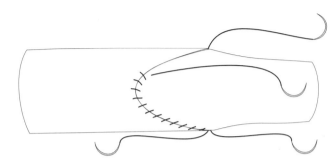

Repeat the same process with the other end of the suture.

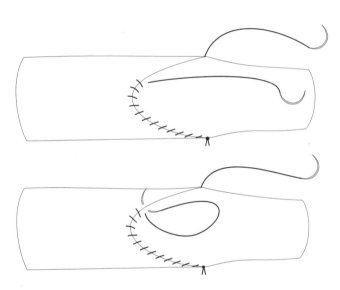

Tie both sutures together.

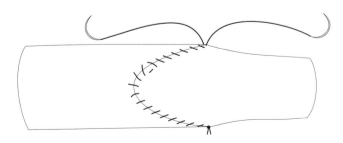

Vessels of Unequal Diameter; Beveled Transection
Combined Technique; Anchor Heel, Parachute Apex

Top view of anastomosis.

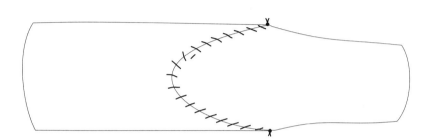

Side view of anastomosis.

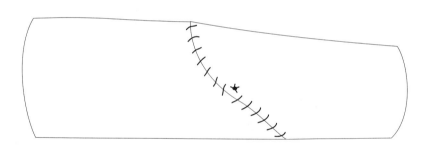

Vessels of Unequal Diameter
End-to-Side; Functional End-to-End

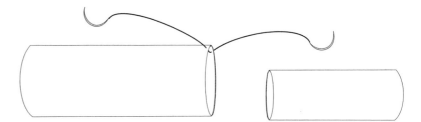

Start one suture in the upper part of the transected vessel.

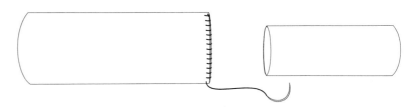

Run the suture towards the base of the vessel.

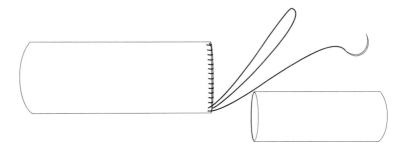

Tie the suture to itself.

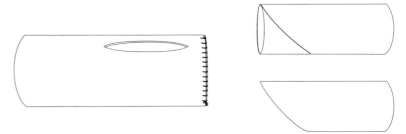

Create an incision in the large vessel and transect the smaller vessel to match the incision site.

Vessels of Unequal Diameter
End-to-Side; Functional End-to-End

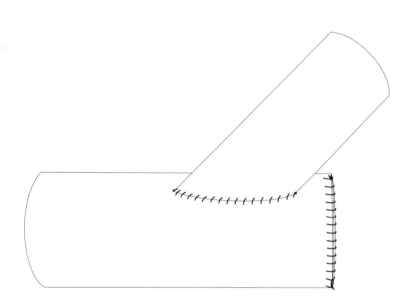

Construct an end-to-side
anastomosis as described in
chapter 9.

Two Vessels of Unequal Diameter
Composite Vein Bypass

When two vein segments of unequal diameters are joined in a reversed manner, the larger end of one segment will be anastomosed to the smaller end of the other vein segment. This anastomosis may be technically challenging and may result in the configuration shown below.

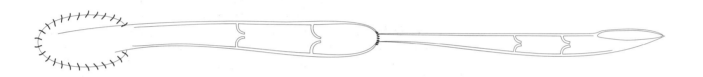

To avoid constructing an anastomosis between two vein segments of unequal diameter, the first segment is attached to the artery in a reversed fashion. The second segment is used in a nonreversed fashion that allows the construction of an anastomosis between the larger ends of the vein segments. The valves in the nonreversed vein segment are disrupted with a valvulotome.

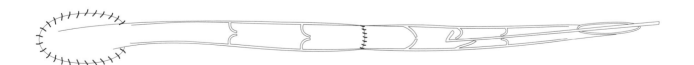

11

Side-to-Side Anastomosis

The conditions in which a side-to-side anastomosis is used include the creation of a side-to-side portocaval shunt in portal hypertension, the creation of a side-to-side radiocephalic arteriovenous fistula for chronic hemodialysis, and the creation of a side-to-side arteriovenous fistula distal to an infrainguinal prosthetic bypass as an adjunctive procedure to decrease the outflow resistance. The side-to-side configuration is also used in the construction of the second anastomosis of a sequential bypass when multiple segments of a limb require revascularization.

A side-to-side anastomosis is infrequently performed because the need for such a reconstruction is rare. Mesocaval interposition shunts are frequently used instead of the side-to-side portocaval shunts because they are considered to be technically less demanding. In addition, these shunts do not violate the hepatic hilum which could increase the difficulty of future liver transplantation. An end-to-side rather than a side-to-side configuration is usually used when creating an arteriovenous fistula for chronic hemodialysis. The end-to-side radiocephalic fistula requires less mobilization of the cephalic vein and the radial artery than the side-to-side configuration, which does not offer in this situation any advantage over the end-to-side reconstruction. The role of an arteriovenous fistula distal to an infrainguinal prosthetic bypass remains controversial, and frequently an end-to-side rather than a side-to-side reconstruction is used.

When a side-to-side anastomosis is being constructed, the vessels are dissected and mobilized to lie adjacent to each other with minimal tension. The anastomosis is created on the part of the vessels where the walls are in direct contact. The posterior part of the anastomosis is constructed first. The anastomosis can be constructed using an anchor technique (Section 1) or a parachute technique (Section 2). The suture line can be started at the midpoint of the incision in the vessel (Section 1) or at either end (Section 2).

Anchor Technique

Start by placing one suture at the midpoint of the venotomy (outside-inside).

Introduce the needle in a corresponding point in the arteriotomy (inside-outside).

Tie down the suture.

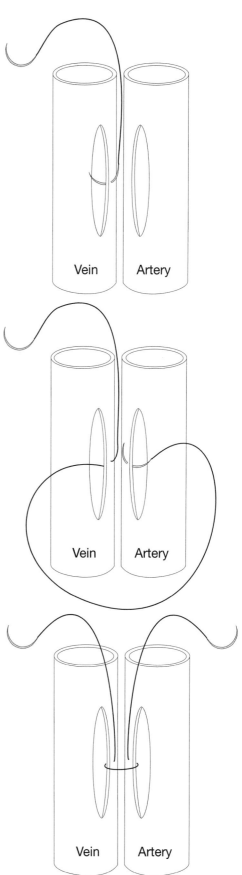

Anchor Technique

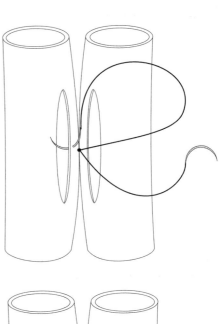

The needle is introduced from the adventitial side of the vein and the intimal side of the artery.

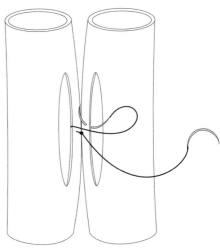

Continue suturing the back wall on one side of the suture.

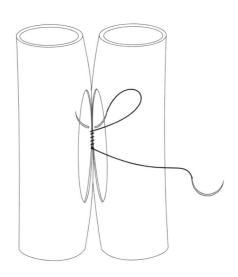

Anchor Technique

Complete the back wall of the anastomosis on one side of the suture.

Complete the back wall on the other side of the suture in a similar manner.

Resume suturing along the anterior wall.
Introduce the needle inside-outside in the artery.

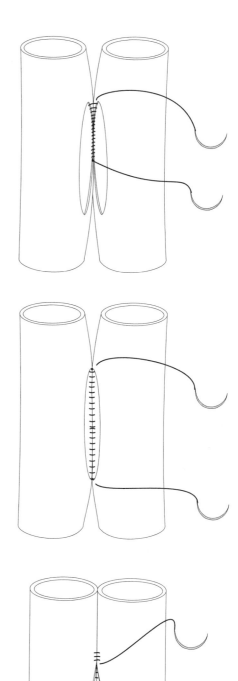

Anchor Technique

Continue running the suture toward the lower
suture.

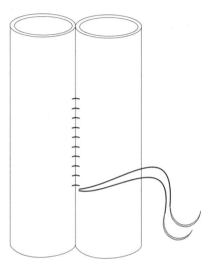

Tie the suture.

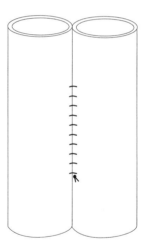

Parachute Technique

Start by placing one suture at the apex of the venotomy (outside-inside).

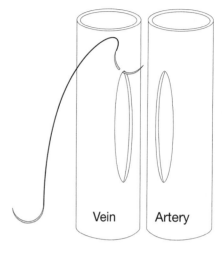

Introduce the needle in the apex of the arteriotomy (inside-outside).

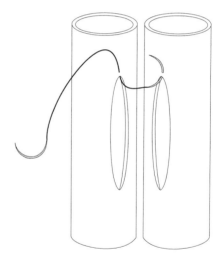

You may tie the suture or continue suturing without tying as shown here.

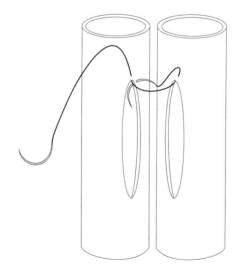

Parachute Technique

The needle is introduced from the adventitial side of the vein and the intimal side of the artery.

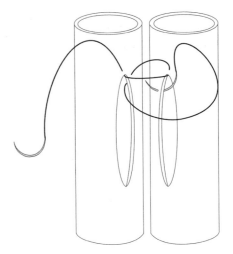

Continue suturing the back wall without tying.

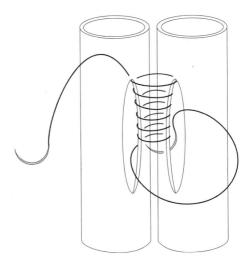

Tighten the suture.

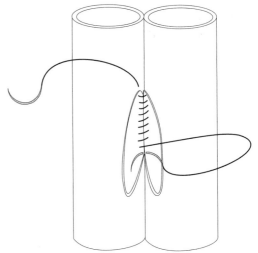

Parachute Technique

Continue placing the sutures until the posterior part of the anastomosis is completed.

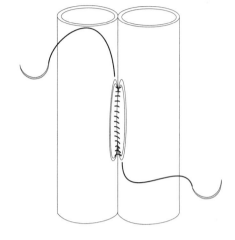

You may continue with the upper suture until it meets the other end.

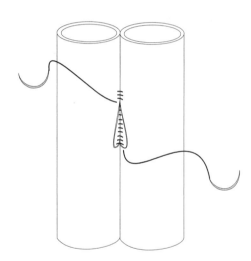

Alternatively, you may start another suture.

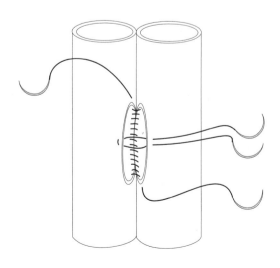

Parachute Technique

Again, introduce the needle inside-outside in the vein and outside-inside in the artery.

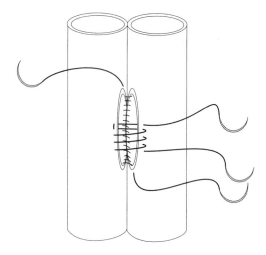

Continue placing the sutures until you reach the inferior apex.

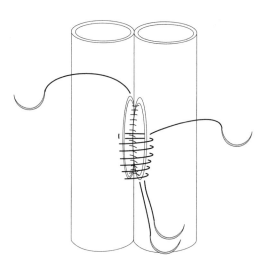

Tie the sutures.

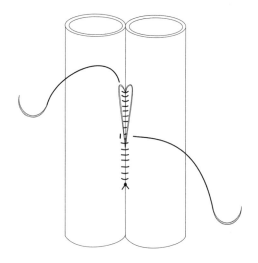

Parachute Technique

Resume suturing with the other end.

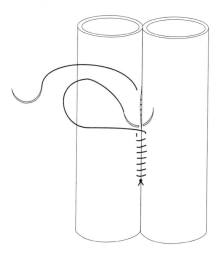

Run the suture toward the upper apex.

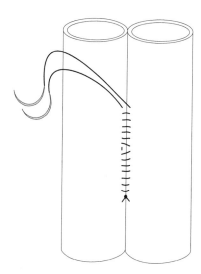

Tie the sutures.

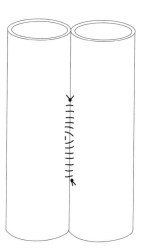

III

Infrainguinal Bypass Surgery

12

Adjunctive Techniques: Proximal Anastomosis of an Infrainguinal Bypass

The main principles of constructing a bypass for infrainguinal occlusive disease include:

1. Identifying a soft arterial segment proximal to the occlusive disease to serve as an inflow source
2. Identifying a soft arterial segment distal to the occlusive disease to serve as a suitable outflow vessel
3. Connecting these two arterial segments with a conduit preferably of autogenous origin

The artery to be used as the inflow vessel is usually selected on the basis of the preoperative angiogram. The inflow vessel may be found to be diseased upon its exposure. The pathology that may be encountered includes heavily calcified plaque or severe thickening of the wall, especially in redo procedures. If dissecting a more proximal segment of the artery is not possible or reveals similar pathology, constructing an anastomosis to a diseased inflow vessel may become unavoidable. In this situation, the proximal anastomosis could become very challenging. Proximal and distal vascular control can be accomplished by occluding the vessels from within using balloon occluding catheters. Even in the presence of heavy calcifications, a soft area in the artery may still be identified and used as the arteriotomy site. If that is not possible, a localized endarterectomy may become necessary. In that situation, it is important to perform the endarterectomy without creating a distal dissection and disrupting valuable collaterals. In addition, because the atherosclerotic disease usually extends distally for a long segment, ending the endarterectomy often requires transecting the plaque and leaving a shelf. Consequently, tacking of the endarterectomy endpoint is often necessary.

SAPHENOFEMORAL JUNCTION
WITH FEMORAL VEIN CUFF

When constructing an anastomosis to an artery with thickened walls, narrowing of the bypass could occur just distal to the heel, especially if the conduit has a small caliber such as with a reversed-vein bypass graft. If a prosthetic conduit is to be used, an 8-mm graft can be selected and the hood can be fashioned to accommodate for the thickening in the arterial wall. If the conduit used is the greater saphenous vein, this narrowing must be avoided. One option is to perform an in situ or a nonreversed free vein bypass. The saphenofemoral junction is used as the hood of the bypass (Section 1). The saphenofemoral junction is dissected freely. A Cooley clamp is applied to the femoral vein in a partially occluding manner. The saphenous vein is transected to include a 1-mm rim of the femoral vein. The venotomy in the femoral vein is then closed with a running suture of 5-0 prolene. The leaflets of the valve at the saphenofemoral junction are excised under direct vision. The hood created will be able to accommodate for the thickening in the arterial wall.

T-JUNCTION

If the saphenofemoral junction is not available, several techniques could be used to assist in performing the proximal anastomosis without creating a narrowing in the bypass. One option involves using the segment of vein with the largest diameter and an associated side branch. The vein is slit along the posterior wall in a fashion to incorporate the side branch. (2,3,5) The shape of the segment of the vein that will be used for the anastomosis will appear as a T. Consequently, this technique is referred to as the T-junction technique (Section 2). The T-junction technique can help prevent the narrowing that could develop just distal to the heel. In addition, it can also be used in the distal anastomosis to prevent undesirable angulation in the bypass. (4) The length of the T-junction can be modified according to the size of the arteriotomy and the length of the side branch.

PATCH ANGIOPLASTY OF THE INFLOW VESSEL

Another option is to perform a vein patch angioplasty of the arteriotomy. An incision is then performed in the patch and used as the new site for constructing the proximal anastomosis. (2) In this technique, the vein bypass is sutured to the soft and thin wall of the vein patch, which could prevent the proximal anastomotic stenosis (Section 3).

PATCH ANGIOPLASTY OF THE HOOD OF THE BYPASS

Another option is to carry the anastomosis in the usual fashion and then perform a vein patch angioplasty if the bypass appears stenotic. The vein patch angioplasty is started in the hood of the graft and may be extended into the bypass as needed (Section 4).

INCORPORATION OF PROFUNDAPLASTY

In the presence of occlusive disease at the orifice of the profunda femoris artery, a profundaplasty may be performed in conjunction with the distal bypass. The arteriotomy in the common femoral artery is extended into the profunda femoris artery. Following the endarterectomy, a vein patch closure of the arteriotomy may be performed. The proximal anastomosis can be carried as described in Section 3. Alternatively, the arteriotomy used for the endarterectomy is incorporated in the proximal anastomosis with the hood of the bypass serving as a patch (Section 5).

SARTORIUS MUSCLE FLAP

The subcutaneous tissues are the only layers separating a femoral anastomosis from the skin. If a wound problem develops, wound debridement can result in exposing the graft and the anastomotic suture line. In this situation, one treatment option is to perform a muscle flap to cover the graft and the anastomosis with vascularized tissue. This can allow adequate debridement without the risk of exposing the graft. The sartorius muscle is readily accessible for use as a rotational muscle flap (Section 6). (1) It can also be used prophylactically in high-risk wounds.

REFERENCES

1. Khalil IM, Sudarsky L. Sartorius muscle "twist" rotation flap; an answer to flap necrosis. J Vasc Surg 1987;6(1):93–94.
2. Linton RR, Darling RC. Autogenous saphenous vein bypass grafts in femoropopliteal obliterative arterial disease. Surgery (St. Louis) 1962;51:62–73.
3. Reinier JAM, Van Dongen MD. T-Junction technique in vein anastomosis. In: Reconstructive Arterial Surgery: New York: Springer-Verlag, 1970:33.
4. Sharp WJ, Shamma AR, Kresowik TF, et al. Use of terminal T-junctions for in situ bypass in the lower extremity. Surg Gynecol Obstet 1991;172:151–152.
5. Taylor LM Jr, Edwards JM, Phinney ES, Porter JM. Reversed vein bypass to infrapopliteal arteries. Ann Vasc Surg 1987;205:90–97.

Saphenofemoral Junction with Femoral Vein Cuff

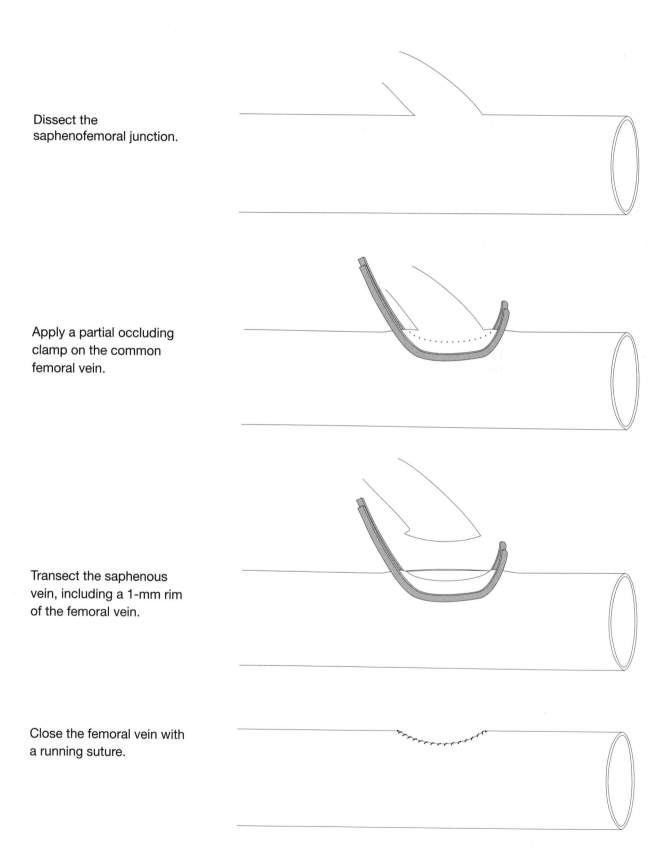

Dissect the saphenofemoral junction.

Apply a partial occluding clamp on the common femoral vein.

Transect the saphenous vein, including a 1-mm rim of the femoral vein.

Close the femoral vein with a running suture.

The vein is harvested with a branch segment 4-mm in length.

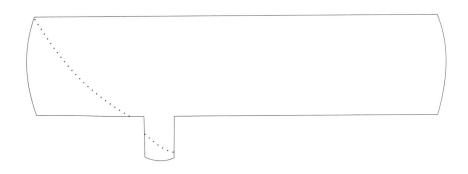

The vein is incised along its posterior aspect toward the branch. The side branch should not be made too long; otherwise, the vein will pivot along its heel.

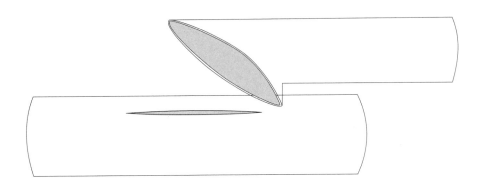

The anastomosis is completed.

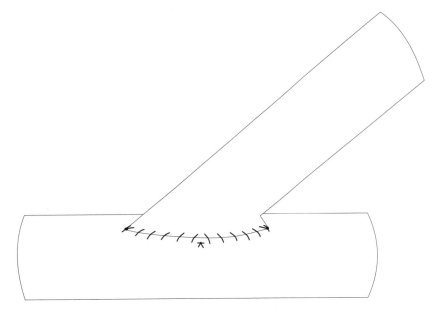

Patch Angioplasty of the Inflow Vessel

Create an arteriotomy in the desired location.

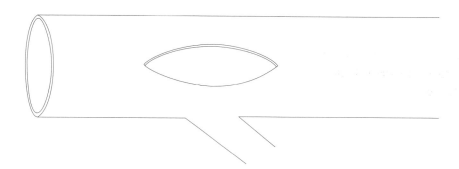

Close the arteriotomy with a vein patch.

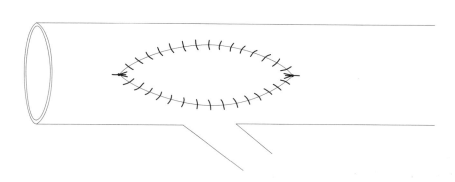

Create a venotomy in the patch.

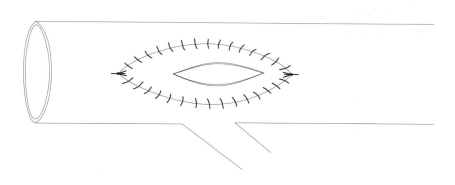

Construct the proximal anastomosis between the vein bypass and the venotomy.

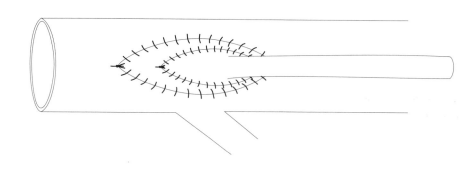

Patch Angioplasty of the Hood of the Bypass

Construct the proximal anastomosis.

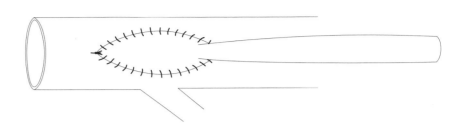

Create an incision in the narrowed segment of the bypass.

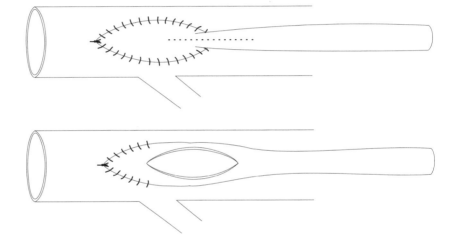

Perform a vein patch angioplasty of the proximal segment of the graft.

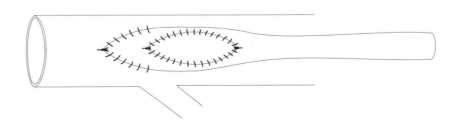

Incorporation of Profundaplasty

Create an arteriotomy
starting in the common
femoral artery and
extending into the profunda
femoris artery.

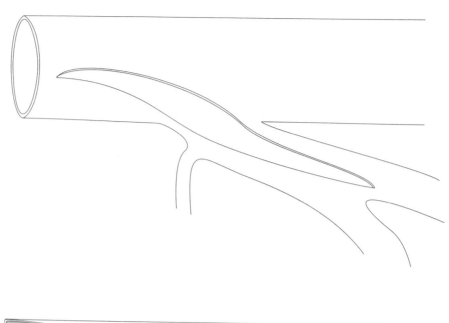

The vein is incised along its
posterior aspect to match
the length of the
arteriotomy.

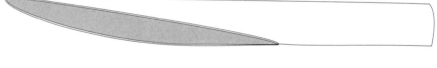

The anastomosis completed
with the hood of the bypass
serving as a patch.

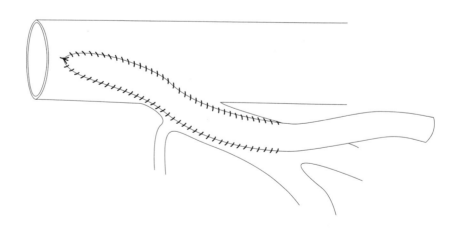

Sartorius Muscle Flap

The skin incision can be extended toward the anterior superior iliac spine. The origin of the sartorius muscle is identified and divided.

The proximal part of the sartorius muscle is mobilized. This usually necessitates division of one or two segmental arterial branches supplying the muscle. The number of transected branches should be kept to a minimum because the blood supply to the sartorius muscle is segmental rather than longitudinal. This is necessary to prevent ischemia of the mobilized muscle segment.

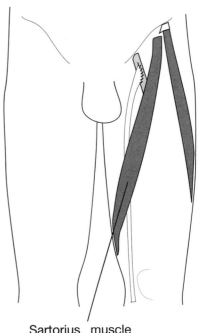

Sartorius muscle

The mobilized sartorius muscle is rotated to cover the anastomosis. The sartorius muscle can be secured to the inguinal ligament and the surrounding tissues with nonabsorbable sutures.

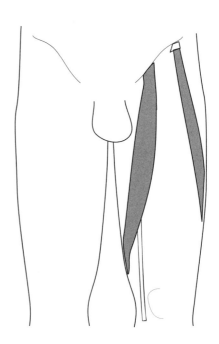

13

Adjunctive Techniques: Distal Anastomosis of an Infrainguinal Prosthetic Bypass

VEIN PATCHES AND CUFFS

Neointimal hyperplasia is a leading cause of bypass failure in the intermediate postoperative period (2–24 months). In prosthetic bypasses, neointimal hyperplasia is most likely to develop at the level of the distal anastomosis. Several techniques have been developed in an attempt to improve the patency of infrainguinal prosthetic bypasses. (1,2,5,6,7,8,9,10) These techniques involve incorporating a segment of vein between the prosthetic bypass and the recipient artery. The theory behind these techniques is that the interposition of the vein segment may ameliorate the future development of neointimal hyperplasia at the level of the distal anastomosis. In addition, incorporating the vein segment could facilitate the construction of the distal anastomosis and improve bypass patency in the immediate postoperative period. Although these techniques are often used, there are very few prospective randomized trials to date that show their efficacy. (1,2,3) Furthermore, there are no prospective randomized trials that compare these various techniques in an attempt to identify which technique is best.

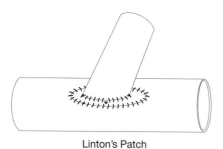

Linton's Patch

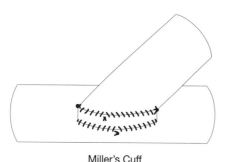

Miller's Cuff

LINTON'S PATCH

In one technique (Section 1a), a vein patch angioplasty is initially performed at the site selected for the distal anastomosis. An incision is created in the patch and used as the new site for constructing the anastomosis. The graft is then sutured to the vein patch. This technique is often referred to as the "Linton's patch" technique. (1,3,4) It is relatively simple to perform and can facilitate the construction of the anastomosis, especially in a heavily calcified vessel.

MILLER'S CUFF

Another technique involves suturing a segment of vein to the arteriotomy at the site selected for the distal anastomosis as a collar or a cuff. The graft is then sutured to the vein cuff. This technique originally described by Siegman is usually referred to as the "Miller cuff technique." (5,7) Several modifications of this technique have been described. The simplest method to perform is illustrated in

Section 1b. St. Mary's boot, another modification of the Miller cuff, is also described in Section 1b. (5)

TAYLOR'S PATCH

Another technique involves constructing the distal anastomosis directly between the graft and the artery. An incision is then created in the graft at the level of the distal anastomosis and extended through the apex for 1–2 cm into the outflow artery. A vein patch angioplasty of the incision is then performed. This method is referred to as the "Taylor patch" (Section 1c). (9) This technique can be technically demanding and requires mobilization of a long segment of artery in order to construct the anastomosis.

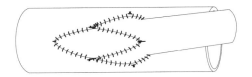

Taylor's Patch

REFERENCES

1. Batson RC, Sottiurai VS, Craighead CC. Linton patch angioplasty; an adjunct to distal bypass with polytetrafluoroethylene grafts. Ann Vasc Surg 1984;199:684–693.
2. Harris PL, Bakran A, Enabi L, Nott DM. ePTFE grafts for femoro-crural bypass-improved results with combined adjuvant venous cuff and arteriovenous fistula? Br J Surg 1983;70(6):377
3. Linton RR, Wilde WL. Modifications in the technique for femoropopliteal saphenous vein bypass autografts. Surgery (St.Louis) 1970;67:234–248.
4. Linton RR, Darling RC. Autogenous saphenous vein bypass grafts in femoropopliteal obliterative arterial disease. Surgery (St.Louis) 1962;51:62–73.
5. Miller JH, Foreman RK, Ferguson L, Faris I. Interposition vein cuff for anastomosis of prosthesis to small artery. Aust NZ J Surg 1984;54:283–285.
6. Raptis S, Miller JH. Influence of vein cuff on polytetrafluoroethylene grafts for primary femoropopliteal bypass. Br J Surg 1995;82:478–491.
7. Siegman FA. Use of the venous cuff for graft anastomosis. Surg Gynecol Obstet 1979;148:930.
8. Stonebride PA, Howlett R, Prestcott R, et al. Randomised trial comparing polytetrafluoroethylene graft patients with and without Miller cuff. Br J Surg 1995;2:555–556.
9. Taylor RS, Loh A, McFarland RJ, et al. Improved technique for polytetrafluoroethylene bypass grafting: long term results using anastomotic vein patches. Br J Surg 1992;79:348–354.
10. Wijesinghe LD, Beardsmore DM, Scott DJ. Polytetrafluoroethylene (PTFE) femorodistal grafts with a distal vein cuff for critical ischaemia. Eur J Vasc Endovasc Surg 1998;15(5):449–453.

Vein Patches and Cuffs
Linton Patch

Create an arteriotomy measuring 1.5–2.0 cm. Suture a vein patch to the arteriotomy as shown in Chapter 8.

Perform an incision in the center of the patch.

Transect the prosthetic graft in a beveled manner to match the incision in the vein patch.

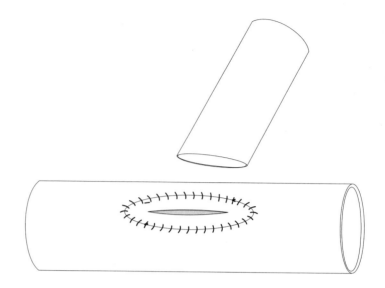

Start one suture at the heel of the graft (outside-inside), and then through the intimal part of the vein patch. Place a similar suture at the apex.

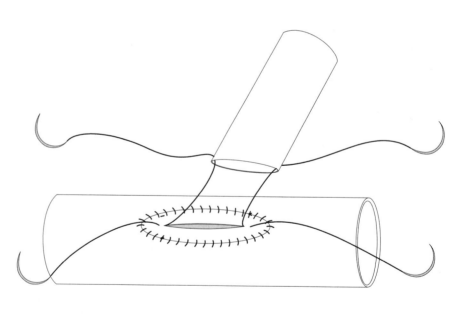

Tie both sutures.

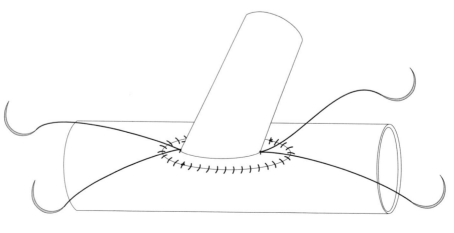

Vein Patches and Cuffs
Linton Patch

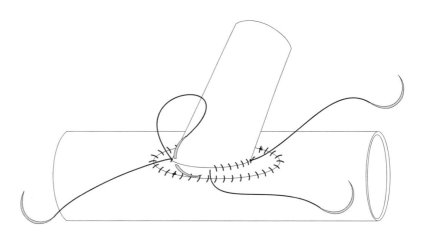

Start suturing with the heel suture. Introduce the needle outside-inside in the graft and inside-outside in the vein patch. Do the same with the apical suture.

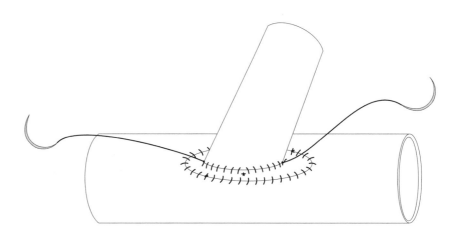

Tie the sutures.

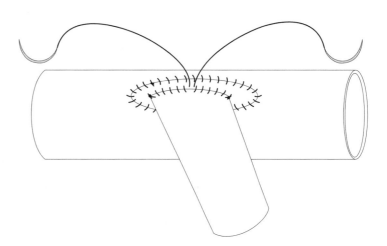

Flip the graft and replicate the suturing process on this side.

Vein Patches and Cuffs
Miller Cuff

Create an arteriotomy measuring 1.5–2.0 cm. Harvest a 4-cm segment of vein and slit the vein to create a patch.

The suture is first started in the center of the vein patch. The needle is introduced from the adventitial side of the vein.

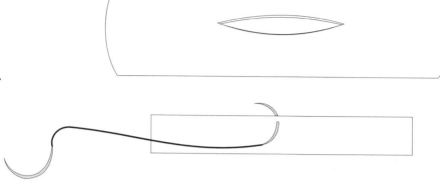

The needle is then introduced from the intimal side of the artery in the middle of the arteriotomy.

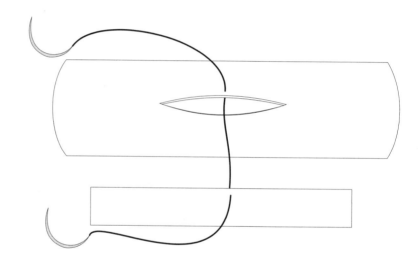

You may continue suturing using a parachute technique.

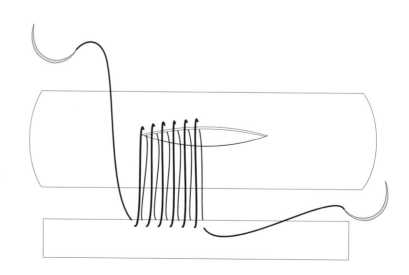

Vein Patches and Cuffs
Miller Cuff

Alternatively, you may tie the suture.

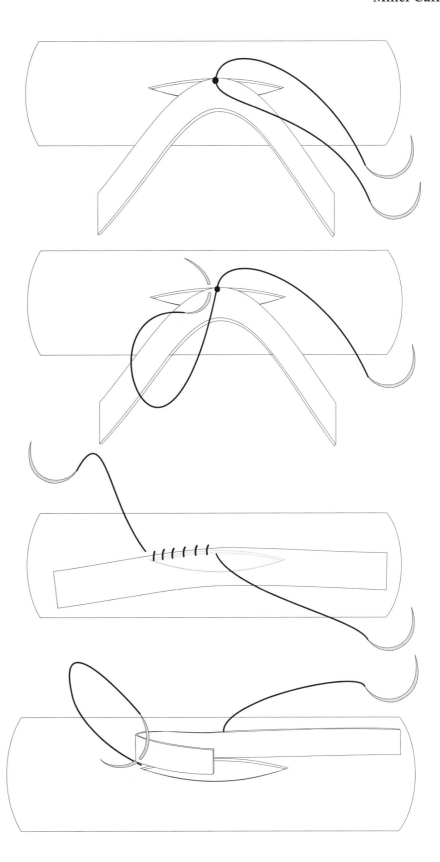

Introduce the needle outside-inside in the vein patch and inside-outside in the artery.

Place several sutures until the apex is reached.

Place an apical bite in the vein.

Vein Patches and Cuffs
Miller Cuff

Introduce the needle through the apex of the artery.

Fold the vein patch.

Continue suturing until you reach one end of the patch.

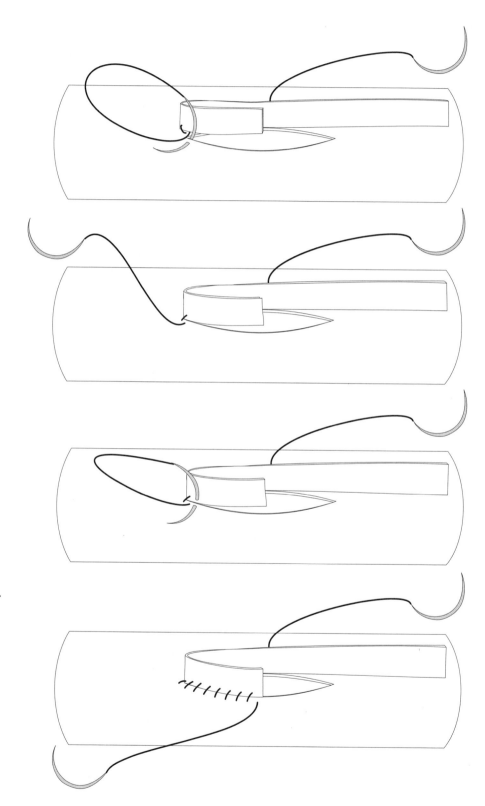

Vein Patches and Cuffs
Miller Cuff

Flip the patch.

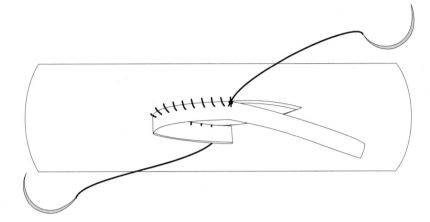

Again, introduce the needle from the adventitial side of the vein patch and then from the intimal side of the artery.

Continue suturing until the heel of the arteriotomy is reached.

Fold the vein.

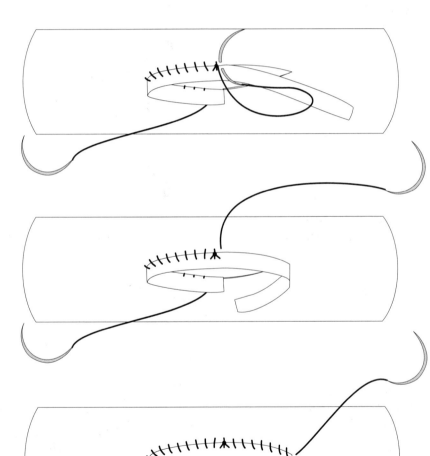

Vein Patches and Cuffs
Miller Cuff

Place the heel sutures. Again, outside-inside in the vein, inside-outside in the artery.

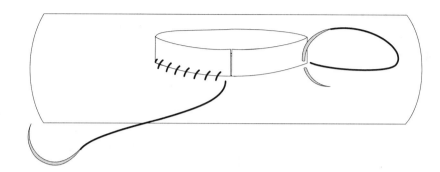

Trim the vein to the appropriate length.

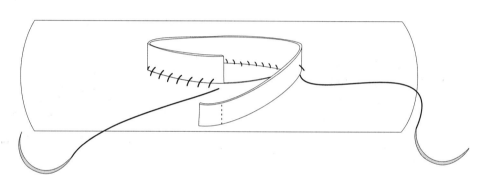

Continue suturing until both ends of the vein patch meet. Tie the sutures and cut one end.

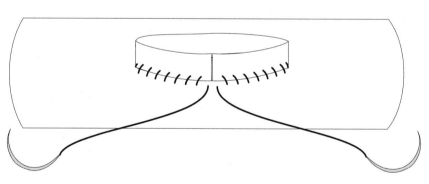

Start another suture at the apex to join the edges of the vein patch.

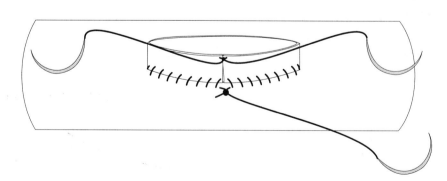

Vein Patches and Cuffs
Miller Cuff

Continue suturing towards the arterial suture line.

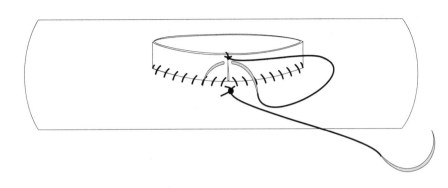

Tie the sutures together.

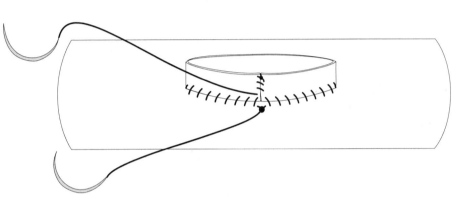

Transect the prosthetic graft in a beveled manner to match the vein cuff.

Construct the anastomosis between the graft and the cuff as described in Chapter 9.

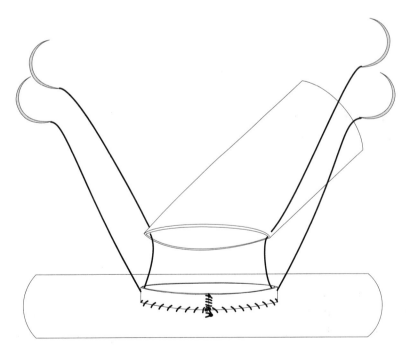

Vein Patches and Cuffs
Miller Cuff Modification
St. Mary's Boot

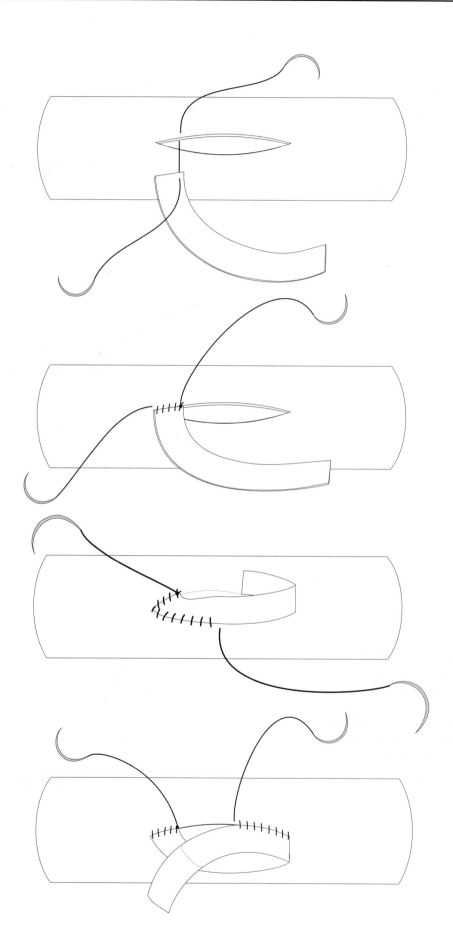

Start suturing from one corner of the vein patch.

Tie the suture. Run one end toward the apex of the arteriotomy.

Fold the vein and continue running the suture toward the heel.

Fold the vein around the heel and continue running the suture toward the apex.

Vein Patches and Cuffs
Miller Cuff Modification
St. Mary's Boot

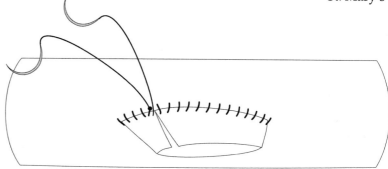

Trim the vein to the
appropriate length.

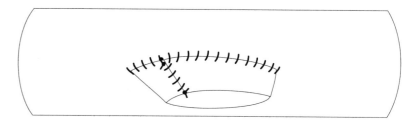

Suture the edges of
the vein patch.

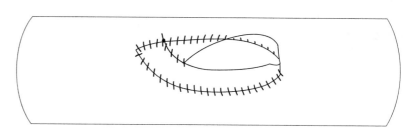

Excise a small wedge of the
vein cuff at the heel.

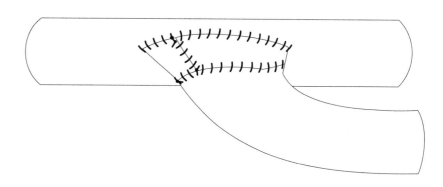

Suture the graft to the
vein cuff.

Vein Patches and Cuffs
Taylor Patch

Construct the heel portion
of the anastomosis using a
parachute or tie-down
technique.

Place one suture on one
side of the center of the
apex. Introduce the needle
outside-inside in the graft,
inside-outside in the artery.

Place an identical suture on
the other side of the apex.

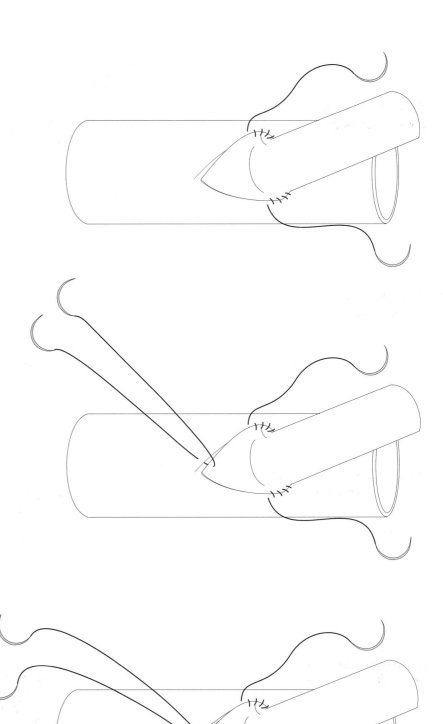

Vein Patches and Cuffs
Taylor Patch

Tie both sutures.

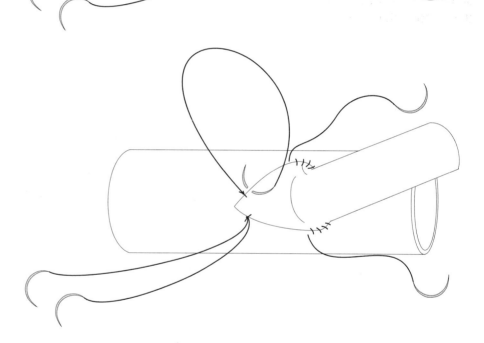

Run one end towards the
heel suture.

Run the other end towards
the heel suture.

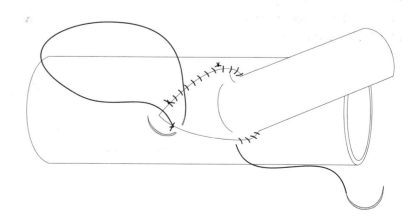

Vein Patches and Cuffs
Taylor Patch

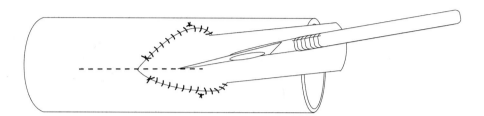

Incise the graft anteriorly
and extend the incision across
the center of the apex.

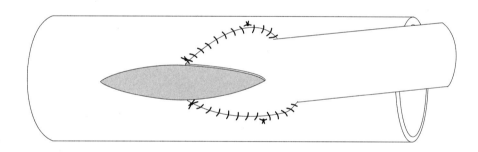

Place two stay sutures
between the incised apices
of the graft and artery.

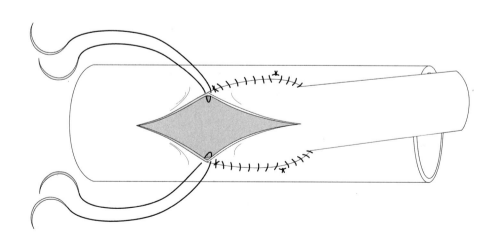

Vein Patches and Cuffs
Taylor Patch

Suture the vein patch starting at the apex. You may use a parachute technique or an anchor technique as shown here. Run each end towards the stay sutures and tie them together.

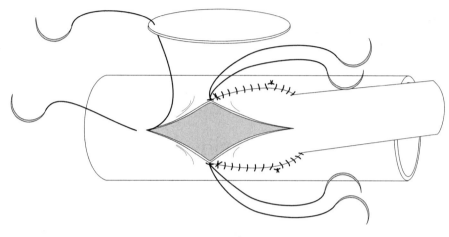

Start another suture in the center of the heel.

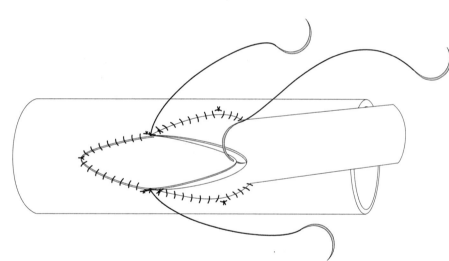

Run each end towards the remaining stay sutures and tie them together.

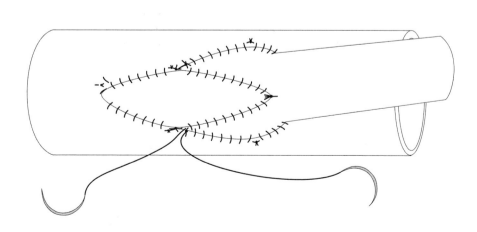

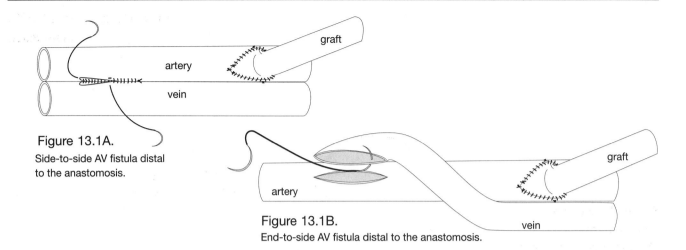

Figure 13.1A.
Side-to-side AV fistula distal
to the anastomosis.

Figure 13.1B.
End-to-side AV fistula distal to the anastomosis.

ARTERIOVENOUS FISTULAE

Poor distal runoff is often cited as a cause of infrainguinal prosthetic bypass failure. Several techniques have been developed in an attempt to improve the patency of prosthetic bypasses with disadvantaged outflow tracts. The main concept of these techniques is the creation of an arteriovenous fistula to improve the outflow and decrease the distal vascular resistance. (3)

In one technique, after constructing the distal anastomosis between the prosthetic graft and the recipient artery, an arteriovenous fistula is constructed a few centimeters distal to the anastomosis. (5) This arteriovenous (AV) fistula can be constructed in a side-to-side fashion (Figure 13.1A) as described in Chapter 11. The arteriovenous fistula can also be constructed by dividing the vein and joining its proximal end to the artery a few centimeters distal to the anastomosis using an end-to-side configuration (Figure 13.1B).

In other techniques, the arteriovenous fistula is incorporated in the construction of the distal anastomosis (Figure 13.2). (3,4) In one variation, the arteriovenous fistula is constructed in a side-to-side fashion (Section 1). An incision is created in the artery at the site selected for the distal anastomosis. A matching incision is created in the vein accompanying the artery. The adjacent walls of the artery and the vein are sutured together, resulting in a combined opening into the artery and the vein. The graft is then sutured to this newly created opening, allowing the blood to flow into the artery and the vein simultaneously. The size of the fistula can be theoretically controlled by changing the length of the venotomy. The longer the size of the venotomy, the larger is the fistula. One advantage of this technique is that it involves adding only one additional suture line between the adjacent walls of the artery and the vein. The disadvantage of this technique is that the prosthetic bypass is connected directly to the artery without the potential theoretical benefit of an interposed vein segment.

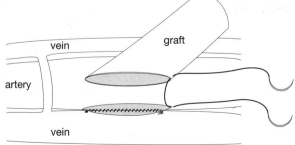

Figure 13.2.
AV fistula incorporated in the anastomosis

Another variation described by Ascer involves incorporating the concept of vein cuff and the concept of arteriovenous fistula together (Section 2). (1) In this method, one of the veins accompanying the artery is mobilized for several centimeters. An arteriotomy is created in the artery at the site selected for the distal anastomosis. The vein is transected and sutured in an end-to-side manner to the artery. It is important to mobilize the vein for a long segment to allow for a gentle curve of the vein over the artery. A venotomy is created in the hood of the vein and will serve as the new site for constructing the anastomosis with the prosthetic graft (Figure 13.3a). The graft is then sutured to the venotomy. Although this technique involves creating an additional anastomosis, it has several attractive features. The anastomosis between the vein and the artery and the anastomosis between the bypass and the vein are conducted by following the same principles of any end-to-side anastomosis. Surgeons are familiar with this type of reconstruction, which can be carried out even in heavily calcified vessels. The anastomosis between the graft and the vein can be accomplished with relative ease and expediency. At the completion of the anastomoses, the flow and the magnitude of the fistula can be controlled by banding of the fistula. The pressure in the graft is measured and compared to the radial artery pressure. Banding is considered unnecessary if the gradient is less than 30 mmHg, or if the pressure in the graft is greater than 100 mm Hg. Banding can be accomplished by placing a 4-mm PTFE ring around the vein (Figure 13.3b).

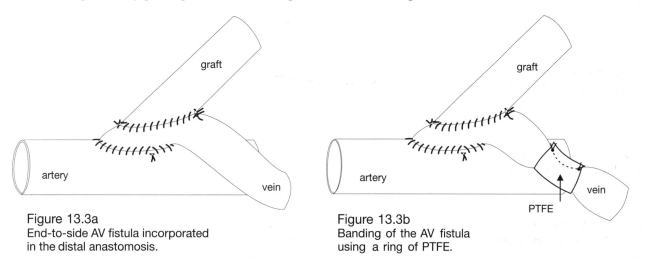

Figure 13.3a
End-to-side AV fistula incorporated
in the distal anastomosis.

Figure 13.3b
Banding of the AV fistula
using a ring of PTFE.

REFERENCES

1. Ascer E, Gennaro M, Polina R, et al. Complementary distal arteriovenous fistula and deep vein interposition: a five-year experience with a new technique to improve infrapopliteal prosthetic bypass patency. J Vasc Surg 1996;24:134–143.
2. Dardik H, Sussman B, Ibrahmin M, et al. Distal arterio-venous fistula as an adjunct to maintaining arterial and graft patency for limb salvage. Surgery (St. Louis) 1983;94(3):478.
3. Dean RE, Read RC. The influence of increased blood flow on thrombosis in prosthetic grafts. Surgery 1964;55:581–584.
4. Harris PL, Campbell H. Adjuvant distal arteriovenous shunt with femorotibial bypass for critical ischaemia. Br J Surg 1983;70(6):377.
5. Paty PSK, Shah DM, et al. Remote distal arteriovenous fistula to improve infrapopliteal bypass patency. J Vasc Surg 1990;1:171–178.

Arteriovenous Fistulae
Side-to-Side

Expose the infrapopliteal
vessels. Select the larger
accompanyimg vein for
creating the AV fistula.

Create an arteriotomy in the
anteroinferior aspect of the
artery, close to the selected
vein.

Create a venotomy in the
selected vein adjacent to the
created arteriotomy. The size
of the venotomy can vary
according to the surgeon's
preference.

Start a horizontal mattress
suture at the apex of the
venotomy. Tie the suture and
cut one end.

Introduce the needle outside-
inside in the vein, close to the
start of the suture.

Introduce the needle in a
corresponding site in the artery
(inside-outside).

Pull the suture. Start suturing
the adjacent arterial and venous
walls together.

The needle is introduced from
the intimal side of the artery
and then from the adventitial
side of the vein.

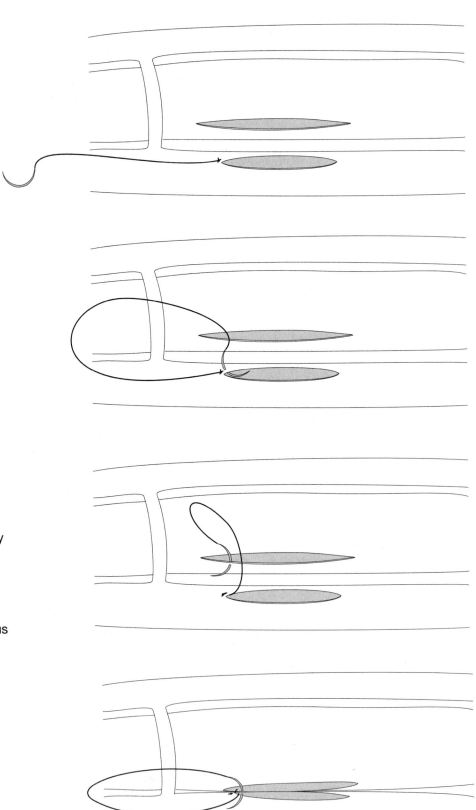

Arteriovenous Fistulae
Side-to-Side

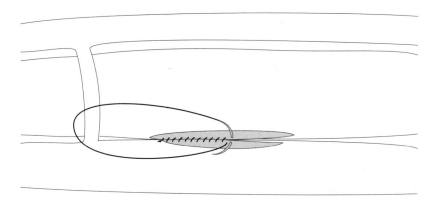

Continue suturing until the adjacent venous and arterial walls are fully approximated.

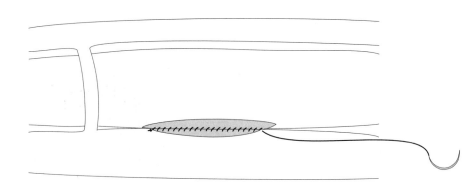

Start another stay suture at the apex of the venotomy and tie the sutures together

Transect the graft to match the size of the arteriotomy.

Start one suture at the center of the heel. Outside-inside in the graft; inside-outside in the artery. You may tie the suture or use a parachute technique as shown here.

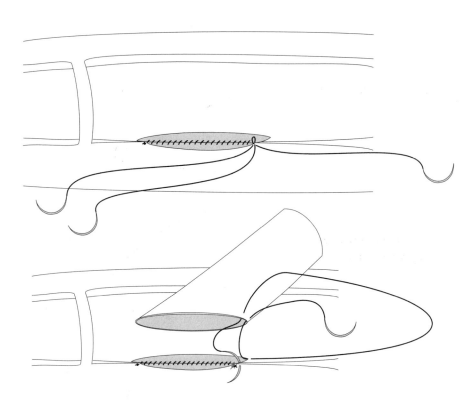

Arteriovenous Fistulae
Side-to-Side

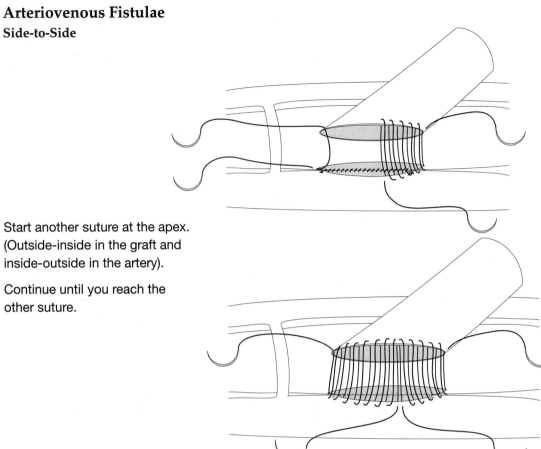

Start another suture at the apex. (Outside-inside in the graft and inside-outside in the artery).

Continue until you reach the other suture.

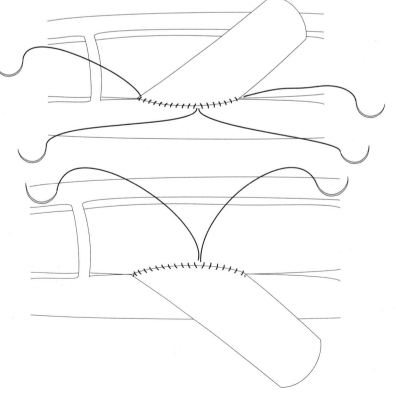

Pull and tighten the sutures.

Flip the graft and replicate the suturing on this side.

Arteriovenous Fistulae
End-to-Side

Expose the tibial vessels
and divide the venae
comitantes.

Dissect a 5 cm segment of
the larger accompanying
tibial vein.

Ligate and transect the vein
as distally as possible.

Perform an arteriotomy in
the tibial artery.

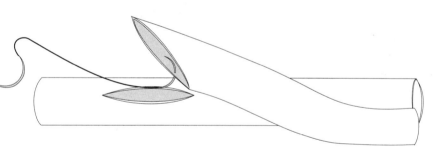

Incise the posterior wall of
the transected vein to match
the size of the arteriotomy.

Make sure to place the vein
on the arteriotomy to accurately
place the incision in the posterior
wall of the vein.

You may perform the anastomosis
using an anchor technique or a
parachute technique as shown here.
Start suturing in the vein a few bites
away from the center of the heel
(outside-inside in the vein,
inside-outside in the artery).

Continue suturing until you
are a few bites beyond the
center of the heel.

Arteriovenous Fistulae
End-to-Side

The anastomosis is completed and checked for hemostasis.

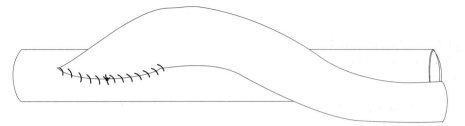

Create a 1–1.5 cm venotomy.

Transect the prosthetic graft in a beveled fashion to match the size of the venotomy.

Construct an end-to-side anastomosis between the graft and the vein as described in Chapter 9.

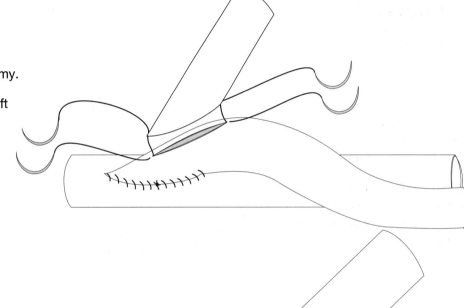

Check the suture lines for hemostasis.

IV

Aortic Surgery

14

Infrarenal Abdominal Aortic Aneurysm Replacement: Proximal Anastomosis

GENERAL PRINCIPLES

During the replacement of an infrarenal abdominal aortic aneurysm, the proximal anastomosis between the graft and the neck of the aneurysm is constructed in an end-to-end fashion. The basic techniques for preparing the neck of the aneurysm for the creation of the proximal anastomosis are illustrated in Section 1. The aneurysm wall is incised longitudinally on its anterior aspect keeping to the right of the origin of the inferior mesenteric artery. The incision in the aorta is carried to the level of the neck of the aneurysm. The incision is then teed off on each side of the neck leaving the posterior wall intact.

INTACT POSTERIOR WALL

The needle will penetrate the aorta approximately 1 cm proximal to the aneurysm neck (Figure 14.1A) and will exit the posterior aortic wall 1.5–2 cm distal to the aneurysm neck (Figure 14.1B). When tension is applied to the suture line, the layers of the aorta just proximal and distal to the aneurysm neck will be pulled together, resulting in a "double-layer" bite (Figure 14.1C). The theoretical advantage of the "double-layer" bite is that the two layers will buttress each other, resulting in a stronger and more hemostatic bite.

The placement of the bites when the posterior aortic wall is left intact can be technically demanding. Occasionally, when the needle is introduced through

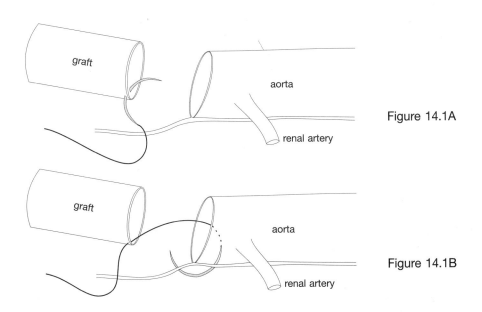

Figure 14.1A

Figure 14.1B

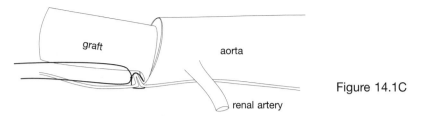

Figure 14.1C

the posterior aortic wall, its tip as it exits distally may not be easily visualized. The temptation to be avoided in such situations is to place a shallower bite. Shallow bites placed in the posterior aortic wall without incorporating the adventitia could tear through the aortic wall. The placement of deep bites and the retrieval of the needle from the aortic wall can be facilitated by using a large needle, such as an MH needle (Ethicon).

The posterior suture line can be carried out using either an anchor or a parachute technique. The parachute technique can be started in the center of the posterior wall or at the beginning of the posterior wall, as shown in Section 2a. When there is a mismatch between the diameter of the graft and the aortic neck, starting at the center could help in better judging the advancement between the bites.

The anchor technique is usually started in the center of the posterior suture line (Section 2b). In general, the placement of the sutures could be facilitated if the surgeon performs his side of the suture line and the first assistant performs the other side. In another modification, the entire or part of the posterior suture line is constructed using an interrupted horizontal mattress suture technique. This technique could be useful when the aortic neck is very diseased. Additional sutures may be needed after the release of the clamps to secure hemostasis, especially with a heavily calcified wall.

TRANSECTED POSTERIOR WALL

Another option is to transect the aortic wall completely.(Section 3) This facilitates the construction of the posterior part of the anastomosis. In this technique, after introducing the needle in the aortic wall, the needle tip can be easily visualized underneath the aortic stump. The transection of the aorta facilitates placing and retrieving the needle. The main disadvantage of this technique is the potential for venous injury during aortic transection. Injury to the vena cava or to a retroaortic renal vein or lumbar veins may result in undesirable bleeding. In addition, after transecting the aorta, the aortic wall may be found to be thinner than expected. In this situation, placement of pledget mattress sutures may be desirable to reinforce the aortic wall for a secure hemostatic anastomosis.

Transection of the aorta is routinely used in the technique of aneurysm exclusion with aortic bypass. It is also used when a transaortic endarterectomy of the renal arteries is contemplated in conjunction with an aortic reconstruction. In the management of aortoiliac occlusive disease, the proximal aorta may be transected when performing an aortobifemoral bypass routinely by some surgeons, especially when the aorta is heavily calcified or when dealing with a chronic aortic occlusion.

When the aortic wall is transected, the posterior suture line may be carried using an anchor or a parachute technique. The anchoring suture is usually started in the center of the posterior wall and may be a simple or a mattress suture. This technique could be ideal when the transected aorta is well exposed in a thin patient. If a parachute technique is used, the suture line may be started in the center of the posterior line or at one end of the posterior wall. Whenever the parachute technique is used, it is most important to check the tightness of the suture line with a nerve hook before tying the final knot.

In general, for right-handed surgeons, the construction of the posterior portion of the anastomosis is facilitated if performed from the opposite side of the table.

General Principles

The aorta can be clamped in a horizontal or transverse manner depending on the presence of plaque in the aortic wall.

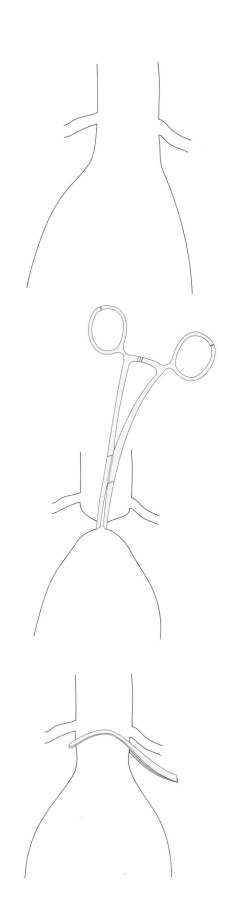

If the aortic wall is free of any palpable plaque or if the plaque is on the lateral wall of the aorta, the aortic clamp is applied in a vertical direction. The clamp is inserted under direct vision and advanced until the tips of the jaws are felt touching the vertebral column. This will ensure that the aorta is completely enclosed between the clamp's jaws.

In the presence of plaque in the posterior wall of the aorta, the aorta is dissected circumferentially and the clamp is applied in a transverse manner to appose the anterior aortic wall against the posterior aortic wall.

General Principles

The aorta is incised along its anterior wall. The incision is carried to the right of the inferior mesenteric artery. This allows for the protection of the IMA should reimplantation become necessary. The sympathetic nerves that run around the origin of the IMA are also preserved.

At the neck of the aneurysm, the incision is carried in a T-fashion from anterior to posterior.

Avoid incising the lateral aspect of the wall in a cephalad direction as this may compromise the placement of posterior sutures.

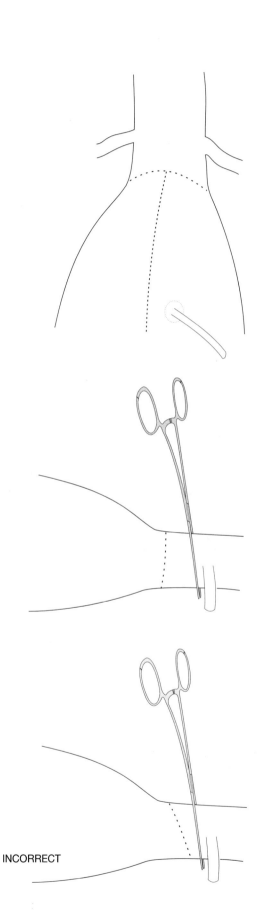

INCORRECT

General Principles

The posterior wall of the aorta can be left intact, which allows placement of a double-layer aortic wall suture. The double-layer sutures of the posterior wall of the aorta may be facilitated by using a large needle.

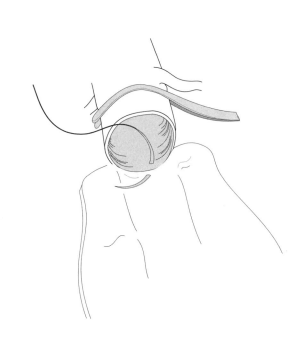

Avoid placing shallow bites in the posterior aortic wall.

General Principles

The needle should be introduced at a right angle to the posterior wall.

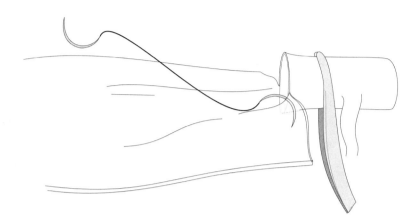

The needle is advanced through the posterior wall while following the curvature of the needle.

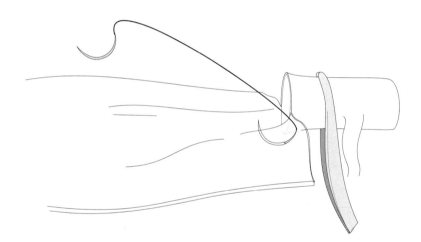

The resulting bite is a deep double-layer bite in the posterior aortic wall.

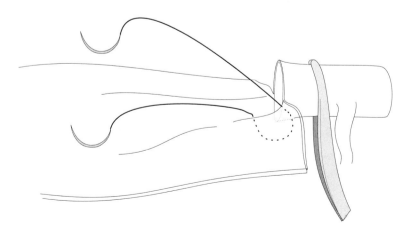

General Principles

Alternatively, the posterior wall may be divided completely.

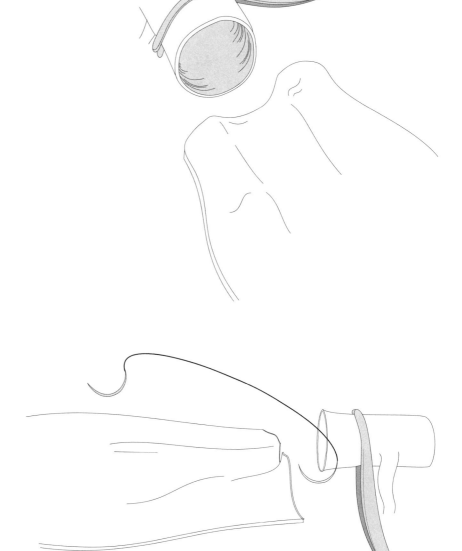

This technique will facilitate placement of the posterior wall sutures. If the wall is relatively thin, reinforcement of the wall with pledget sutures may be necessary.

Intact Posterior Wall
Parachute Technique
Starting on the lateral aspect of the aorta

Start by introducing the needle (outside-inside) in the graft.

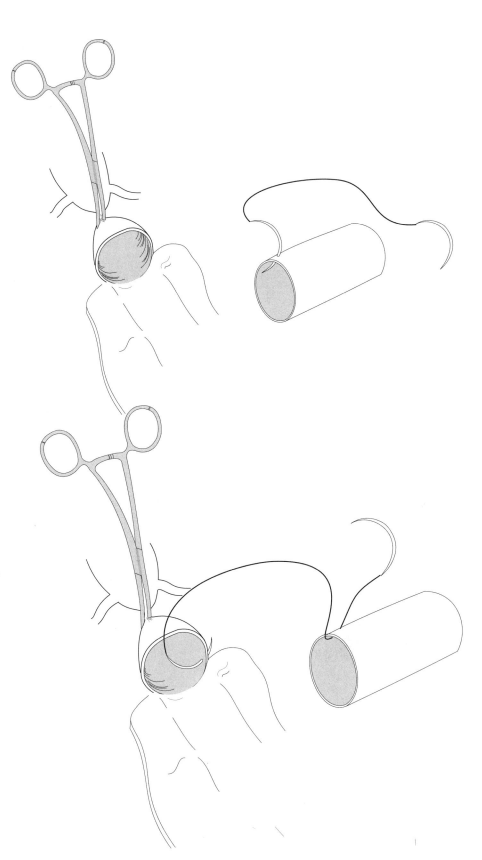

Place the next suture in the aortic wall very close to the line of division of the lateral wall. This bite is a single-layer bite in the aortic wall. Make sure that the suture line is not crossed by grabbing the needle from underneath the loop.

Intact Posterior Wall
Parachute Technique
Starting on the lateral aspect of the aorta

Place the next bite in the graft. Make sure that the suture line, again, is not crossed.

Place a double-layer suture in the aortic wall.

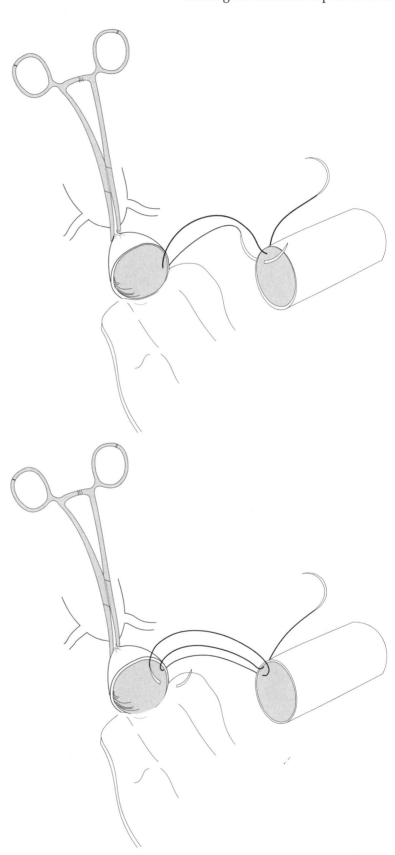

Intact Posterior Wall

Parachute Technique

Starting on the lateral aspect of the aorta

Introduce the needle in the graft.

Continue suturing the back wall of the aorta with double-layer sutures. Make sure the sutures are placed deeply through the posterior wall of the aorta.

Continue suturing until the posterior wall of the anastomosis is completed.

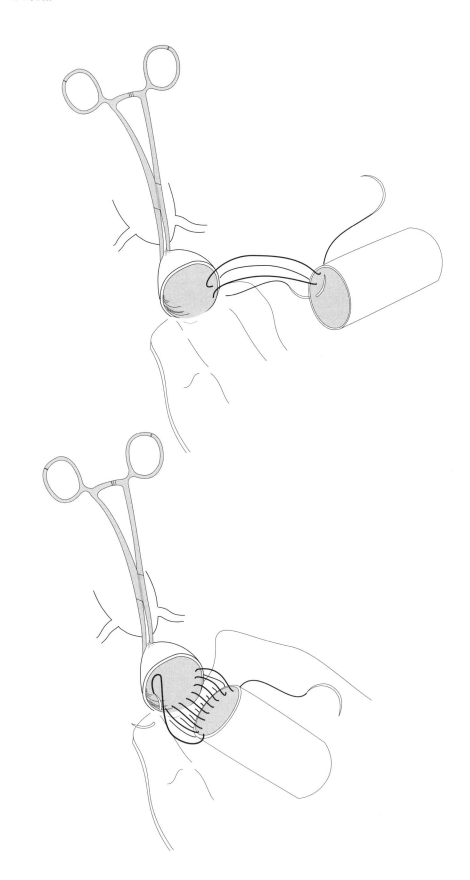

Intact Posterior Wall
Parachute Technique
Starting on the lateral aspect of the aorta

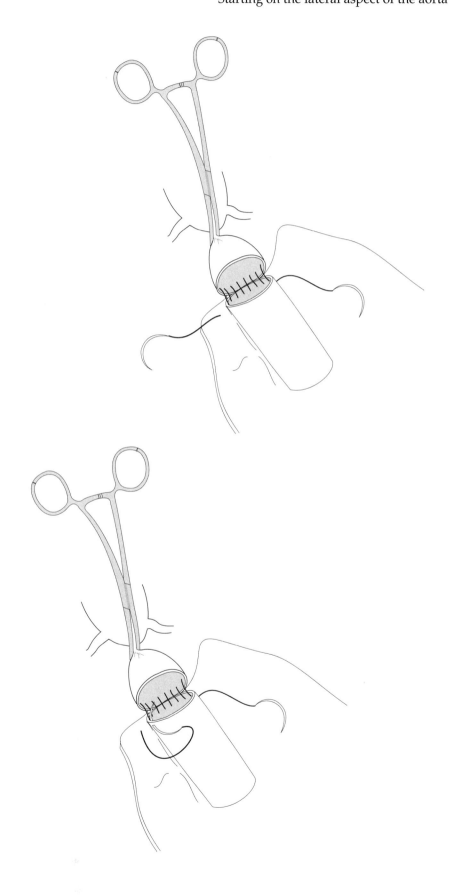

Bring down the graft to the aortic wall by pulling and tightening the suture. Use a nerve hook to ensure that the suture line is tight.

You may complete the entire anastomosis with one suture as shown below.

Introduce the needle in the graft.

Intact Posterior Wall

Parachute Technique
Starting on the lateral aspect of the aorta

Introduce the needle in the
single-layer aortic wall.

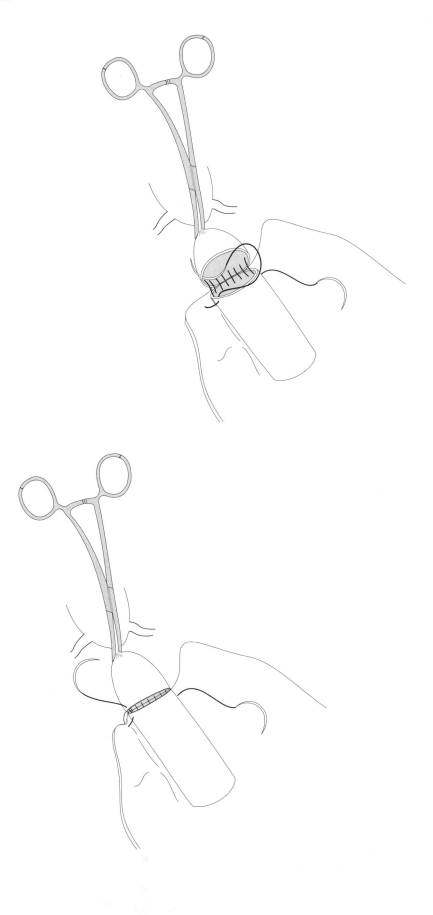

Pull and tighten the suture.

Intact Posterior Wall
Parachute Technique
Starting on the lateral aspect of the aorta

Continue running the suture all the way along the anterior aortic wall.

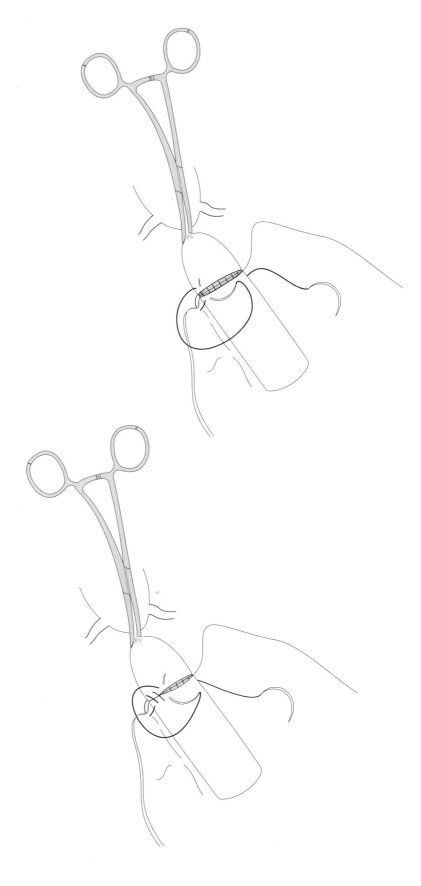

Intact Posterior Wall

Parachute Technique

Starting on the lateral aspect of the aorta

Pull and tighten the suture line on the anterior wall and the posterior wall. Use a nerve hook again to ensure that the suture line is not loose.

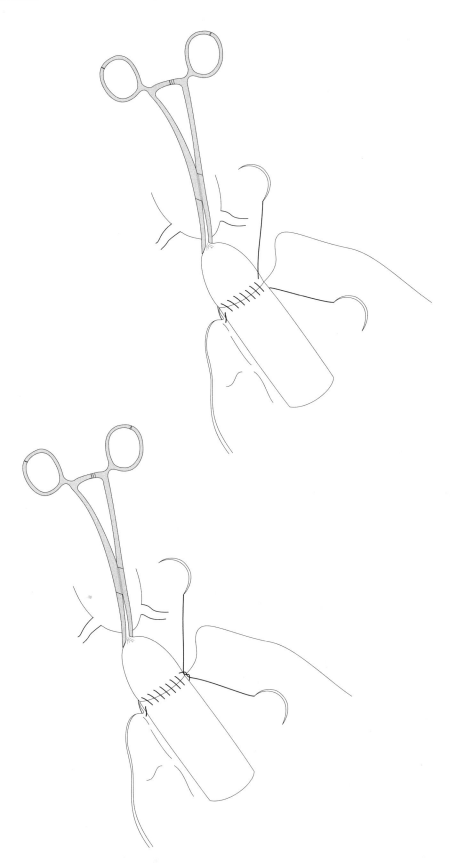

Intact Posterior Wall
Parachute Technique
Starting on the lateral aspect of the aorta

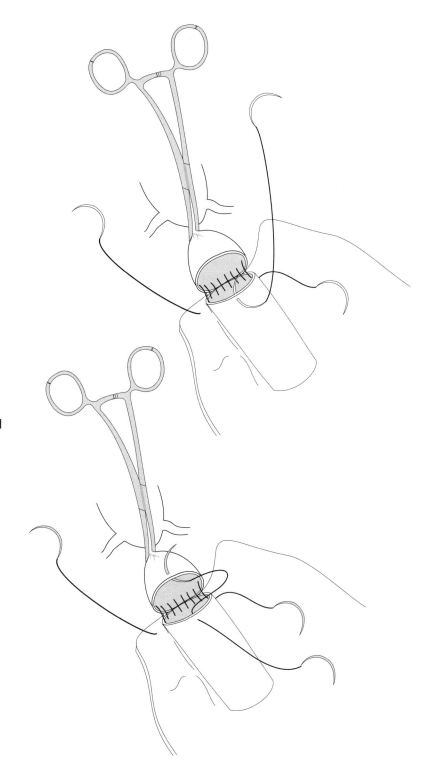

Alternatively, you may start another suture in the center of the anterior wall of the graft.

You may use a parachute technique for the anterior wall or an anchor technique as shown here.

Introduce the needle in a corresponding site in the aorta. This suture may be a horizontal mattress or a simple suture as shown here.

Intact Posterior Wall
Parachute Technique
Starting on the lateral aspect of the aorta

Introduce the needle
outside-inside in the graft,
inside-outside in the aorta.

Continue suturing with one end
of the suture towards the
posterior wall of the aorta.

Tighten the suture.

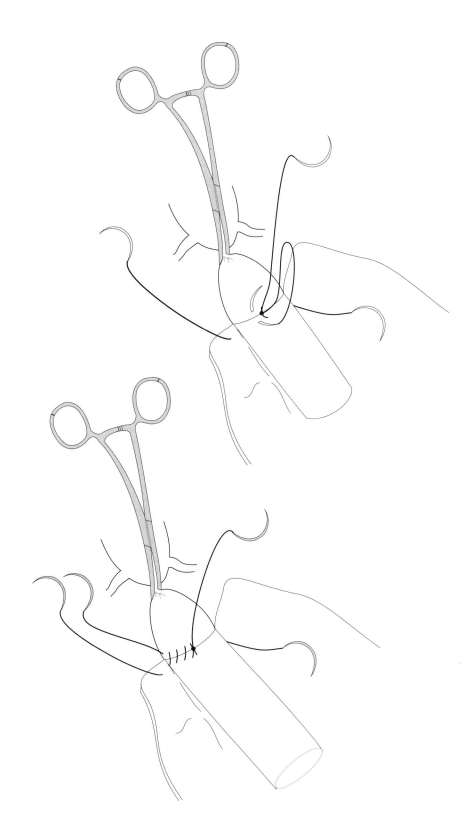

Intact Posterior Wall
Parachute Technique
Starting on the lateral aspect of the aorta

Start suturing with the other end towards the posterior wall of the aorta.

Introduce the needle outside-inside in the graft, inside-outside in the aorta.

Continue suturing until you reach the other suture.

Pull and tighten the suture line.

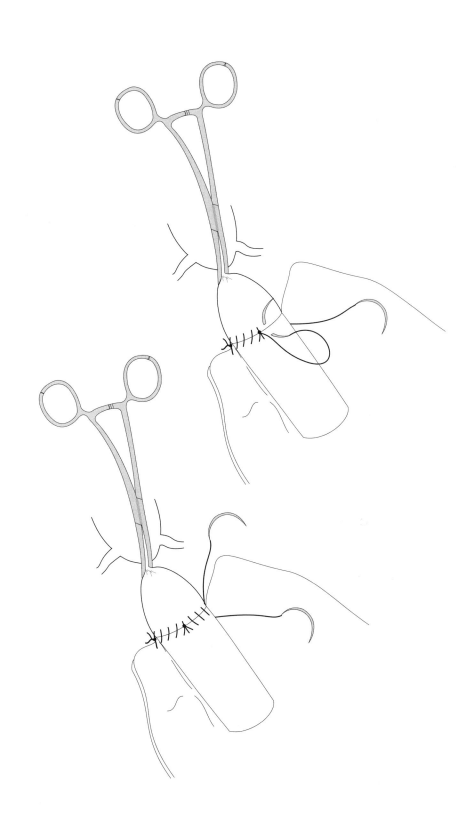

Intact Posterior Wall
Anchor Technique
Continuous sutures

Introduce the needle
outside-inside on the graft.

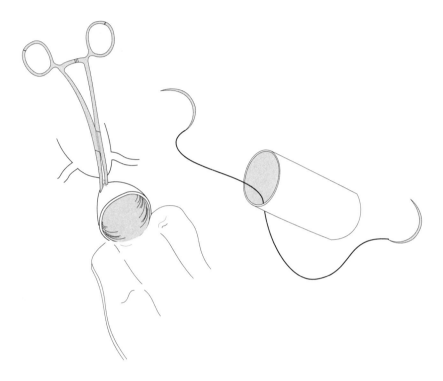

Introduce the needle in the
back wall of the aorta.
Make sure that the bite in
the aortic wall is deep and
is incorporating the full
thickness of the wall.

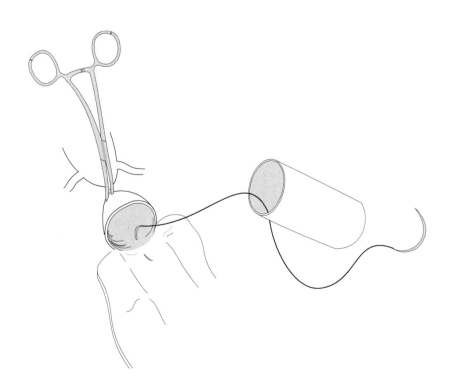

Intact Posterior Wall
Anchor Technique
Continuous sutures

Introduce the needle 2–3 mm
away from the previous suture.

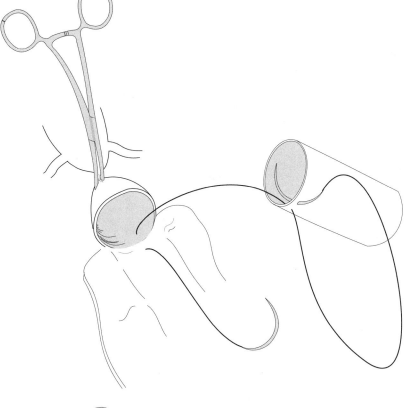

Repeat the same in the
back wall of the aorta.

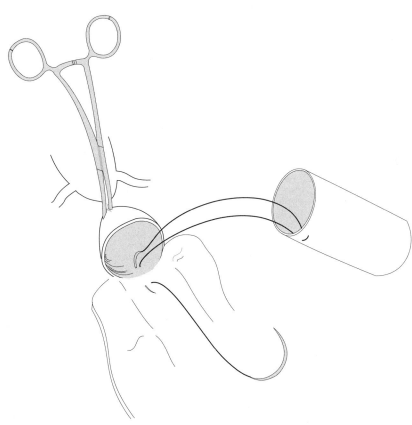

Intact Posterior Wall
Anchor Technique
Continuous sutures

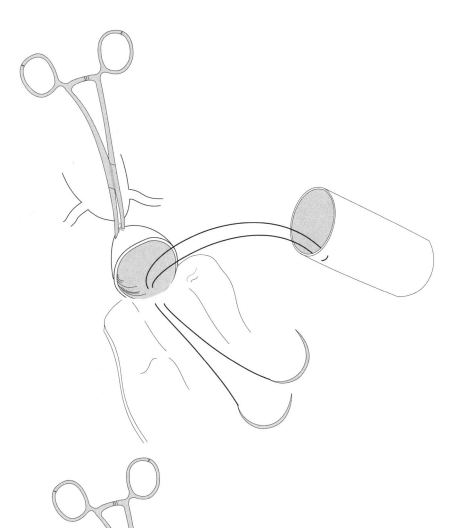

Tie the suture.

Intact Posterior Wall
Anchor Technique
Continuous sutures

Start running the suture on one side. Again, outside-inside in the graft and inside-outside in the aorta.

When performing a transabdominal aortic replacement, these bites are best placed with a forehand movement when the surgeon is standing on the right-hand side of the patient.

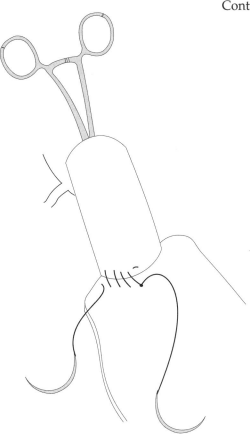

Start running the suture toward the other side.

The placement of the bites on this side will be facilitated if placed by the assistant using a forehand motion or using a backhand movement by the surgeon.

Intact Posterior Wall
Anchor Technique
Interrupted mattress sutures

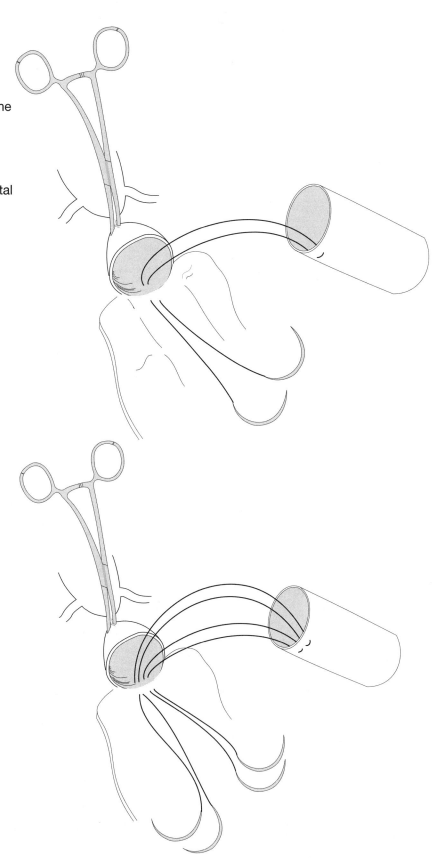

Alternatively, the posterior suture line is constructed using interrupted mattress sutures.

This technique may be used in a calcified aorta. Interrupted horizontal mattress sutures will be used for suturing the entire or part of the posterior wall suture line.

Start by placing a horizontal mattress suture in the graft and in the center of the back wall of the aorta.

Place additional horizontal mattress sutures in the graft and the back wall of the aorta on either side of the center.

Intact Posterior Wall
Anchor Technique
Interrupted mattress sutures

You may construct part of the posterior wall with interrupted mattress sutures.

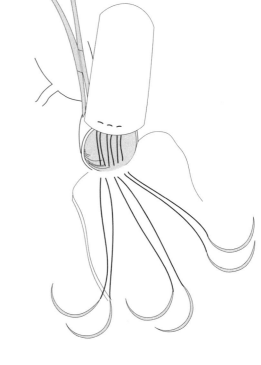

Tie the sutures. Construct the remaining part of the posterior anastomosis using a continuous running suture.

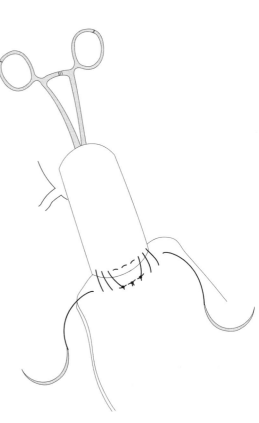

Intact Posterior Wall

Anchor Technique

Interrupted mattress sutures

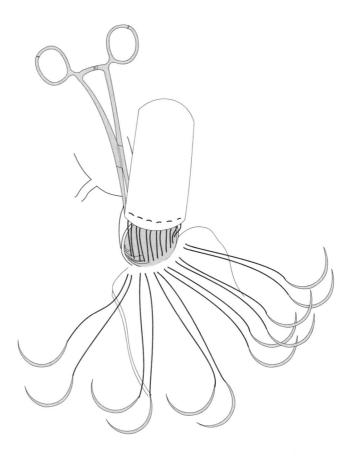

Alternatively, you may construct the entire posterior wall with interrupted horizontal mattress sutures.

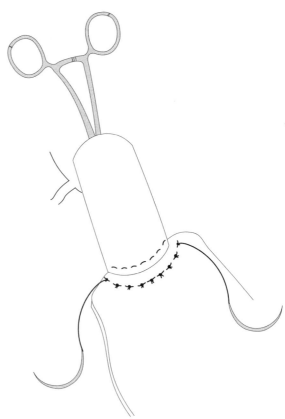

Transected Posterior Wall
Parachute Technique; Anchor Technique

Transecting the aortic wall can facilitate placement of the posterior wall sutures. Care should be taken to avoid injury to any retroaortic, lumbar, or renal vein branches.

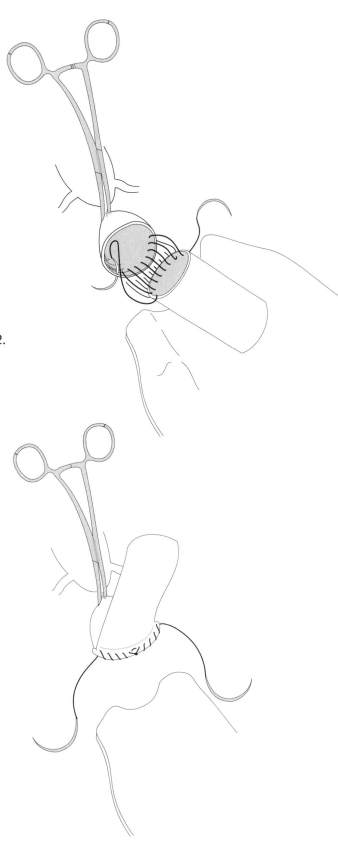

The entire posterior suture line can be performed in a running parachute fashion. Suturing is started from the end away from the surgeon and then progressing towards the surgeon's side as illustrated in Section 2.

Alternatively, the entire posterior suture line can be constructed using an anchor technique as illustrated in Section 3.

Transected Posterior Wall
Interrupted Mattress Sutures

Alternatively, the entire posterior wall can be performed using interrupted sutures.

Place the horizontal mattress sutures as previously illustrated (outside-inside on the graft, inside-outside on the aorta).

If the aortic wall appears attenuated, pledget sutures can be placed to reinforce the suture line.

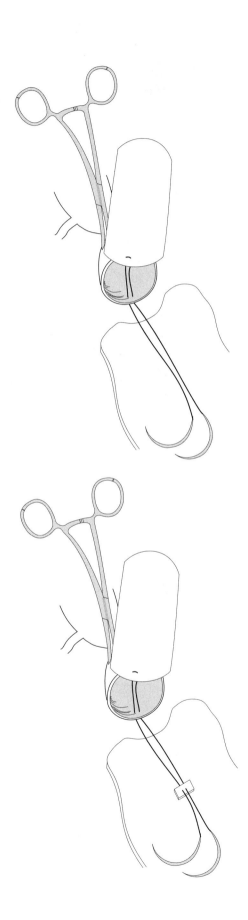

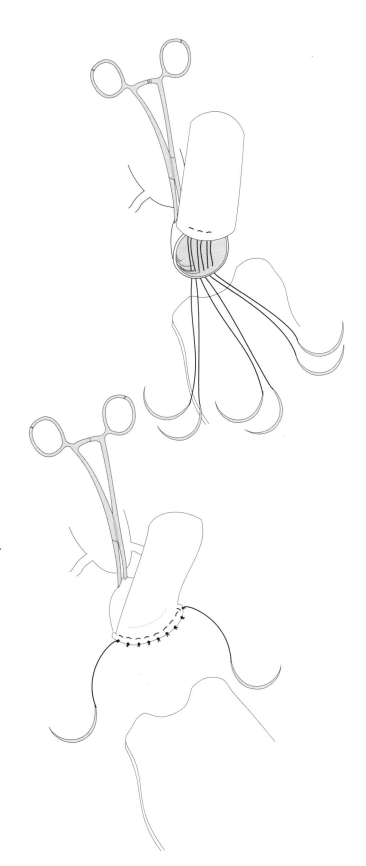

Place as many horizontal mattress sutures
as necessary.

Pull and tie the sutures.

The entire anastomosis can be constructed
with interrupted mattress sutures.
Alternatively, the anterior wall is constructed
with a continuous suture as previously illustrated.

You can inspect the posterior suture line by
gently lifting the graft. This could allow
accurate placement of any additional
sutures to correct bleeding from the suture line.

15

Thoracoabdominal Aortic Aneurysm Replacement: Proximal Anastomosis

The technique utilized for construction of the proximal aortic anastomosis in a patient with a thoracoabdominal aortic aneurysm depends on the extent of the aneurysmal pathology and the relationship of the aneurysm to the orifices of the celiac, superior mesenteric, and the right and left renal arteries.

PROXIMAL ANASTOMOSIS INCORPORATING THE CELIAC, SUPERIOR MESENTERIC AND RIGHT RENAL ARTERIES

When the aneurysmal disease starts at the level of the celiac artery and the aorta becomes normal just proximal to the celiac artery (Crawford type IV), one option is to incorporate the orifices of the celiac, superior mesenteric, and both renal arteries in the proximal anastomosis. The anastomosis is appropriately tailored depending on the distance between the right and left renal arteries. In the presence of significant aneurysmal pathology between the right and left renal arteries, only the celiac, superior mesenteric, and right renal arteries are incorporated as a tongue of aortic tissue into the proximal anastomosis. The left renal artery will have to be reimplanted separately.

REIMPLANTATION OF THE CELIAC, SUPERIOR MESENTERIC AND RIGHT RENAL ARTERIES ON AN AORTIC PATCH

When the aneurysmal pathology extends several centimeters proximal to the origin of the celiac artery, the visceral vessels cannot be incorporated in the proximal anastomosis. The proximal anastomosis is performed at the level where the aortic wall is normal. The celiac, superior mesenteric, and renal arteries will be reimplanted as an island. Frequently the left renal artery cannot be included in the island and is to be reimplanted separately. After completion of the distal anastomosis, a partial occluding clamp is then applied on the aortic graft in preparation for the reimplantation of the left renal artery. It is important to avoid placing the clamp very close to the suture line as it may cause an excessive stress on the suture line, resulting in bleeding. Another factor one must consider is to accommodate for the return of the left kidney to its normal anatomical position when selecting the site for the left renal artery reimplantation.

Proximal Anastomosis Incorporating the Celiac, Superior Mesenteric, and Right Renal Arteries

This picture shows the incision line of the procedure as performed through a thoracoabdominal approach or medial visceral rotation with the left kidney remaining in its posterior location.

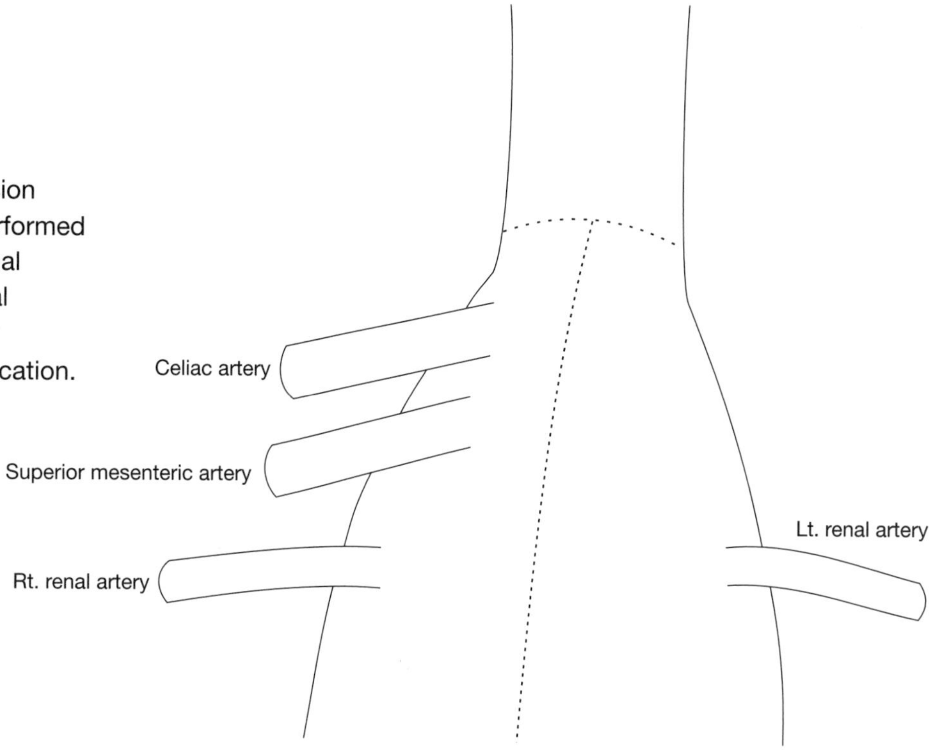

Celiac artery

Superior mesenteric artery

Lt. renal artery

Rt. renal artery

This picture shows the incision line if the procedure is performed through a medial visceral rotation, thoracoabdominal or retroperitoneal approach with the left kidney being mobilized anteriorly.

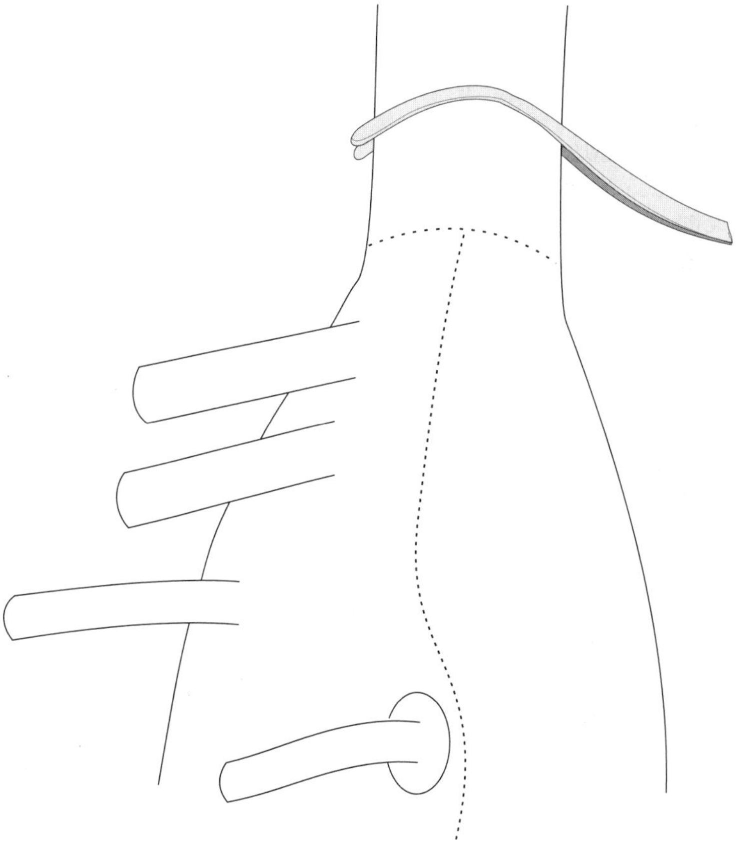

Proximal Anastomosis Incorporating the Celiac, Superior Mesenteric, and Right Renal Arteries

After opening the aortic aneurysm, the orifices of the celiac, superior mesenteric, and renal arteries are inspected to check if they can all be incorporated together in one tongue.

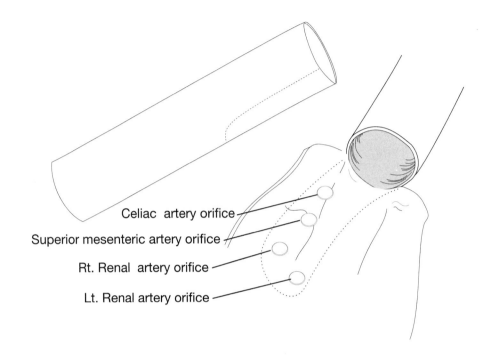

Celiac artery orifice

Superior mesenteric artery orifice

Rt. Renal artery orifice

Lt. Renal artery orifice

Most often, however, the celiac, superior mesenteric, and right renal arteries are close to each other and can be incorporated as one island, leaving the left renal artery to be reimplanted separately.

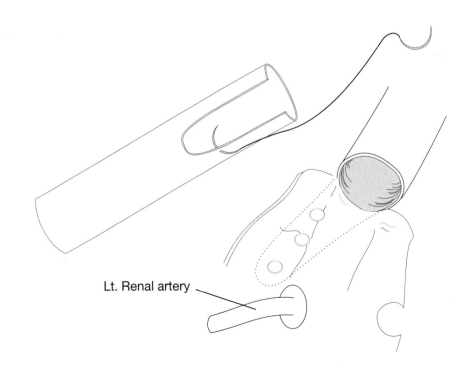

Excise a rectangular piece of the graft as shown here. Start placing the suture a few bites away from the center of the heel.

Lt. Renal artery

Proximal Anastomosis Incorporating the Celiac, Superior Mesenteric, and Right Renal Arteries

Introduce the needle in a matching location in the aorta using a double-layer bite.

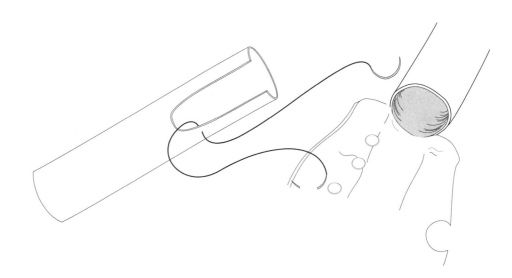

Introduce the needle in the graft (outside-inside)

Proximal Anastomosis Incorporating the Celiac, Superior Mesenteric, and Right Renal Arteries

Introduce the needle in the aorta using a double-layer aortic bite.

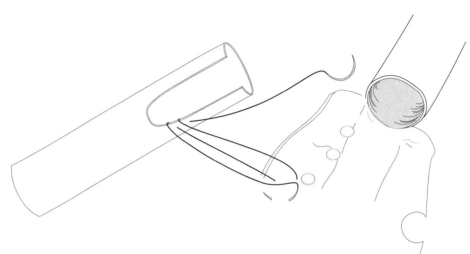

Continue running the suture until you are a few bites away from the center of the heel. Avoid wide advancement on the posterior suture line as bleeding in that area can be difficult to control.

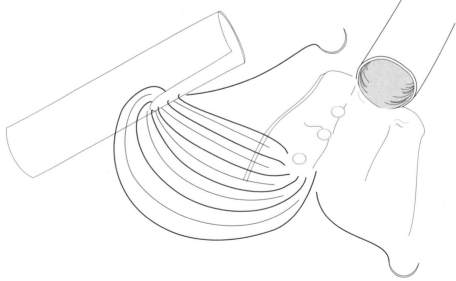

Proximal Anastomosis Incorporating the Celiac, Superior Mesenteric, and Right Renal Arteries

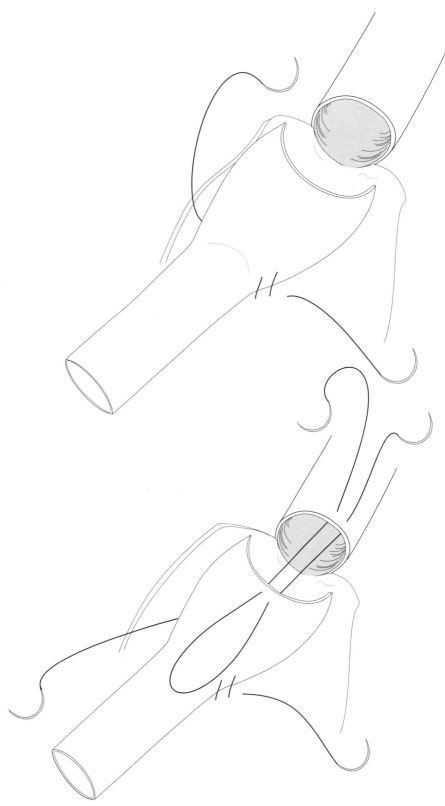

Tighten the suture line. Use a nerve hook to make sure that the suture line is not loose.

Start another suture in the graft in the center of the apex.

Introduce the needle in a matching point in the aorta.

This suture may be a simple or a mattress suture as shown here.

Proximal Anastomosis Incorporating the Celiac, Superior Mesenteric, and Right Renal Arteries

Tie the suture.

Start running one end of the suture toward the heel.

The needle is introduced outside-inside in the graft, inside-outside in the aorta.

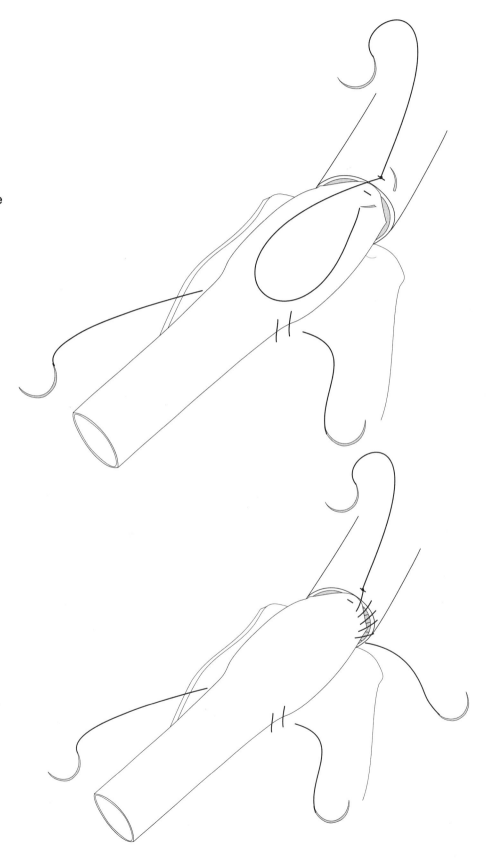

Proximal Anastomosis Incorporating the Celiac, Superior Mesenteric, and Right Renal Arteries

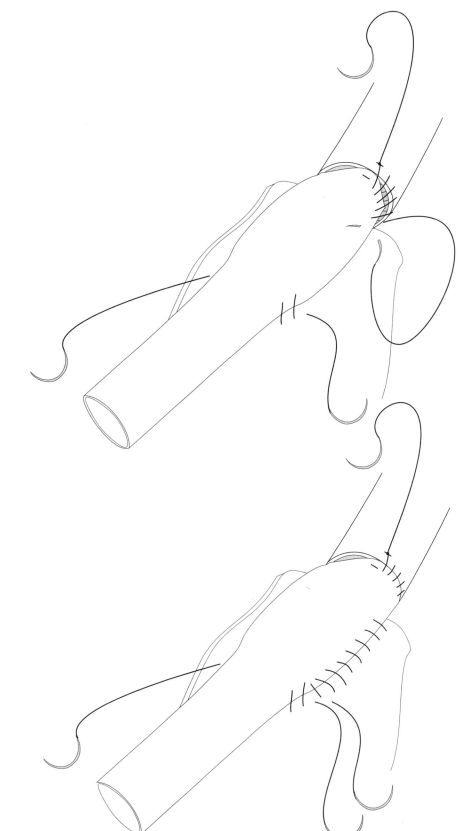

The aorta is usually free of any significant plaque at this level. Placing the sutures outside-inside in the aorta and inside-outside in the graft may be performed if the angle of suturing is more favorable.

Tighten the suture line and tie the sutures together. Use a nerve hook to ensure that the suture line is not loose.

Proximal Anastomosis Incorporating the Celiac, Superior Mesenteric, and Right Renal Arteries

Start running the other end of the apical suture.

Keep running the suture toward the heel.

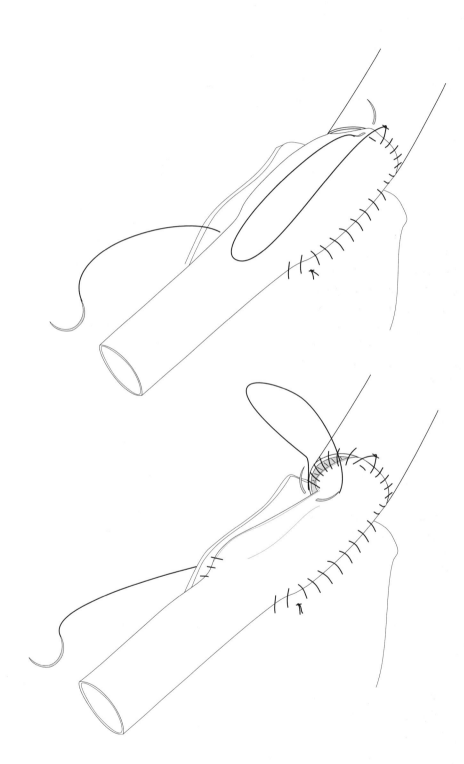

Proximal Anastomosis Incorporating the Celiac, Superior Mesenteric, and Right Renal Arteries

Tighten the suture line and
tie the sutures.

Reimplant the left renal
artery as described in the
inferior mesenteric artery
reimplantation section
(Chapter 17).

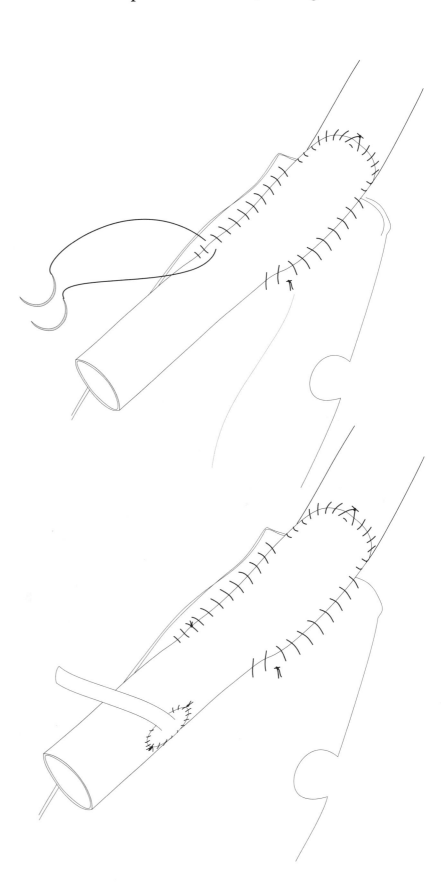

Reimplantation of the Celiac, Superior Mesenteric, and Right Renal Arteries on an Aortic Patch

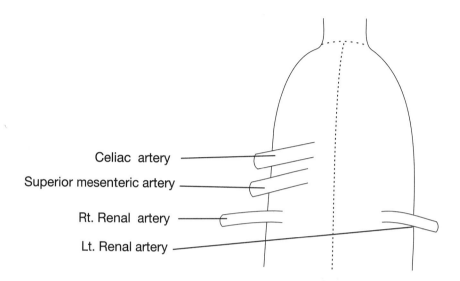

Celiac artery
Superior mesenteric artery
Rt. Renal artery
Lt. Renal artery

When the aneurysmal disease starts several centimeters proximal to the origin of the celiac artery, the proximal anastomosis will have to be performed first followed by reimplantation of the mesenteric and renal vessels. The celiac artery, superior mesenteric artery, and the right renal artery will be incorporated as one island. The left renal artery will be implanted separately.

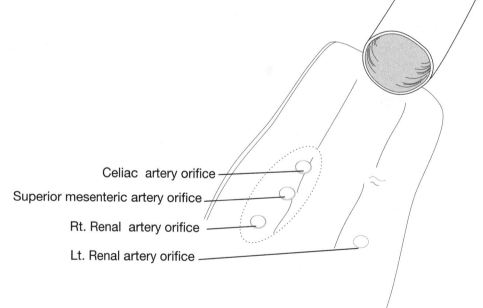

Celiac artery orifice
Superior mesenteric artery orifice
Rt. Renal artery orifice
Lt. Renal artery orifice

Reimplantation of the Celiac, Superior Mesenteric, and Right Renal Arteries on an Aortic Patch

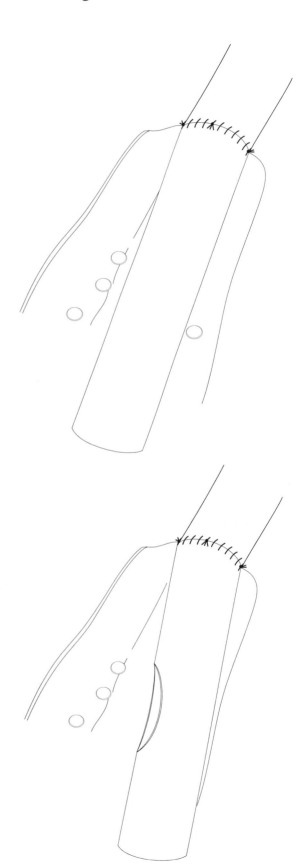

Construct the proximal aortic anastomosis as previously described in the infrarenal abdominal aortic aneurysm replacement (Chapter 14).

Excise an elliptical piece of the graft that matches the size of the island. The ellipse should not be too wide.

Reimplantation of the Celiac, Superior Mesenteric, and Right Renal Arteries on an Aortic Patch

Start the suture in the graft. Introduce the needle in the center of the apex (outside-inside)

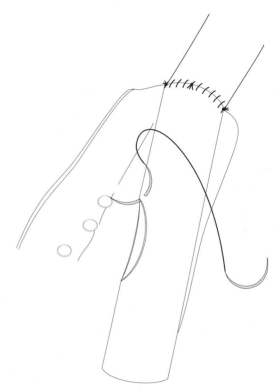

Introduce the needle in a matching location in the artery using a double-layer bite.

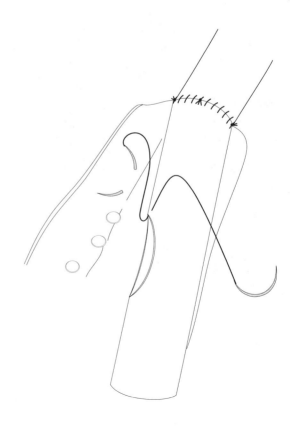

Reimplantation of the Celiac, Superior Mesenteric, and Right Renal Arteries on an Aortic Patch

The posterior part of the anastomosis is constructed first. Introduce the needle in the graft, inside-outside to facilitate the construction of the suture line.

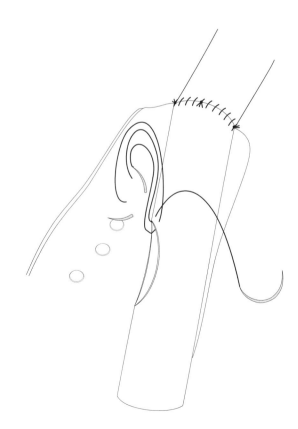

Place a double-layer bite in a matching location in the aorta.

Reimplantation of the Celiac, Superior Mesenteric, and Right Renal Arteries on an Aortic Patch

Continue running the suture line until you have completed the posterior part of the anastomosis.

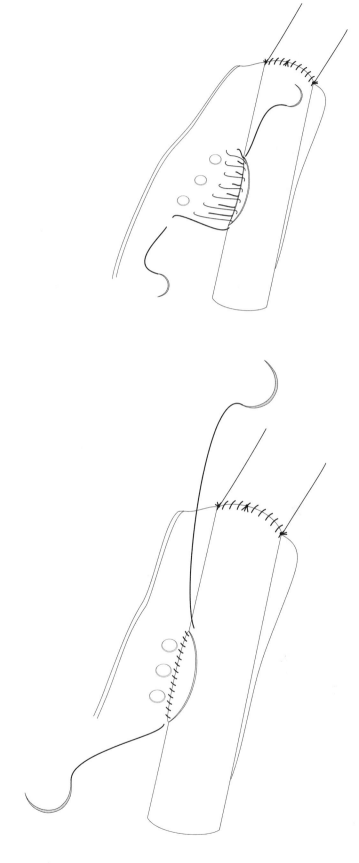

Pull and tighten the suture line.

Reimplantation of the Celiac, Superior Mesenteric, and Right Renal Arteries on an Aortic Patch

Start a new suture at the apex very close to the starting point of the previous suture.

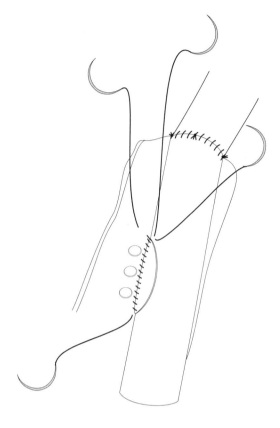

Tie the suture.

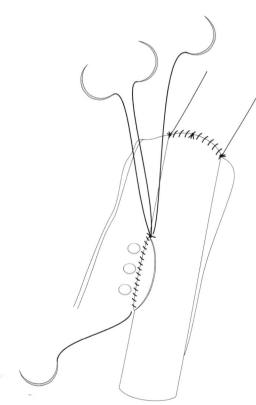

Reimplantation of the Celiac, Superior Mesenteric, and Right Renal Arteries on an Aortic Patch

Tie one end of the suture to the posterior suture.

Start running the suture along the anterior part of the anastomosis.

Introduce the needle in the graft.

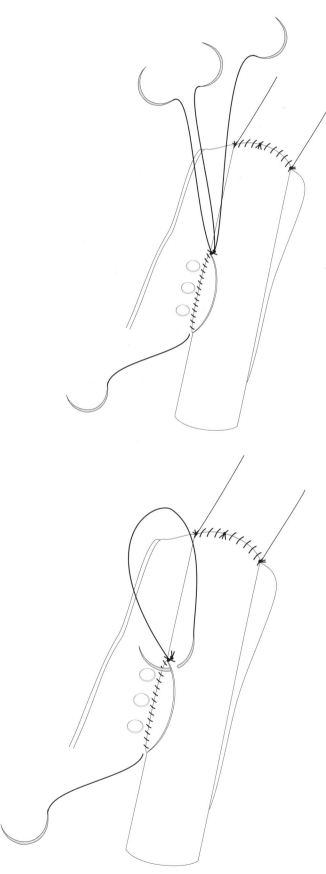

Reimplantation of the Celiac, Superior Mesenteric, and Right Renal Arteries on an Aortic Patch

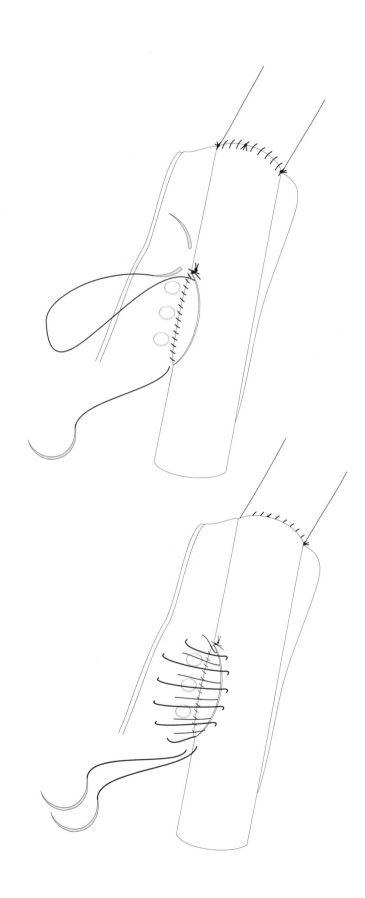

Introduce the needle in a matching location in the aorta.

Keep running the suture along the anterior wall until you reach the other suture.

Reimplantation of the Celiac, Superior Mesenteric, and Right Renal Arteries on an Aortic Patch

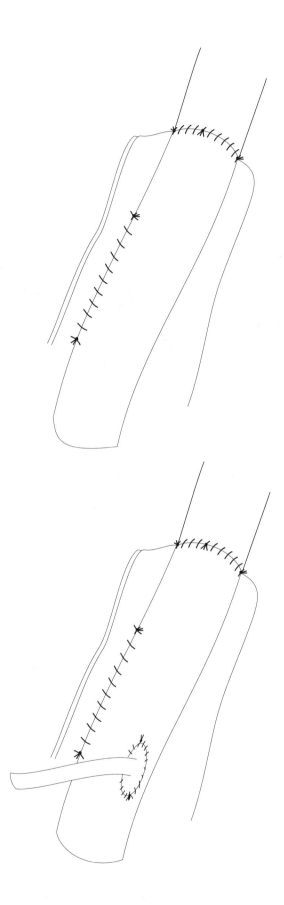

Pull and tie the suture.

The left renal artery is reimplanted as previously described.

16

Pelvic Revascularization During Aortic Reconstruction

Preservation of pelvic perfusion should be an integral part of any aortic reconstructive procedure. Pelvic ischemia is an important complication that may, on occasion, be fatal. The clinical manifestations of pelvic ischemia include buttock claudication, buttock necrosis, rectosigmoidal ischemia, cord ischemia resulting in urinary and fecal incontinence, and sexual dysfunction. A knowledge of the pelvic blood supply is essential to understanding and planning the preservation of pelvic perfusion during aortic reconstruction.

The pelvic blood supply is derived from several sources. The right and left internal iliac arteries provide the major blood supply to the pelvis. In addition, the pelvis receives some blood supply from branches of the external iliac artery. These branches include the inferior epigastric and the deep external iliac circumflex arteries. The inferior mesenteric artery (IMA) can also contribute to the pelvic blood supply. The inferior mesenteric artery divides into three main

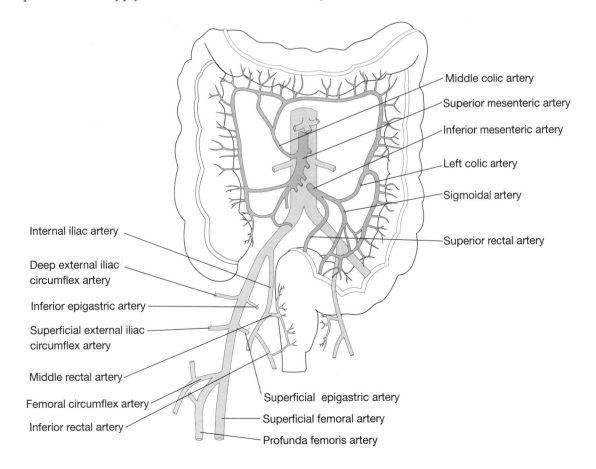

branches: the left colic artery, the sigmoidal artery, and the superior rectal artery. The contribution of the IMA to the pelvic blood supply is usually through the superior rectal artery, which communicates with the middle and inferior rectal arteries. The pelvis can also receive some blood supply from the superior mesenteric artery through its middle colic artery branch. The middle colic artery communicates with the left colic artery, which in turn connects with the superior rectal artery. The pelvis may also acquire further blood supply from the common femoral arteries through the superficial epigastric and superficial iliac circumflex arteries. In addition, the profunda femoris artery through its femoral circumflex branches can also contribute to the pelvic blood supply. Thus, the collateral blood flow to the internal iliac artery may originate from the contralateral internal iliac, the ipsilateral external iliac, the inferior mesenteric, the superior mesenteric, the common femoral, and the profunda femoris arteries.

An important principle of aortic reconstruction is to maintain the perfusion of at least one internal iliac artery to avoid the possible complication of pelvic ischemia. (1,4) However, the perfusion of both internal iliac arteries is desirable if it can be safely accomplished without excessive prolongation of the duration of the procedure.

AORTOILIAC OCCLUSIVE DISEASE

In a patient with aortoiliac occlusive disease, the proposed reconstruction is usually an aortobifemoral bypass. The proximal anastomosis can be carried out in an end-to-end (Section 1a) or end-to-side configuration (Section 1b). Pelvic perfusion may be maintained by constructing the proximal aortic anastomosis in an end-to-side fashion. This type of anastomosis is especially necessary when the external iliac arteries are heavily involved with occlusive disease. In this situation, an end-to-end aortofemoral bypass could not provide retrograde perfusion to the internal iliac arteries due to the disease in the external iliac arteries. If an end-to-side aortobifemoral bypass cannot be performed, pelvic revascularization may still be achieved by constructing a side-to-side anastomosis between the graft limb and the common iliac artery bifurcation. (Section 1c) (2) It is important during the aortobifemoral bypass procedure to perfuse the profunda and preserve its branches. A profundaplasty should be performed if necessary.

AORTOILIAC ANEURYSMAL DISEASE

In aortic aneurysmal disease, the extent of replacement is usually governed by the extent of the aneurysmal disease and the anatomy of the pelvic circulation. If the aneurysmal disease is limited to the infrarenal aorta, a tube graft replacement is usually performed (Section 2a). The perfusion of the internal iliac arteries is then restored to the preoperative status. Similarly, if the aneurysmal disease extends into the common iliac arteries but does not involve the iliac bifurcation, the preoperative internal iliac perfusion can be maintained by the placement of an aortobiiliac bypass graft (Section 2b).

When the aneurysmal disease extends to the level of the iliac bifurcation, several options may be available. One option is to transect the common iliac artery approximately 1.5 cm proximal to the bifurcation. An arteriotomy is created into the origin of the external iliac artery for 1–1.5 cm. The limb of the graft is transected in a beveled fashion and sutured in an end-to-end manner to the transected common iliac artery (Section 2c). When constructing the posterior part of the anastomosis, the needles usually are introduced close to the orifices of the internal iliac and external iliac arteries that are not involved by the aneurysmal pathology. The advantage of this technique is that it provides direct antegrade flow into the internal and external iliac arteries. In addition, it involves performing one single anastomosis. However, if the iliac arteries are heavily calcified, this anastomosis may be quite challenging. A localized endarterectomy may need to be performed with tacking of the endarterectomy endpoint.

Another option to preserve internal iliac artery flow is to transect the common iliac artery approximately 1.5 cm from the iliac bifurcation. The transected common iliac artery is oversewn without obliterating the orifices of the external and internal iliac arteries (Section 2d). The arteriotomy is then created in the external iliac artery. A limb of the aortobiiliac graft is sutured in an end-to-side manner to the external iliac artery. The perfusion into the internal iliac artery is provided by retrograde flow from the external iliac artery. This technique may be ideal when the iliac bifurcation is calcified and the plaque extends into the proximal part of the external iliac artery. In this situation, the distal external iliac artery is mobilized and the arteriotomy is created in the disease-free distal segment of the external iliac artery.

The aneurysmal disease may extend beyond the iliac bifurcation into the internal iliac artery with sparing of the external iliac artery. If the disease is limited to the proximal part of the internal iliac artery, one possible technique involves suturing the limb of the graft to the internal iliac artery in an end-to-end manner. (3) The external iliac artery is then reimplanted into the limb of the graft (Section 2e). If the aneurysmal disease extends into the proximal part of the external iliac artery, the limb of the graft can be connected to the external iliac artery in an end-to-end fashion. A separate graft is then sutured to the internal iliac artery (Section 2f). This graft may originate from the body or limb of the aortic graft. If the aneurysmal disease extends into the distal part of the internal iliac artery, an anastomosis may not be technically possible. In this situation, ligation of the internal iliac artery becomes necessary.

Infrequently, perfusion of at least one internal iliac artery is not possible because of extensive involvement by aneurysmal or occlusive disease. In this situation, the pelvic blood supply may be maintained by preserving the collateral blood supply of the internal iliac artery. This can be accomplished by reimplanting the inferior mesenteric artery. In addition, the blood flow into the external iliac artery and the profunda femoris artery and their branches should be maintained. (4)

REFERENCES

1. Connolly JE, Ingegno M, Wilson SE. Preservation of the pelvic circulation during infrarenal aortic surgery. Cardiovasc Surg 1996;4:65–70.
2. Cronenwett JL, Gooch JB, Garrett E. Internal iliac artery revascularization during aortofemoral bypass. Arch Surg 1982;117:838–839.
3. Hoballah JJ, Chalmers RTA, Nazzal MM, Mohan CR, Corson JD. Internal iliac revascularization during aortic aneurysm replacement: A review and description of a useful technique. Am Surg 1997;63:970–974.
4. Iliopoulos JI, Hermreck AS, Thomas JH, Pierce GE. Hemodynamics of the hypogastric arterial circulation. Journal of Vasc Surg 1989;9:637–642.

Aortoiliac Occlusive Disease
End-to-End Aortobifemoral Bypass

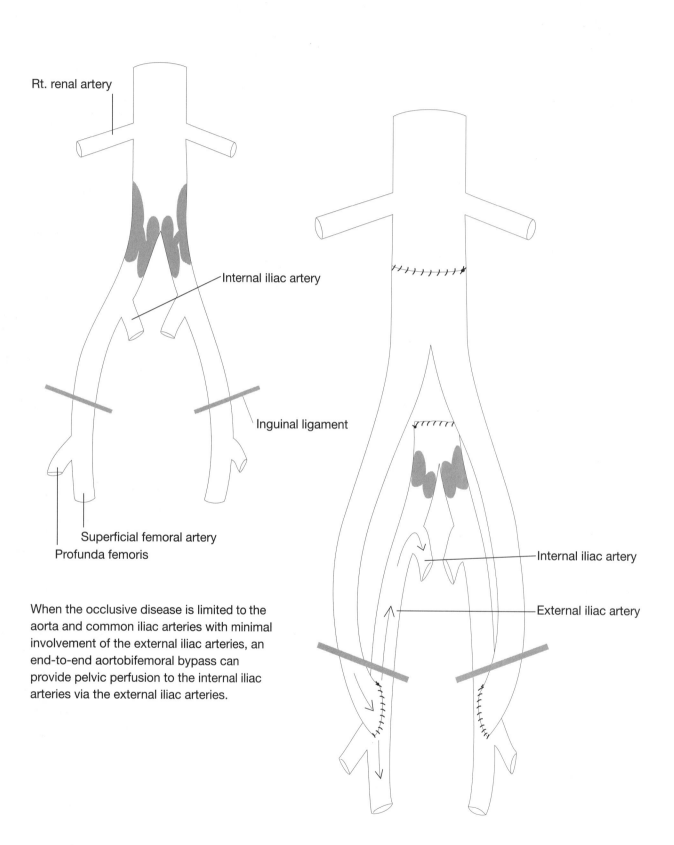

Rt. renal artery

Internal iliac artery

Inguinal ligament

Superficial femoral artery

Profunda femoris

Internal iliac artery

External iliac artery

When the occlusive disease is limited to the aorta and common iliac arteries with minimal involvement of the external iliac arteries, an end-to-end aortobifemoral bypass can provide pelvic perfusion to the internal iliac arteries via the external iliac arteries.

Aortoiliac Occlusive Disease
End-to-Side Aortobifemoral Bypass

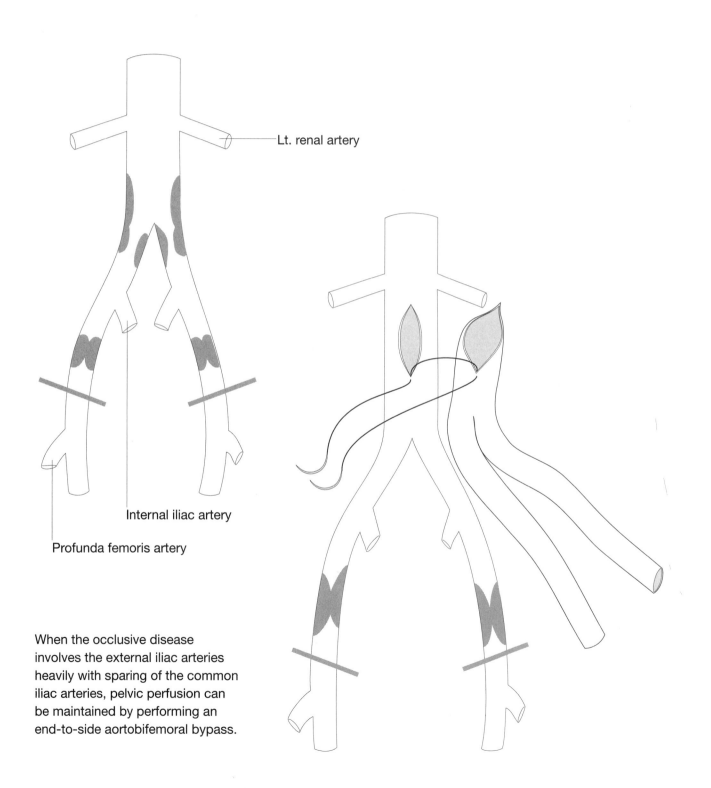

Lt. renal artery

Internal iliac artery

Profunda femoris artery

When the occlusive disease
involves the external iliac arteries
heavily with sparing of the common
iliac arteries, pelvic perfusion can
be maintained by performing an
end-to-side aortobifemoral bypass.

Aortoiliac Occlusive Disease
End-to-Side Aortobifemoral Bypass

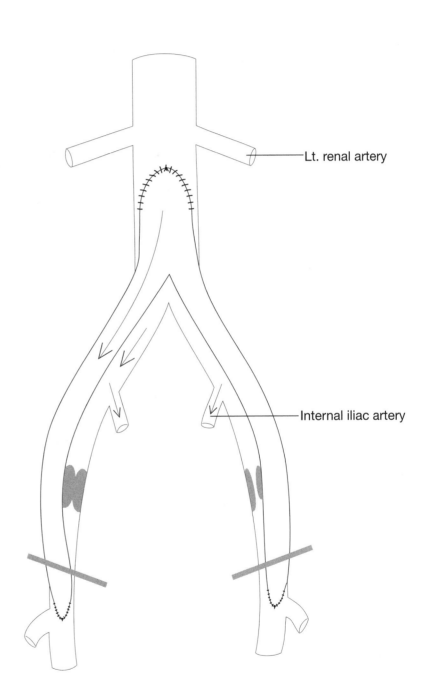

Lt. renal artery

Internal iliac artery

In the end-to-side reconstruction, the native circulation is usually left undisturbed.

Aortoiliac Occlusive Disease
End-to-End Aortobifemoral Bypass

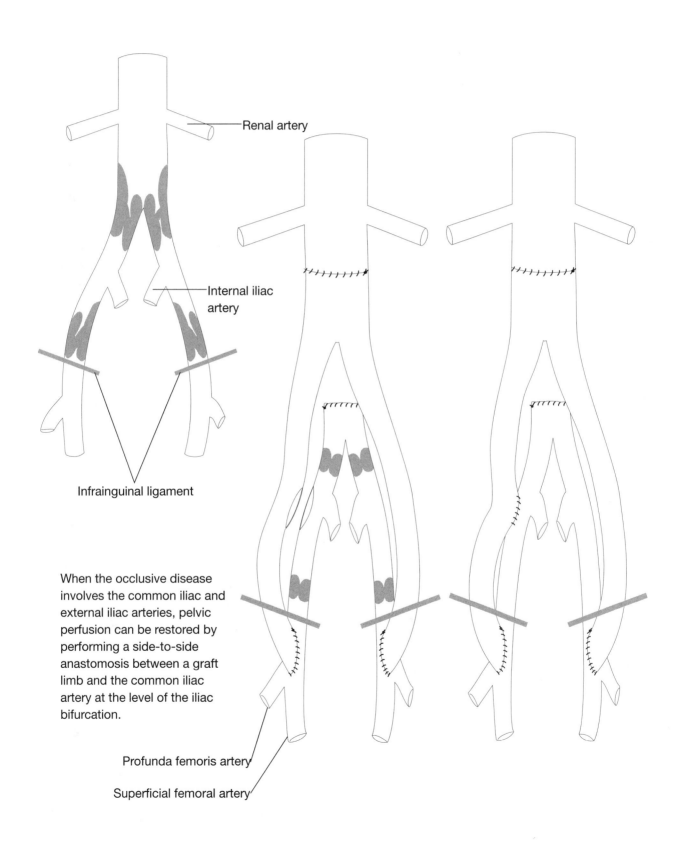

Renal artery

Internal iliac artery

Infrainguinal ligament

When the occlusive disease involves the common iliac and external iliac arteries, pelvic perfusion can be restored by performing a side-to-side anastomosis between a graft limb and the common iliac artery at the level of the iliac bifurcation.

Profunda femoris artery

Superficial femoral artery

Aortoiliac Aneurysmal Disease
Distal Anastomosis to the Aortic Bifurcation

When the aneurysmal pathology is limited to the aorta and does not involve the common iliac arteries, a tube graft replacement is performed.

When performing a tube graft replacement, the distal anastomosis can be very challenging because of calcifications or the absence of a well-defined neck at the level of the aortic bifurcation.

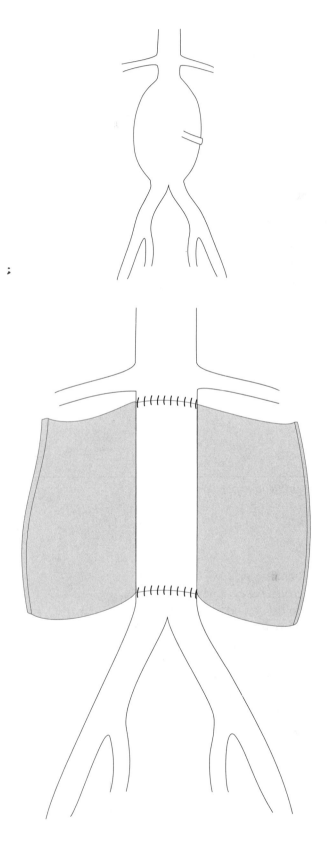

Aortoiliac Aneurysmal Disease
Distal Anastomosis to the Aortic Bifurcation

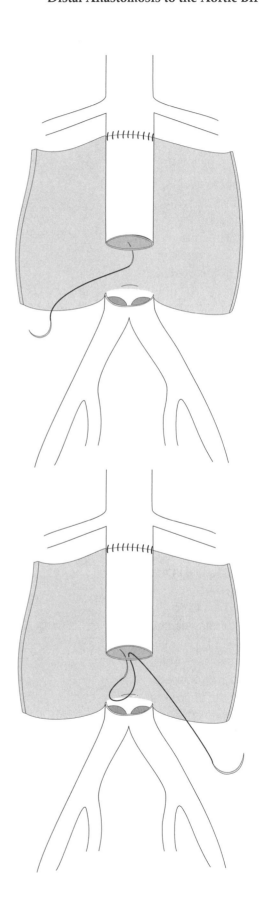

The same principles discussed in the construction of the proximal aortic bifurcation apply here as well. The suture can be started at the center of the posterior suture line or on either side. However, when the neck is ill defined, starting at the center of the posterior wall can help to establish even progression on either side, as shown here.

Start by placing a horizontal mattress suture in the center of the posterior wall of the graft.

Aortoiliac Aneurysmal Disease
Distal Anastomosis to the Aortic Bifurcation

It is preferable to avoid excessive advancement when constructing the posterior wall because of the difficulty in controlling bleeding from the posterior suture line.

Introduce the needle in the center of the posterior aortic wall. The site of introduction of the needle should be free of aneurysmal disease. The needle can be introduced very close to the orifices of the common iliac arteries.

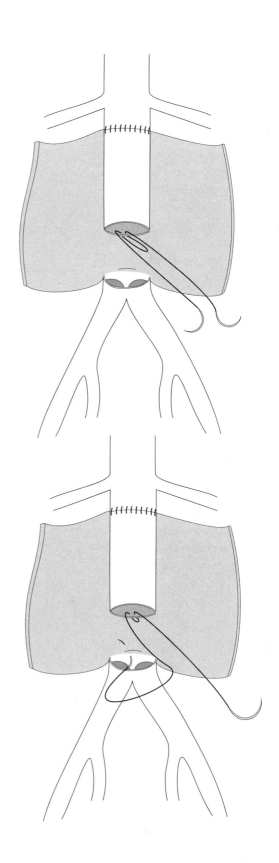

Aortoiliac Aneurysmal Disease
Distal Anastomosis to the Aortic Bifurcation

Place a matching horizontal mattress suture in the center of the posterior aortic wall.

You may tie this suture or continue using a parachute technique as shown here.

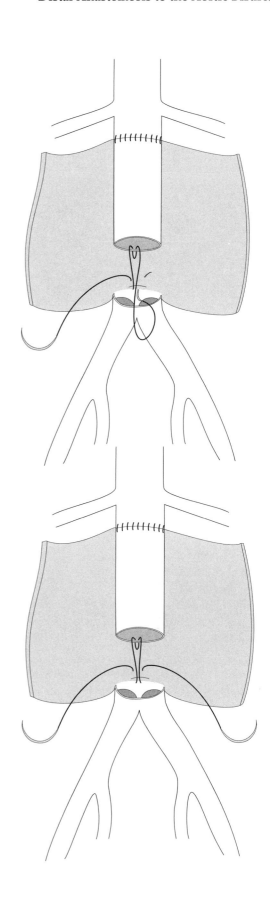

Aortoiliac Aneurysmal Disease
Distal Anastomosis to the Aortic Bifurcation

Introduce the needle in the
graft.

Complete suturing the
posterior part of the suture
line on one side.

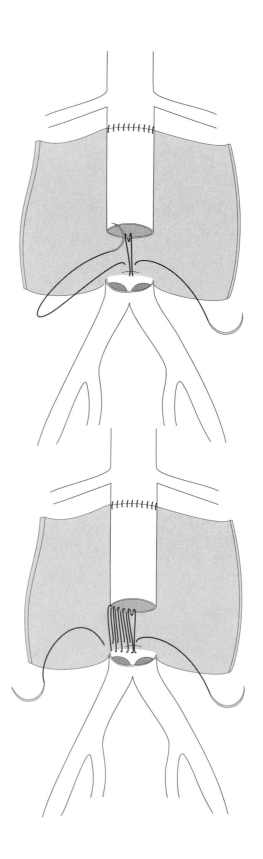

Aortoiliac Aneurysmal Disease
Distal Anastomosis to the Aortic Bifurcation

Do the same on the other side. Introduce the needle in the graft, outside in.

Complete the posterior suture line on the other side.

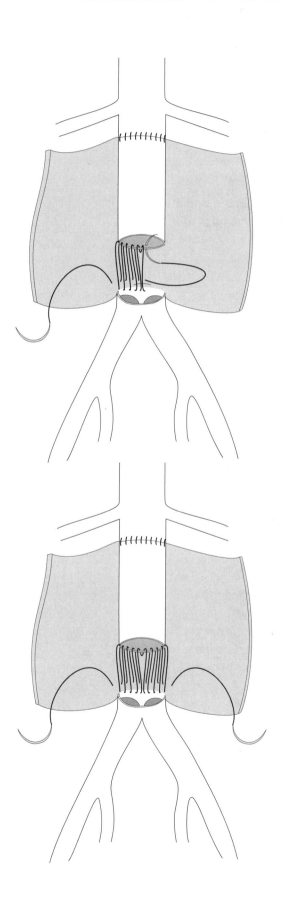

Aortoiliac Aneurysmal Disease
Distal Anastomosis to the Aortic Bifurcation

Pull and tighten the suture line. Use a nerve hook to ensure that the suture line is not loose.

You may start another suture for the anterior part of the anastomosis. Alternatively, you may continue with the same suture to complete the anastomosis as shown here.

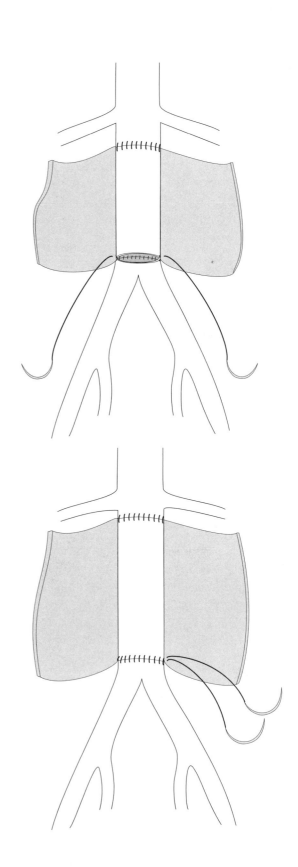

Aortoiliac Aneurysmal Disease
Distal Anastomosis to the Common Iliac Artery

When the aneurysmal pathology extends to the proximal portion of the common iliac arteries, a bifurcated graft replacement to the level of the distal common iliac arteries is performed.

The posterior wall of the common iliac artery may be transected or left intact. Be careful to avoid injury to the iliac veins, which could occur during the transection of the common iliac arteries. In addition, make sure that the bites in the transected iliac artery include the adventitia. On the left side, the graft can be tunneled through the aneurysmal iliac artery.

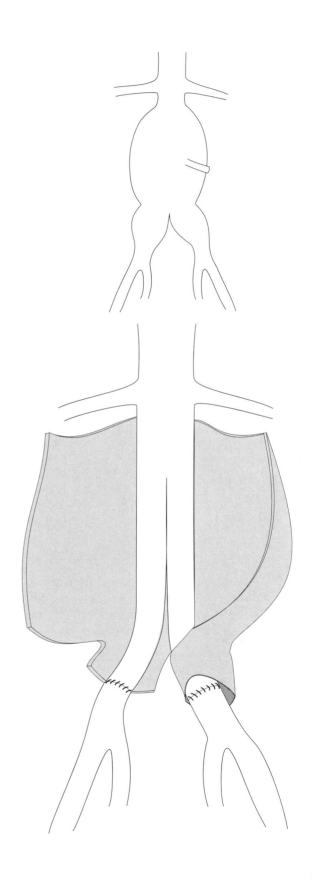

Aortoiliac Aneurysmal Disease
Distal Anastomosis to the Iliac Bifurcation

When the aneurysmal
disease extends to the iliac
bifurcation, several options
are available depending on
the quality of the common
iliac artery at the bifurcation.

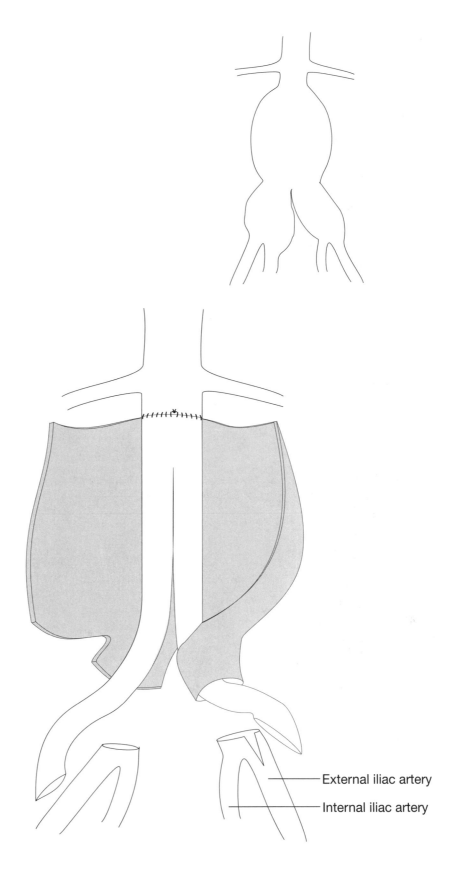

If the iliac bifurcation is not
heavily calcified, the
arteriotomy can be
extended into the orifice of
the external iliac artery as
shown on the left side.

External iliac artery

Internal iliac artery

Aortoiliac Aneurysmal Disease
Distal Anastomosis to the External Iliac Artery

If the iliac bifurcation is heavily calcified, or if the first part of the external iliac artery is involved with occlusive pathology, the transected common iliac artery is oversewn as shown on the right side.

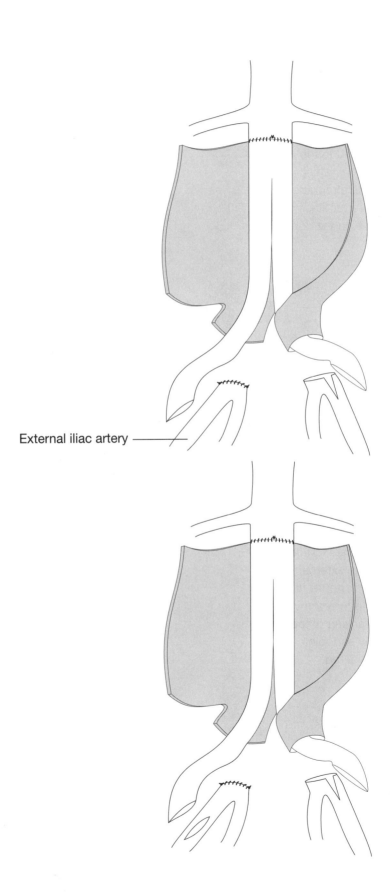

External iliac artery

A soft area is then chosen in the external iliac artery for constructing the distal anastomosis.

Aortoiliac Aneurysmal Disease
Distal Anastomosis to the External Iliac Artery

An end-to-side anastomosis is then constructed to the external iliac artery, which will also provide retrograde flow into the internal iliac artery as shown on the right side.

The reconstruction on the left side provides antegrade perfusion into the external and internal iliac arteries. If a localized endarterectomy is performed, tacking of the endarterectomy endpoint should be considered.

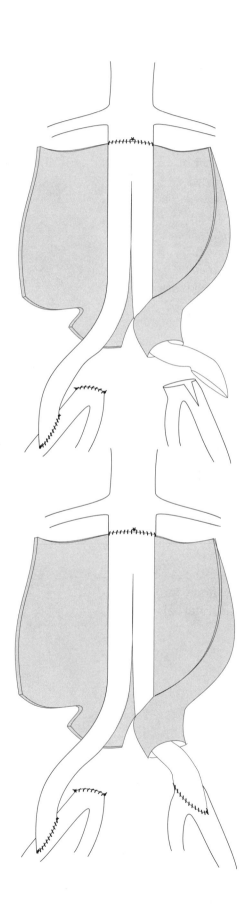

Aortoiliac Aneurysmal Disease
Distal Anastomosis to the Internal Iliac Artery with Reimplantation of the External Iliac Artery

When the aneurysmal disease extends beyond the iliac bifurcation into the proximal part of the internal iliac artery, revascularization of at least one internal iliac artery should be attempted.

If the aneurysmal disease is limited to the very proximal part of the internal iliac artery, one option is to transect the external iliac artery at the level of the iliac bifurcation.

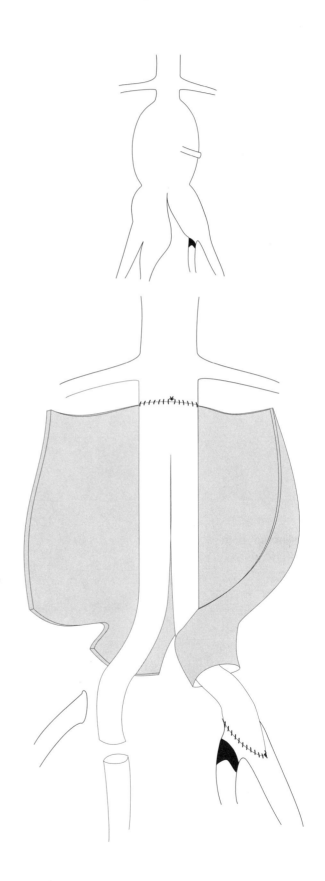

Aortoiliac Aneurysmal Disease
Distal Anastomosis to the Internal Iliac Artery with Reimplantation of the External Iliac Artery

The graft is anastomosed to the internal iliac artery using an end-to-end configuration as shown on the right side.

The external iliac artery is then reimplanted into the limb of the graft.

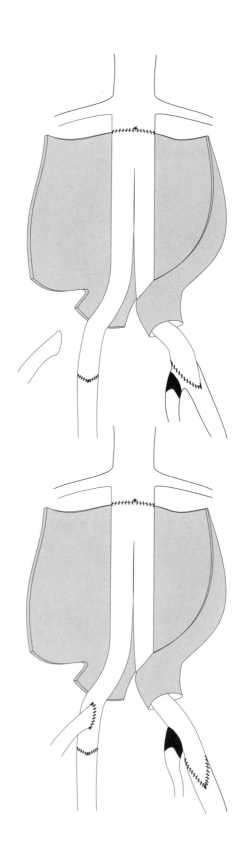

Aortoiliac Aneurysmal Disease
Distal Anastomosis to the Internal Iliac Artery with Reimplantation of the External Iliac Artery

Another option to revascularize the pelvis in the situation shown on the right side involves constructing a separate bypass to the internal iliac artery.

The graft is anastomosed to the external iliac artery.

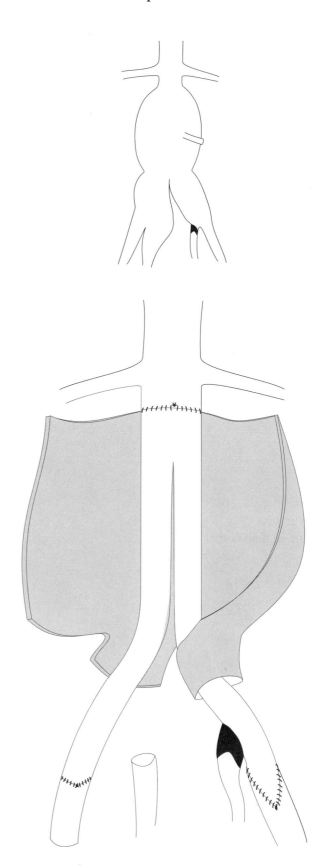

Aortoiliac Aneurysmal Disease
Distal Anastomosis to the External Iliac Artery with a Bypass to the Internal Iliac Artery

A separate graft is then sutured to the body of the graft or to one of its limbs as shown here.

The bypass is then anastomosed to the internal iliac artery.

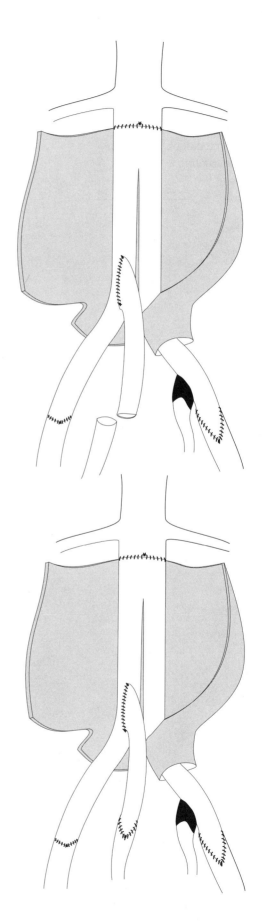

17

Inferior Mesenteric Artery (IMA) Reimplantation

MANAGEMENT OF THE INFERIOR MESENTERIC ARTERY (IMA) DURING AORTIC ANEURYSM REPLACEMENT

When the aortic aneurysm is entered, the orifice of the inferior mesenteric artery should be inspected. If pulsatile backbleeding is noted, it is usually safe to oversew the origin of the inferior mesenteric artery. The orifice is suture ligated from within the aneurysmal lumen to avoid injury to its branches, especially at the junction of the left colic to the sigmoidal and superior rectal branches.

If the backbleeding from the inferior mesenteric artery is poor, the orifice is occluded by a Fogarty catheter. Alternatively, the inferior mesenteric artery may be carefully dissected and controlled close to its origin by a vessel loop. After completing the distal part of the aortic reconstruction and reestablishing distal flow, the backbleeding from the IMA is reassessed. If the backbleeding is brisk and pulsatile, the IMA is ligated from within. Occasionally, the backbleeding may not be impressive due to the presence of an orificial atherosclerotic plaque and will improve following endarterectomy of the origin of the IMA. If after completing the aortic reconstruction the backbleeding from a patent IMA is still weak, reimplantation of the IMA may be necessary. If the backbleeding from the IMA is questionable, back pressure measurements can help determine the need for IMA reimplantation. IMA back pressure can be measured by inserting a blunt-tip needle through the IMA orifice; a vessel loop is pulled around the needle to prevent bleeding around the needle. Reimplantation of the IMA is considered if the back pressure is less than 35 mmHg.

Other reasons for reimplanting the IMA include inability to perfuse at least one internal iliac artery, previous colonic resection that may have interrupted the collaterals between the left colic artery and the middle colic artery, and a widely patent IMA as seen by angiogram with stenotic pathology in the superior mesenteric artery.

The incision in the aortic
aneurysm is placed to the
right side of the inferior
mesenteric artery at least
1.0 cm from its origin in
anticipation of the need of
reimplanting the IMA.

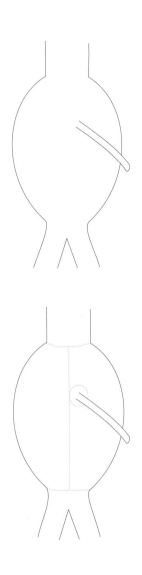

When reimplantation of the
inferior mesenteric artery is
deemed necessary, a
circular button of aortic wall
is then created around the
orifice of the inferior
mesenteric. Occasionally
an eversion endarterectomy
of the orifice of the inferior
mesenteric artery will be
necessary.

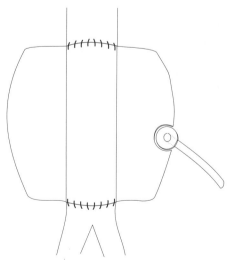

After completion of the
aortic replacement, a side-
biting clamp will be applied
to the aortic graft, thus
maintaining the blood flow
into the lower extremities.

Proper positioning of the
clamp is essential to avoid
excessive tension on the
suture lines. An incision in the
graft is then performed and
the suture line is started at
the apex of the aortic graft
incision. A small wedge of
the graft may be excised
to facilitate the construction
of the anastomosis.

The needle is introduced
into the Carrell patch of the
mesenteric artery in a
corresponding location.
The suture can be tied at
this level or continued in a
parachute fashion as shown
here.

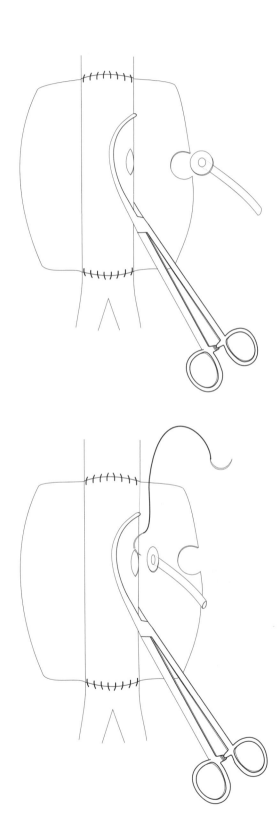

The posterior portion of the anastomosis is sutured first.

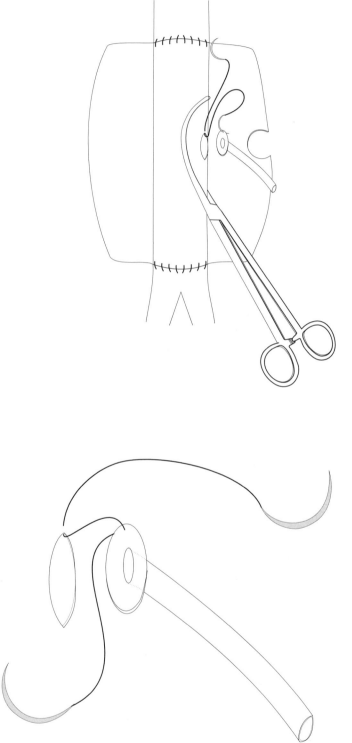

The needle is then introduced into the aortic graft. Multiple bites are placed until one side of the anastomosis has been completely sutured.

Again the needle is
introduced inside-outside in
the IMA patch and outside-
inside in the graft.

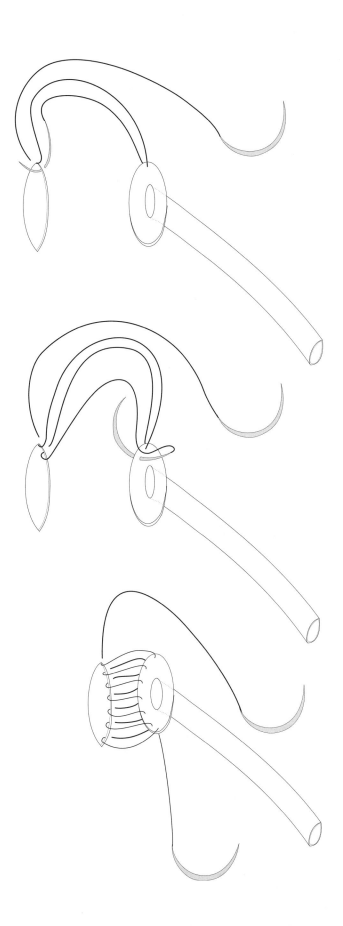

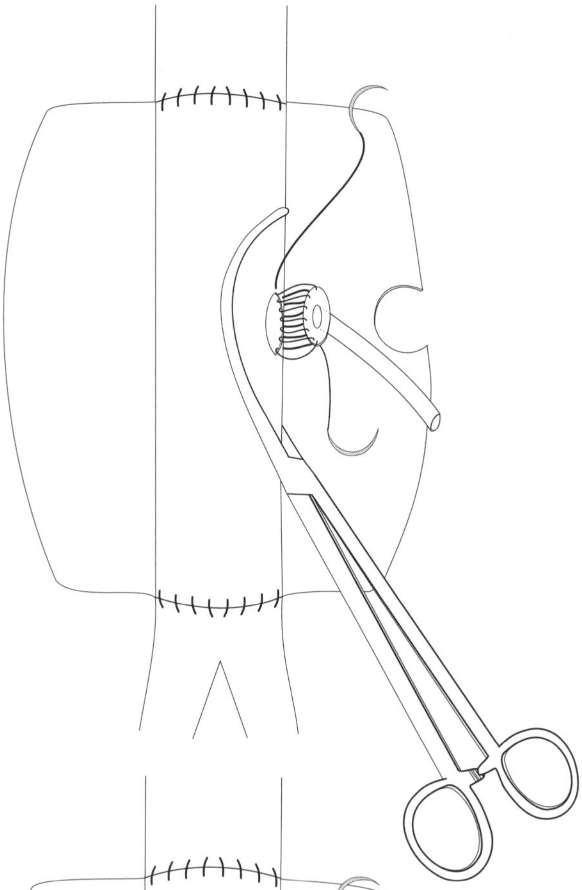

The suture line is then
tightened. The upper suture
may then be used to
complete the suture line all
the way down on the
anterior portion of the
anastomosis.

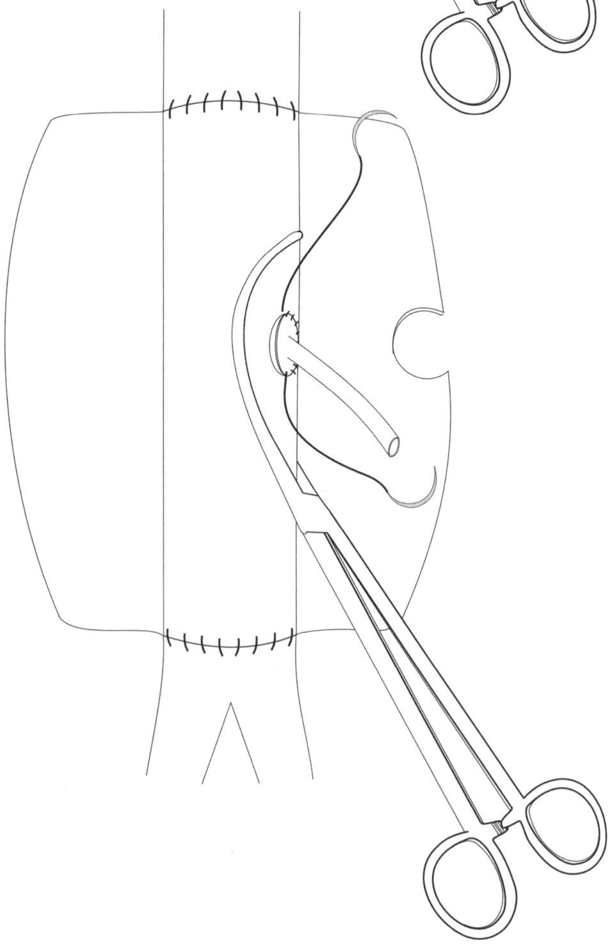

Alternatively, another suture may be started at the apex as shown here.

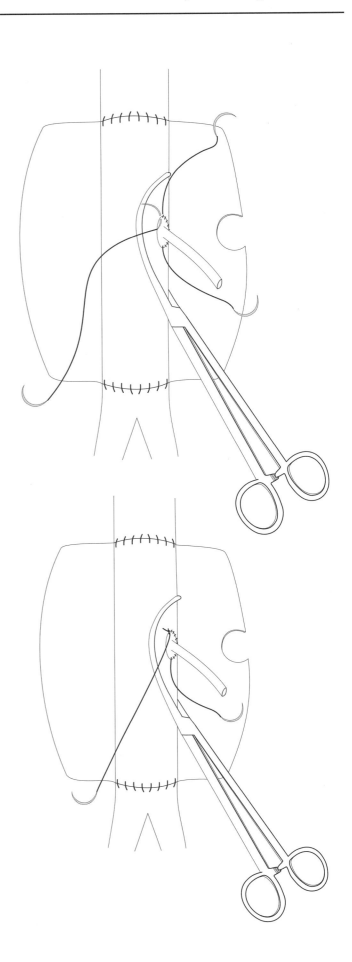

The suture is tied to itself. One end of the suture is tied to the original apical suture.

The new suture is then used to complete the anastomosis.

In this part of the anastomosis, the needle may be introduced outside-inside in the IMA patch and then inside-outside in the graft.

Run the upper suture
toward the lower suture.

Tie the sutures.

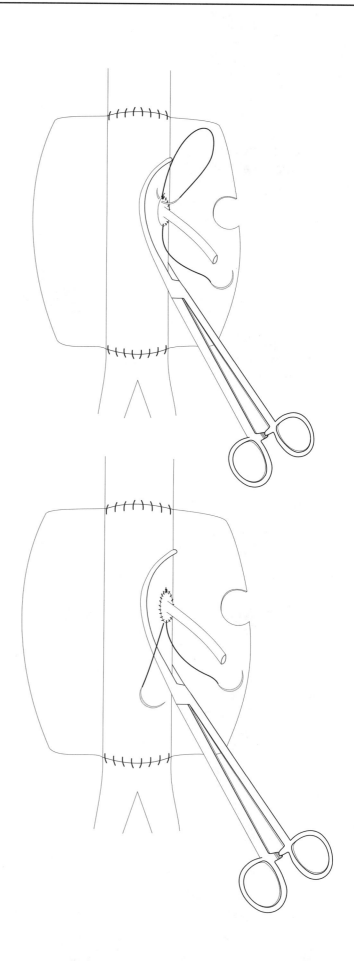

18

Coverage of Abdominal Aortic Grafts

The interposition of viable tissue between an aortic graft prosthesis and the posterior wall of the duodenum has long been recognized as an important technique to limit the incidence of graft enteric erosions and fistulae. In patients with aortoiliac occlusive disease, the periaortic tissue is approximated over the aortic prosthesis to insulate the graft from the adjacent bowel.

ANEURYSM WALL WRAP

In patients with aneurysmal disease, the redundant aneurysm wall is wrapped around the implanted aortic graft before approximating the periaortic tissue. The redundant aneurysmal wall is usually closed over the graft with an attempt to minimize the dead space between the aortic prosthesis and the aortic wrap. In the presence of a very large aneurysmal sac, a vest-over-pants closure of the excessively redundant aortic wall may be necessary.

OMENTAL FLAPS

Occasionally, the aneurysmal aortic wall or the periaortic tissue cannot adequately cover the aortic prosthesis, especially at the level of the proximal anastomosis. This can be encountered in patients with small aneurysms or in thin patients with aortoiliac disease where an end-to-side aortobifemoral graft has been placed. Similarly, in patients in whom an aortorenal bypass or an aortomesenteric bypass has been performed in addition to an aortic reconstruction, coverage of the bypass grafts with periaortic tissue may be hard to perform without compressing the aortorenal or aortomesenteric bypass. In these situations, omental flaps can be developed and used to cover the aortic prosthesis. (1,2,3) Omental flaps have also been used in the management of infected aortic grafts to wrap the transected aortic stump.

The omental flap can be based on any patent omental artery. In thin patients, the entire omentum may have to be used as a flap. To cover the aortic prosthesis, the omental flaps are placed in either an anticolic or a retrocolic position. When using the anticolic position, there is a potential for the development of an internal hernia between the omentum and the colon mesentery. (2) Securing the omentum with a running suture along its edges can be effective in closing any potential hernia defects. The retrocolic position of the omental flap can avoid the creation of a potential hernia defect. However, this method usually requires the mobilization of the omentum from the colon and then creating a defect in the mesocolon to pass the omental flap to the desired location.

A simple technique is to create a flap based on the left omental artery, which is usually a constant anatomical finding. (3) The flap is created by dividing the omentum in an avascular plane in a direction perpendicular to the transverse colon. The splenic flexure will serve as the base of the flap, which usually measures 10–15 cm in width. The graft to be covered is exposed. The flap is allowed to fold gently over the transverse colon mesentery and is placed over the aortic prosthesis. The flap is first secured in place with few interrupted 3-0 silk sutures. A running 3-0 silk suture is also utilized to secure the edges of the flap to the mesocolon to prevent any herniation between the transverse colon and the omentum. In this technique, the omentum is divided in only one plane. The major part of the omentum supplied by the right and middle omental arteries is left intact and can still be placed under the midline abdominal incision.

REFERENCES

1. Bunt TJ, Doerhoff CR, Haynes JL. Retrocolic omental pedicle flap for routine plication of abdominal aortic grafts. Surg Gynecol Obstet 1984;158:591–592.
2. Foy H, Fay S, Johansen K. Bowel obstruction following omental patching of aortic grafts. Am Surg 1985;51:661–663.
3. Hoballah JJ, Mohan CR, Nazzal MM, Corson JD: The use of omental flaps in abdominal aortic surgery: a review and description of a simple technique. Ann Vasc Surg 1998;12:292–295.

Aneurysm Wall Wrap

Start one suture in the edge of the proximal aneurysmal wall.

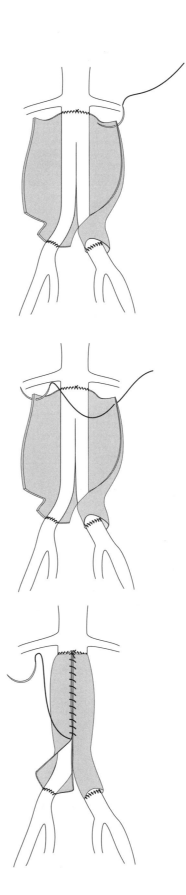

Tie the suture and run it toward the aortic bifurcation. This suture will help control bleeding from the edges of the aneurysmal wall.

Aneurysm Wall Wrap

Start another suture in the wall of the right
common iliac artery.

Run the suture cephalad.
Tie the sutures together.

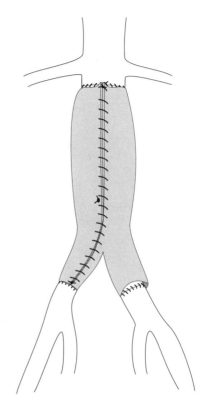

In the presence of excessive redundant
aneurysmal wall, a vest-over-pants closure may
help eliminate excessive dead space between the
aortic prosthesis and the aortic wrap.

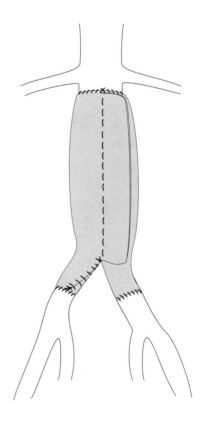

Omental Flaps

When developing an omental flap, the blood supply to the greater omentum is first evaluated.

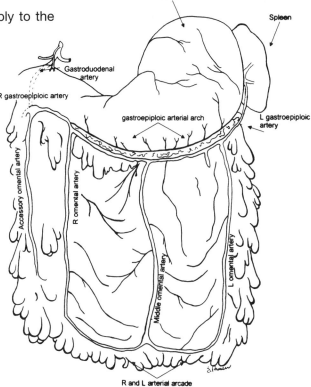

The omental flap is created by dividing the omentum perpendicular to the transverse colon. The longer flap can be developed by dividing the inferior part of the omentum parallel to the transverse colon.

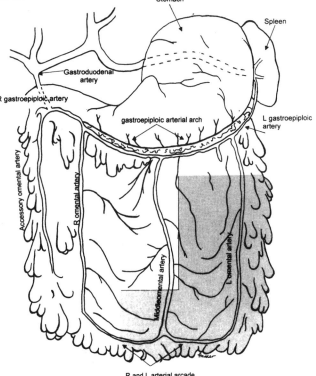

Omental flap

Omental Flaps

The graft to be covered is exposed.

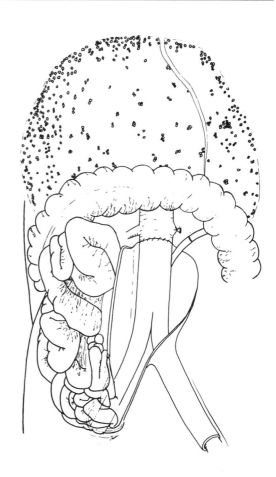

The omental flap is folded gently over the transverse colon mesentery and is placed over the aortic prosthesis. The flap is secured in place with a few interrupted sutures. The edge of the flap is secured with a running silk suture to the mesocolon.

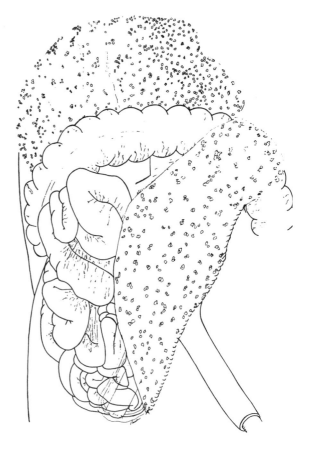

Appendix

Vascular Anastomosis Workshop

PURPOSE

The purpose of this workshop is to expose the participant to commonly used basic vascular reconstructions. The participant is expected to learn new skills during the workshop and be able to review and practice what was learned at a later convenient date. It is hoped that this workshop will improve the surgical residents' performance in the operating room when rotating on the vascular surgery service.

DESCRIPTION

The workshop will have a structured format with flexible applications. The participant will be asked to perform a series of technical exercises of increasing complexity. Participants can skip the exercises that may be too simple for their level of training.

At the completion of the workshop, the participant should be familiar with

1. Primary closure of an arteriotomy using an interrupted or continuous suture technique
2. Patch angioplasty closure of an arteriotomy using an "anchor" or "parachute" technique
3. End-to-side anastomosis using an "anchor" or "parachute" technique
4. End-to-end anastomosis in a straight or beveled fashion
5. End-to-end anastomosis between two grafts of different diameters

WORKSHOP TOOLS

Each participant will be provided with

    1 suture board
    1 needle holder
    1 forceps
    1 scissors
    (2) 8-mm grafts
    (2) 6-mm grafts
    Vascular sutures
    Workshop manual (Part II)

Part II will provide guidance through detailed illustrations on the various techniques used to perform the required exercises. The workshop supervisor can add his/her suggestions and recommendations to the instructions provided in Part II. Even with minimal supervision, the participant should be able to benefit from the workshop and identify any shortcomings in understanding the technical aspects of the reconstruction. A workshop video demonstrating the exercises to be performed can also be supplemented for review before or after the workshop.

EXERCISES TO BE PERFORMED IN THE WORKSHOP

For the purpose of this workshop, assume that the 8-mm graft is an artery.
The 6-mm graft will serve as a conduit to be used for creating a bypass.

Create a transverse arteriotomy.
Close the arteriotomy with interrupted sutures.

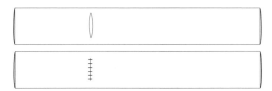

Create a longitudinal arteriotomy.
Close the arteriotomy with a running suture.

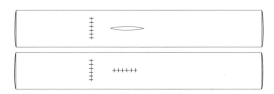

Create a longitudinal arteriotomy.
Transect a 2-cm segment of the distal part of the
6-mm graft. Create a patch from that segment.
Use that patch to close the arteriotomy.

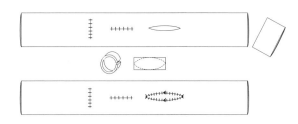

Create a 1-cm longitudinal arteriotomy in the 8-mm
graft near the left end. Construct an end-to-side
anastomosis with one end of the 6-mm graft using an
anchor technique.

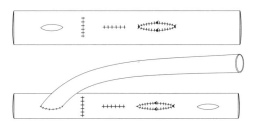

EXERCISES TO BE PERFORMED IN THE WORKSHOP

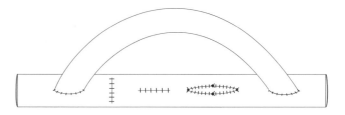

Create a 1-cm longitudinal arteriotomy in the 8-mm graft close to its right end. Construct an end-to-side anastomosis with the free end of the 6-mm graft using a parachute technique.

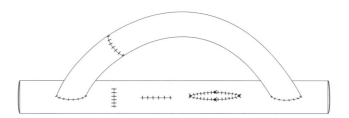

Transect the 6-mm graft and suture it back together in a straight fashion.

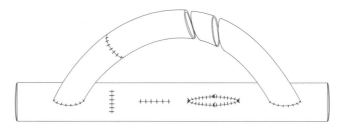

Excise a 4-cm segment of the 6-mm graft and suture the ends back together in a beveled fashion.

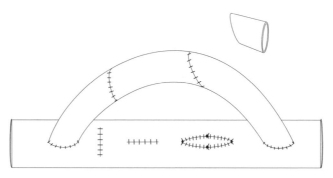

Construct an end-to-end anastomosis between the 6-mm graft segment and the 8-mm graft.

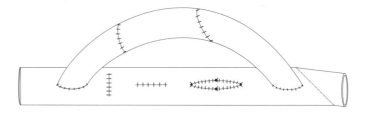

Index

of the iliac arteries, 72
of the juxtarenal aorta and renal arteries, 54-57
of the superior mesenteric artery, 64-65
of the supraceliac aorta, 63
    blind dissection, 62-63
Transverse arteriotomy, primary closure of, 167
    continuous sutures, 169-71
    interrupted sutures, 172
Trapdoor thoracotomy, 30
Trauma, avoiding in thrombectomy-embolectomy, 150-51
Tunneling, 109-16
Tying guidelines, for vascular reconstruction, 133

U

Ulnar artery, anatomy and exposure of, 39
Ultrasonography, for intraoperative evaluation of vascular reconstruction, 134
Umbilical vein grafts (UVG), 20
Upper abdominal aorta, thoracoabdominal exposure of, 71
Upper extremity, veins of, exposure of, 101

V

Valve cutting procedure, using valvulotomes, 6
Valvulotomes, 6, 16
    Bush, 6
    Fogarty, 6
    Gore Eze-Sit, 6
    Hall, 6
    LeMaitre, 6
    Mills retrograde, 9

Vascular clamps
    for blood vessel control, 117-18
    partially occluding, specifications and common use, 4
    self-compressing, specifications and common use, 5
    totally occluding, specifications and common use, 4
Vasculare reconstruction, basic steps in, 107-35
Vascular grafts, 17-22
Vascular patches, 22-23
Vascular sutures, permanent, 23-25
Vein patches and cuffs
    distal anastomosis of an infrainguinal prosthetic bypass, 276-77
    Linton patch, 278-79
    Miller cuff, 280-85
    Miller cuff modification, St. Mary's boot, 286-87
    Taylor patch, in distal anastomosis of an infrainguinal prosthetic bypass, 288-91
Veins
    cryopreserved, 20
    superficial femoral-popliteal, 18-19
    of the upper and lower extremities, 100-104
    See also Basilic veins; Cephalic veins; Greater saphenous vein; Lesser saphenous vein; Superficial femoral vein
Vertebral artery
    anatomy of, 27-28
    exposure of, 34-35

W

Workshop, vascular anastomosis, 383-86